SHOCK

A Physiologic Basis for Treatment

ALAN P. THAL, M.D., Ph.D.

Professor of Surgery
University of Kansas Medical Center

E. B. BROWN, Jr., Ph.D.

Professor and Chairman, Department of Physiology
University of Kansas Medical Center

ARLO S. HERMRECK, M.D.

Resident Surgeon, USPHS Postdoctoral Fellow in Physiology
University of Kansas Medical Center

HUGH H. BELL, M.D.

Assistant Professor of Medicine, Section of Cardiology
University of Kansas Medical Center

With a Foreword by

OWEN H. WANGENSTEEN, M.D., Ph.D.

Regents' Professor of Surgery and Chairman Emeritus
University of Minnesota

SHOCK

A Physiologic Basis for Treatment

YEAR BOOK MEDICAL PUBLISHERS, INC.

35 EAST WACKER DRIVE · CHICAGO

Library of Congress Catalog Card Number: 72-119580

International Standard Book Number: 0-8151-8788-2

Foreword

THIS PAINSTAKING, informative and discerning monograph by Dr. Thal and his associates of the University of Kansas mirrors the complex technology and the expertise and sophistication of earnest modern-day students of the shock problem. It also reflects the increased awareness of today's clinicians of their dependence upon the basic biologic disciplines.

In World War I the Harvard physiologist, Walter B. Cannon, took his laboratory to the front lines to try to bring enlightenment and understanding into the shock problem. The work of Cannon and his associates did succeed in setting aside the thesis of a diffuse vasomotor paralysis in shock, which theory had long been current prior to that time, despite the work of Seelig and Lyon (1909, 1910) and of Mann (1914), which had shown very definitely that peripheral vasomotor constriction was in large measure responsible for the "lost blood" in traumatic shock. Alert surgeons of the third decade of this century gave saline solution and blood to increase the cardiac output, depending solely on reestablishment of functional equilibrium to correct peripheral vasomotor constriction. Shock which fails to respond to restoration of blood volume has come to be known as irreversible shock. Today's surgeon-physiologist has at his command a number of effective vasodilator agents, corticosteroids and antibiotics to hasten reestablishment of normal vasomotor tone in endotoxin shock and to combat existing sepsis, conditions that fail to respond to restoration of blood volume. Successes with this type of management characterize the progress that current-day studies are lending surgery's advance in an area previously surrounded by an aura of hopelessness.

In his lecture "The New Physiology" before the Harvey Society in New York City (1916) Haldane predicted that understanding the normal physiologic processes would come to make a great impact upon medicine, a theme already stressed by Claude Bernard (1865) half a century earlier. In 1952 (Proc. Staff Meet. Mayo Clinic, 27:537), this writer expressed the hope that the time would not be far off when physiologists would be as active on the wards as the pathologist. Dr. Thal and his associates have taken the laboratories of the physiologist and biochemist to the patient's bedside to recognize the physiologic and biochemical changes attending the shock syndrome, enabling physicians to keep a running account of necessary corrective measures to be invoked.

As a junior medical student in 1920 at the Minneapolis General Hospital, I observed one of my teachers, Dr. J. Frank Corbett, recently returned from a period of military service in France and a student of shock and "adrenal exhaustion," treat a patient with avulsion of the shoulder girdle by repetitive injections of large doses of epinephrine. The patient's pallor increased despite momentary rise in blood pressure and within an hour he was dead. Corbett (1914, 1915) was persuaded that adrenal exhaustion dominated the picture. Less than a year later, I was a junior intern in the same hospital and was in the emergency admitting ward when a pulseless and cyanotic patient, with a crushing injury of neck and upper thorax sustained in the nearby railroad yard, was brought in during early hours of the morning. The overworked and tired resident was called and he examined the patient and remarked that the situation was hopeless and left. Not capitulating so readily to a sense of utter futility I performed my first tracheostomy, and with help from the nurse on duty administered two liters of saline solution. By the time the multiple wounds had been satisfactorily dealt with, the patient had become conscious and eventually left the hospital. I tell this story only to indicate that this episode terminated the treatment of shock by injections of epinephrine in this area.

It is to be remembered that whereas a few clinicians had advised intravenous infusions as early as the mid-1880s, a precept which Rudolph Matas early adopted, hypodermoclysis, save in emergencies, continued to be the standard manner of giving fluids postoperatively up into the mid-1920s. Blood transfusion had come into being, but the only available donors were patients on the wards known to have group O blood.

Today's surgical house officers, too often unfamiliar with the trials of their predecessors of the late nineteenth and early twentieth centuries in meeting the emergencies of traumatic shock, probably little appreciate how much they are beholden to the studies of George W. Crile, Walter B. Cannon, Alfred Blalock, and to a number of investigators who made blood transfusion a practical reality. Blood banks and accurate fluid and electrolyte replacement have done much to improve the surgeon's record in dealing with trauma and what surgeons of a century ago often alluded to as the "shock" of operation.

When Sir Frederick Treves wrote the second edition of his *Intestinal Obstructions* (1899), the only fluid administered to patients dehydrated from vomiting was an occasional enema, apart from small quantities of hot water or ingested tea. Paget (Lancet 1:148, 1863) recommended and employed subcutaneous injections of morphine after operation as an antidote to shock. One of Treves' distinguished countrymen, O'Shaughnessey, 60 years earlier (1831-32) had shown how the collapse from the diarrhea of cholera could be assuaged by the intravenous administration of fluids containing the electrolytes sodium and potassium in the same concentration as observed in diarrheal stools. We constantly need to be mindful of the admonition of the Preacher in Ecclesiastes I:11 concerning "remembrance of former things."

As early as 1867, a *Practical Treatise on Shock,* a monograph of 88 pages, was authored by the London surgeon, Edwin Morris. He described shock as a "peculiar effect on the animal system, produced by violent injuries from any cause, or from violent mental emotions." Groeningen's (1885) monograph professed to be a critical study of the physiologic basis of shock. He advised rest, alcohol, strychnine, and digitalis as the best remedial agents and concluded with the hope that future studies, characterizing the nature of shock, would find a better name for the condition.

Prior to Cannon's studies (1923), a goodly segment of the blood lost from the circulation was presumed to be in the veins of the abdominal viscera, though the English surgeon Malcolm (Lancet 2:579, 1905) had pointed out that the intestines were pale in shock. As early as 1879 the Irish surgeon Mapother (Brit. M. J. 2:1023) had suggested that shock was owing to "contraction of arterioles"; the vasodilator nerves he postulated were paralyzed. Cannon believed the stagnant blood to be in the capillaries. Blalock (1930) stressed the loss of blood and plasma in the injured tissues in shock. Modern-day students of the problem cite the venules as an additional site of the trapped blood. Great military surgeons had long advised bleeding for gunshot wounds when bleeding was not prominent. Ambroise Paré (1634) stated that phlebotomy is "required in great wounds where there is fear of deflexion, paine, Delirium, Raving and unquietness" (1968 reprint, p. 326).

Le Dran (1743) spoke of "the shock* and agitation which commonly follows gun-shot wounds. . . . Bleeding is of prodigious advantage here; nay it is absolutely necessary, if no considerable haemorrhage has preceded."

The British surgeon Ranby (1776, p. 121) endorsed phlebotomy for gunshot wounds and wrote "where the wounded person has not suffered any great loss of blood it will be advisable to open a vein immediately, and take from the arm a very large quantity and to repeat bleeding, as circumstances may require."

John Hunter in his *Treatise on the Blood, Inflammation and Gunshot Wounds* (1796, vol. 2, p. 287) endorsed, though somewhat unenthusiastically, bleeding for gunshot wound if spontaneous hemorrhage had not accompanied the injury.

MacLeod (1862, p. 251), writing of the Crimean War, stated that in the management of compound fractures of thighs he followed the advice of

---

*Le Dran had used the word *secousse* or *saisissement* (*Traite . . . sur les playes d'armes a feu,* 1740, pp. 2, 74). His unnamed English translator (1743) interpreted it as "shock" (pp. 2, 48–50).

Ravaton (1768, p. 323) in such injuries, who recommended removal of fragments from wounds and early bleeding, none of which "could protect him against inevitable death." Larrey (1832, Rivinus translation, p. 38) recommended bleeding for gunshot wounds only when complications developed. In the first decade of the nineteenth century, Philip Syng Physick, usually referred to as the Father of American Surgery, introduced phlebotomy for the reduction of dislocations and fractures, bleeding the patient in the erect posture until limp, thus providing at least as effective relaxation as with inhalation of anesthesia. In the War of the Rebellion (1861-1865) Mitchell, Morehouse, and Keen (Surgeons Generals' Circular No. 6, 1864) described reflex paralysis of peripheral nerves as a result of severe trauma.

In reporting upon *Surgical Experience in the Boer War of 1899-1900*, George Makins (1901, p. 110) related that shock was treated by administration of stimulants, hypodermic injection of strychnine, and in severe cases, when operation was necessary, by the intravenous injection of saline solution and stimulants.

This brief recital serves to indicate that only when physiologic techniques were applied at the front by the physiologist Cannon was notable progress made in military circles in the solution of the shock problem. Three centuries of experience was not the equal of physiologic assessment in appraising the nature of traumatic shock.

In his Harvey Lecture of 1919 (vol. 15, p. 30, 1921) Henry Dale emphasized the importance of secondary wound shock as a very significant factor in mortality. A number of the case histories of patients related by Dr. Thal and his associates obviously fall into this category. The cause of the death is often a mystery. Is there a dialyzable toxic factor as suggested by Cannon in his shock monograph (1923, pp. 160-162), whether of tissue or bacterial origin? Is there still an unrecognized factor not adequately dealt with? Are lapses in therapy responsible for the mortality? Certainly in late deaths infection is often the significant factor.

The *why* still continues to be as important as the *how* in the baffling shock syndrome. The interdependence of organ function and systems is well brought out in this penetrating study by Dr. Thal and associates, which should find eager readers among house officers, surgeons, and physicians who deal with the complex problems of shock. Moreover, these scientific explorations and achievements, in the hands of the University of Kansas investigators, point the way to solution of other bewildering and knotty clinical problems.

OWEN H. WANGENSTEEN, M.D.

Regents' Professor of Surgery
University of Minnesota

Preface

To THE beginning medical student, many of the preclinical disciplines may appear to lack relevance for his urgent goal of patient care. Too often, the basic sciences are merely regarded as a necessary barrier which, once surmounted, may be forgotten. But, with the development of the intensive care unit (ICU) and its attendant laboratory, modern surgical care has become an exercise in applied physiology. Quantitative measurements formerly obtainable only by the investigator are now rapidly available and allow the surgeon to interpret a problem in terms used by the physiologist and biochemist, and thus, in some measure, to bridge the gap between the preclinical and clinical years.

Over the past several years we have developed a combined course, Intensive Care of Critically Ill Patients, for junior medical students. Since the course formed the stimulus for writing this book, its design may have some interest for the reader. Three students are assigned full-time for one week to the surgical ICU, rotating night and weekend schedules. They are responsible, under supervision, for the care and study of all patients in the unit and make rounds with the staff surgeons and residents as indicated. Attached to the ICU is a small laboratory staffed by a single technician and equipped to provide measurements of blood gases, coagulation, and hematocrit. Within the unit there is also equipment for measuring inspired and expired oxygen concentrations and CO_2 concentrations as well as a densitometer and recorder to measure cardiac output by dye dilution. Aside from direct patient responsibility, the students have daily tutorials aimed at integrating physiologic and biochemical measurements with clinical observations. Students learn to make their own measurements of blood gases, under supervision, and to use the values to calculate the pulmonary shunts and physiologic dead space.

In addition, they have a weekly meeting in the ICU with Dr. E. B. Brown (Physiology) to review pulmonary and metabolic problems from the physiologic viewpoint. Dr. Dante Scarpelli (Pathology) examines current cases in terms of ultrastructure and cellular biochemistry. Dr. Dan Azarnoff (Clinical Pharmacology) reviews the basis for drug therapy, and Dr. Marjorie Sirridge discusses acute coagulopathies in trauma or shock patients. Finally, Dr. Donald Greaves (Psychiatry) discusses the emotional problems of the patient and the physician in relation to critical illness. Pertinent references are filed in a small library in the laboratory.

By and large, this course has been favorably received by both students

and faculty, It is, in essence, a course in applied physiology of the acutely
ill patient. For the superior student, it offers an exciting integration of
basic and clinical knowledge. Even for the average student, the concentration of acute clinical material and the practical instruction in the use
of ventilators, in tracheostomy care, and in cardiac support offers definite
advantages. An unanticipated benefit of this course has been the opportunity it has offered faculty members from the preclinical and clinical
areas to exchange ideas and gain a broader insight into the patient faced
with life-threatening injury.

This book is designed to provide a physiologic basis for the care of the
shock patient and to answer some of the questions raised by our students
and residents. Major attention has been focused on the lung, the cardiovascular and renal systems, and acid-base balance. Clearly the liver, gut,
muscle masses, and the reticuloendothelial system are of great importance
in the response to shock, but measurements of their function in the shock
patient are at the moment largely in the realm of the investigator.

The material gathered here utilizes the phenomenon of shock as a basis
for crossing traditional departmental boundaries along the lines of the integrated curricula now being proposed in several medical schools. In the
opening sections, the concept of shock is reviewed and the physiologic
principles upon which diagnosis is made and treatment prescribed are developed. The common clinical entities with which shock is often associated
are reviewed. Measurements now considered vital in proper patient care
are described, and calculations that have clinical or didactic value are
given. Finally, therapy is stressed as a series of logical steps aimed at vital
organ support and based upon repeated measurement.

ACKNOWLEDGMENTS*

We wish to thank our many colleagues for helpful advice and criticism,
and for permission to use their data and illustrations. We are especially
indebted to Dr. Marjorie Sirridge for contributing the section on coagulation. Drs. Kenneth Goetz, Francis Cuppage, Lawrence Sullivan, Carl
Teplitz, Frank Scamman, and Douglas Voth gave liberally of their time
and expert knowledge. Mr. Robert Pruett, Mrs. Carol Boettcher, and Mrs.
Ann Lyons contributed valuable technical and secretarial help. The dia-
grams were drawn by Mrs. Blanche Lenon.

Finally, and most importantly, we owe our interest in teaching surgery
as a form of applied physiology to Dr. Owen H. Wangensteen, who pio-
neered the concept.

---

*These studies were supported by USPHS Grant #5R01HE12678.

Table of Contents

11

1

Growth of the Concept

SHOCK IS, in essence, a story of survival, a struggle by the organism in an adverse environment to preserve the life of its most vital tissues. It is a story of attack and defense, of gain and loss, of a kaleidoscope of defensive maneuvers to preserve the most vital organs. As such it is encountered in virtually all the clinical disciplines, and for treatment it needs an understanding of circulatory dynamics and cellular physiology.

The term *shock* has been applied for more than two centuries to many conditions in which the initiating injuries seemed disproportionately and mysteriously small when compared with the immediate or gradual collapse of the vital processes. The enigma was well brought out by Sir Astley Cooper in his "Commentary on War Injuries" when he drew attention to the fact that many soldiers had died without significant blood loss, severe pain, or gross injury. Then and now, the term was loosely applied to a wide variety of life-threatening states in which the pathologic findings failed to supply a reasonable cause of death.

The word *shock* was first used medically in the English language in 1743 in a translation of Henri François Le Dran's second French edition of "A Treatise of Reflections Drawn from Experience with Gunshot Wounds." The translator used the word to convey the impression of a jolt or a blow followed by progressive deterioration, loss of consciousness, and death. To John Collins Warren (Fig. 1-1), shock was "A momentary pause in the act of death." This concept embraces much that is currently acceptable, particularly the notion that shock is not an entity in itself but rather an adaptive response to life-threatening injury of varying origin and marked by temporary or permanent damage to vital organ function.

The report of Thomas Latta, in 1831, describing his treatment of the hypovolemic state in cholera is a classic in therapeutics. "Having no precedent" to direct him, he proceeded with caution to infuse 330 ounces of saline intravenously into a patient in a 12-hour period with dramatic clinical improvement.

With the advent of the era of experimental physiology in the nineteenth century, measurements of the response of mean blood pressure to various

17

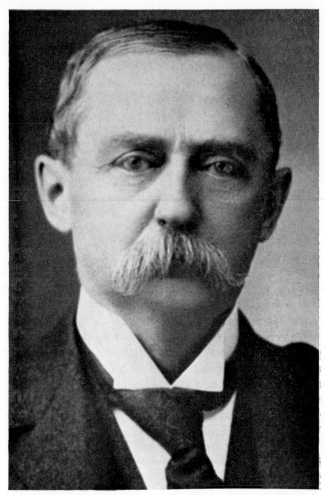

Fig. 1–1.—John Collins Warren (1842–1927). Moseley Professor of Surgery, Harvard University, 1889–1907. Among his many contributions, Warren's clinical descriptions of shock, culminating in his definition, "A momentary pause in the act of death," have had considerable historical importance and represent the era of observation and speculation. (Used by permission of the University of Kansas Medical Center, Department of History of Medicine.)

stimuli were continuously recorded on the kymograph. The inhibitory effect of the vagus nerve on the heart was described, and the existence of a vasomotor center which controlled the circulatory system through the autonomic nervous system was established. Experiments demonstrating the reflex inhibition of heart action by peripheral stimuli, such as tapping the frog belly or by introducing abrupt gravitational changes in the rabbit, suggested that an experimental analogue of human shock had been developed. As a result of these studies, the concept arose that shock was the result of inhibition of the vasomotor center which produced weakening of the heart beat and peripheral pooling of blood. This neurogenic concept of shock developed during the era when interest in experimental and clinical neurology flourished under the stimulus of Claude Bernard, Brown-Sequard, and Charcot.

George W. Crile (Fig. 1-2), who worked originally in the laboratory of Victor Horseley at University College, London, later contributed a detailed monograph, published in 1899, describing the first extensive experimental study of shock. Crile used the recording tambours, manometers, and kymograms of the physiologist to measure reactions to injury in a large number of animal experiments. Many of his observations have considerable bearing on our present concept of shock. He emphasized the relationship between increased duration of operation and the likelihood of inducing shock. He noted that a small hemorrhage preceding an operation impaired the animal's ability to withstand injury, and he defined the role of hypothermia, anesthesia and, in particular, blood and fluid loss. Crile also delineated the acceleration and deepening of respiration following hemorrhage and the portal venous hypertension associated with a falling central venous pressure. In describing the response of the animal in shock to an infusion of warm saline, he wrote: "What has the saline done? It has increased the venous pressure which in turn filled the heart; this, in its turn, beat strongly and sent out larger quantities of saline blood which in turn fed the exhausted and starving centers, and carried the over-charged blood to the lungs for the respiratory changes."

The response of the heart to saline infusion led Crile to conclude that cardiac action was the last of the vital functions to fail. His concepts of the importance of the venous pressure as a determinant of cardiac output, his recognition that the venous pressure in hemorrhagic shock is low, that it can be raised by infusion of warm saline and that the heart responds with an increased output, are ideas highly acceptable to the modern clinician. He ascribed the ultimate determinant of shock to exhaustion of the vasomotor center. Later a good deal of evidence suggested that, quite to the contrary, the vasomotor center was hyperactive and that denervation of an organ resulted in prompt increase in blood flow.

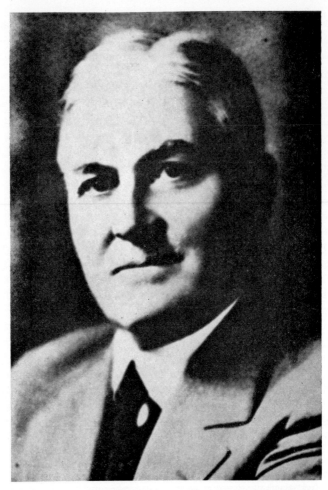

Fig. 1-2.—George W. Crile (1864–1943). This imaginative investigator and master surgeon conducted pioneering experiments in animals and in a prophetic way defined the importance of venous pressure and the responses to volume loading. These concepts are summarized in his book, *Surgical Shock*, published in 1897. (From Surgery 14:4, 1943. The C. V. Mosby Co., St. Louis.)

Nine years later, Yandel Henderson also stressed the importance of venous return to the heart. "Venous pressure is, so to speak, the fulcrum of circulation. Shock, as surgeons use the word, is due to failure of the fulcrum. Because of the diminished venous supply, the heart is not adequately distended and full during diastole." Again and again in the present work, mention will be made of the fundamental concept of the decreased venous return in the understanding and therapy of shock. Interestingly, the deleterious effects of hypocapnea, stressed by Henderson, are again coming into vogue, although Henderson was also the center of controversy as a result of his suggestion that hypocapnea was "a causative mechanism" rather than a result of shock.

Interest in the mechanisms and treatment of shock has always been stimulated by war. World War I, for the first time, brought physiologists into contact with the battlefield. In 1917, Archibald and McLean, after considerable firsthand experience in the treatment of shock in the wounded, summarized their opinions regarding the value of blood pressure measurements: "While a low blood pressure is one of the most constant signs of shock, it is not the essential thing, let alone the cause of it . . . we have focused our attention far too much on blood pressure."

The work of Crile and, in particular, Henderson, had supported the concept that failure of venous return was the prime determinant in shock in that the heart maintained its ability to pump until the terminal stages. Accordingly, attention was focused on the peripheral small vessels. The wartime experience was most enlightening in view of the then current controversies regarding the use of vasoconstrictor and vasodilator drugs. At that time, the debate was between those who believed that vasomotor exhaustion with pooling of blood in the great veins was the cause of shock and those who believed that vasoconstriction was the cause of deterioration. In treating war casualties, surgeons noted the pallor of the tissues of patients in shock, the disappearance of peripheral pulses at a time when femoral and carotid pulses were palpable, and the constriction of peripheral veins. Ducastaing provided further evidence of vasoconstriction in shock when he observed that peripheral pulses became palpable after the use of the vasodilator amyl nitrite.

The collaborative efforts of American and British physiologists and clinicians, led by Cannon (Fig. 1-3) and Bayliss, created an important precedent for future battlefield studies by investigative groups. The broad perspectives of their study—the clinical descriptions by front-line medical officers and the measurements of physiologic and biochemical phenomena in patients in shock and in parallel studies of animals—set a standard for similar investigative units. From these observations in the field and in the laboratory, Cannon attempted to explain hypotension in terms of cardiac failure, loss of vasomotor tone, fall in blood volume, or stagnation in venous reservoirs.

In the summer of 1917, at Bethune, Cannon used the then new Van Slyke apparatus and documented a correlation between low blood pressure and reduction in alkali reserve. He surmised that the fall in alkali reserve was due to the accumulation of fixed acids (such as lactic acid)

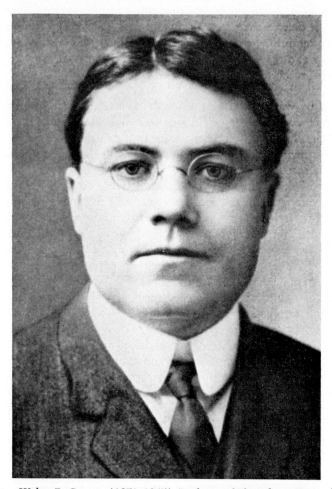

Fig. 1–3.—Walter B. Cannon (1871–1945). Professor of Physiology, Harvard Medical School, 1906–1942. His classic work, *Traumatic Shock*, published in 1923, summarized studies conducted with the English physiologist Bayliss on battle casualties in World War I. This work represents one of the first quantitative studies of shock patients. (Used by permission of the University of Kansas Medical Center, Department of History of Medicine.)

as a result of impaired oxygen transport. He recognized the acidosis as a secondary phenomenon, and he noted the striking improvement in shock patients after the administration of sodium bicarbonate.

During this period Keith studied blood volume in the war-wounded by means of dye dilution methods and showed clearly that the severity of shock correlated with the reduction in blood volume. Cannon thereupon defined wound shock as a discrepancy between blood volume and vascular capacity. The finding of a reduction in blood volume without external evidence of bleeding required explanation, however. Also at that time many interesting observations were made concerning the nature of crush injuries among the war-wounded. There were many descriptions of wounded soldiers who lay, apparently in good condition, with their limbs pinned under fallen timbers. Within minutes after removal, however, rapid de-

Fig. 1–4.—Carl J. Wiggers (1883–1963). Director, Department of Physiology, School of Medicine, Western Reserve University, Cleveland. Wiggers developed a standard shock preparation which, in modified form, has become accepted as the hemorrhagic shock model in animals. This preparation gave rise to the concept of irreversibility. (From Circulation 4:482, 1951. Used by permission of the American Heart Association, Inc.)

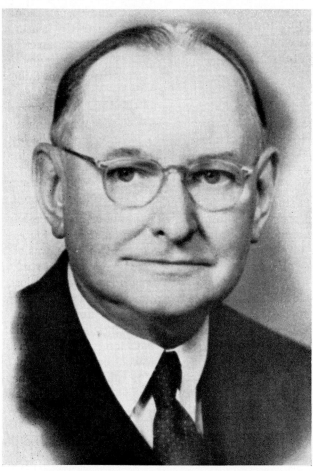

terioration in the patient's condition followed. Similarly the removal of tourniquets which had isolated crushed limbs was often followed by all the signs of progressive shock leading to death. On the other hand, amputation of the limb before removing the tourniquet often resulted in survival. This observation led to the concept of traumatic toxemia and stimulated Cannon and Bayliss to create an experimental model in the laboratory. The question they sought to answer was whether death following crushing injury was caused by toxic agents liberated from the damaged tissues or was due to loss of fluid at the site of injury.

The experiments of Cannon and Bayliss, interpreted in the light of the work of Dale and Richards on the toxic effects of histamine, led to the conclusion that the dominant factor in traumatic shock was the release of toxic materials into the systemic circulation. Substances such as histamine appeared to supply a basis for loss of vasomotor tone producing sequestration of blood and failure of venous return to the heart. While these conclusions were seriously questioned later, Cannon nevertheless clearly documented that the most important phenomenon in traumatic shock was the loss of circulating blood volume and the subsequent failure of venous return. To this phenomenon he applied the term *exemia*.

In 1930, Phemister and Blalock (Fig. 1-5), working independently, challenged the Cannon concept of a generalized vascular injury and loss of vasomotor tone. They demonstrated conclusively that the lost blood and plasma had accumulated in and around the wound and infiltrated the tissue spaces far beyond the area of local injury.

During World War II units were established by the United States and England to study battle casualties and air-raid victims. A board, headed by H. K. Beecher, was formed for the study of the severely wounded in the Mediterranean theaters of operation of the United States Army. This board, by taking the laboratory close to the front line, was able to obtain the first early biochemical studies of war-wounded. Their studies indicated that the major cause of shock was hemorrhage and fluid loss, which led to metabolic acidosis when the condition was severe and protracted.

Many of Cannon's concepts, which lack the documentation of modern technology, were later confirmed by Cournand, Richards, and their associates, who carried out the first cardiac output measurements in shock. Finding a standard animal for shock studies continues to be a problem. Differences in the responses of dog and man to injury, especially the necrotizing enterocolitis in the dog, further prevent ready transfer of canine experimental data to the human. When endotoxin became commercially available, its lethal effect in animals was studied as the prototype of human septic shock. Today this assumption is often challenged, especially when the dog model is used.

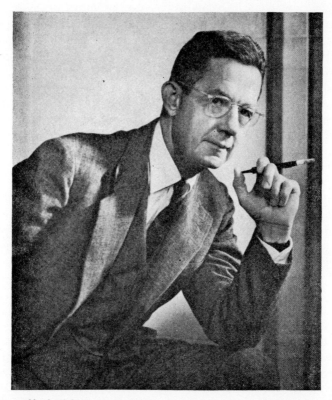

Fig. 1–5.—Alfred Blalock (1899–1964). Best known for his pioneering work in cardiac surgery, Alfred Blalock performed some of the classic studies in traumatic and hypovolemic shock. He demonstrated the importance of fluid loss into injured tissue and measured the partition of blood flow during hypovolemia. (Courtesy of Dr. William P. Longmire, Jr.)

The experiences of the two world wars were augmented by information gained during the Korean conflict when the standards of medical care were clearly outstanding. During this campaign specialized investigative groups undertook studies that led not only to the better care of battlefield casualties but also to subsequent application of this care to civilian practice. Thoracic surgical teams, renal support units, and groups of highly trained vascular surgeons were available for early treatment of battle casualties. Afterward, interest in the investigation of civilian shock was maintained and stimulated by the Shock Committee of the National Academy of Science. Arising out of the work of this group were plans to foster the development of shock study units in various parts of the country. From these studies came the first extensive measurements of hemodynamic, biochemical, and clinical events in the various forms of civilian shock. Recently, the Vietnam conflict and civilian experience have emphasized the importance of a peculiar form of lung injury which follows shock and massive tissue damage, leading to a progressive failure of oxygenation. *Shock-lung, posttraumatic wet lung,* and a host of other terms have been used to identify this syndrome, but its origin and pathogenesis are largely obscure. Similar functional changes and comparable histologic findings occur after a variety of insults such as burns, blast injuries, rapid overtransfusion, fat embolism, oxygen toxicity, and head injury. Regardless of their origin, these severe changes in lung function are currently one of the major problems in the salvage of the critically ill patient. The recent interest in giving appropriate ventilatory support has grown out of a frustrating inability to provide oxygenation when other indicators point toward the likelihood of survival. While much investigation remains to be done in the laboratory and at the bedside in elucidating its mysteries, the scientific study of shock has changed the care of the critically ill patient from an empirical approach to one based upon physiologic measurement.

Clinical, Hemodynamic, and Biochemical Considerations in Shock

Shock may be defined as a state of reduced tissue perfusion leading to generalized cellular hypoxia and vital organ damage. Before considering altered organ function in shock, it is necessary to evaluate any particular case in clinical, hemodynamic, and biochemical terms. The dynamic nature of the problem requires collection of these data at repeated intervals in order to define the course of the illness, to recognize the extent of vital organ damage, and to assess the effects of therapy.

Clinical Evaluation

The original definitions of shock were purely descriptive, and to this day an evaluation by the experienced clinician offers important, if at times intuitive, impressions regarding the over-all response of the patient and the prognosis in a given case. The age of the patient, the past history, the evidence of severe underlying disease, and the function of vital organs are almost preconsciously appraised by the clinician. This information, which is not readily quantitatable nor transferable from one patient to another, is vital in the interpretation and analysis of data in shock. Aside from traumatic and some cases of hemorrhagic shock, the illness almost invariably complicates a chronic underlying disease process. Septic shock, for example, is often associated with genitourinary disease or disease of the biliary tract and liver or with the late stage of burns. Shock in the aged patient, regardless of its causation, may bring out otherwise latent deficiencies in myocardial, pulmonary, and renal reserve which greatly influence the outcome of the illness.

Hypotension in a young patient, even when of long duration, may be responsive to therapy. In the aged patient with sclerotic blood vessels and peripheral venous stasis, early impairment of cardiac function and embolization of the lungs may rapidly complicate the illness and change a simple problem of hypovolemia into a complex one of cardiac failure and impaired pulmonary gas exchange. For these reasons, cases of shock under study may require individual consideration or, when considered collectively, should be categorized into comparable matching groups by the *age of the patient*, the *underlying disease process*, and the *depth and duration of the shock episode*.

The importance of defining shock in clinical terms lies also in recognition of the early impressions of impending disaster that may be apparent for some time before blood pressure and metabolic changes become evident. The astute clinician notes these evidences of increased sympathetic activity: constriction of the blood vessels of the skin; rapid, thready pulse; beads of sweat on the forehead extending progressively to the extremities; pale, mottled, clammy skin; falling urine output; increase in rate and depth of respiration; and change in the state of consciousness which may herald beginning cerebral hypoxia by restlessness, and increasing hypoxia by apathy and diminished responsiveness. Sometimes the correlation between the bedside evaluation and the quantitative physiologic and biochemical measurement is poor, however. Blood pressure, vascular resistance, and cardiac output may be manipulated within the normal range without true improvement in the patient's condition.

Unfortunately, clinical information is often randomly collected, varies in quality, and cannot be retrieved readily. To provide a better definition of shock, standardized methods are necessary for collecting clinical data so that they may be meaningfully interrelated with hemodynamic and biochemical information. Although essential, clinical examination of the patient in shock reveals but part of the complex picture to be analyzed.

HEMODYNAMIC CRITERIA

Traditionally clinicians have regarded shock from the circulatory viewpoint; this approach gives only a partial view of the whole problem, however. Blood pressure, heart rate, and venous pressure are the most readily and most commonly measured variables, but measurements of cardiac output and calculations of peripheral vascular resistance and myocardial function provide the most important means of understanding the hemo-dynamic problem in shock.

ARTERIAL BLOOD PRESSURE.—Shock is often considered as a problem in arterial blood pressure when in fact a more satisfactory common denominator appears to be cellular damage from inadequate capillary blood flow. While it is true that a falling blood pressure of greater or lesser degree is an almost invariable occurrence, hypotension may be a relatively late development in the course of the illness. Similarly, while the degree of hypotension often correlates with the severity of the shock, there are many notable exceptions.

Perhaps the most striking example of hypotension which may be well tolerated for considerable periods of time, as long as other excessive demands are not present, is that seen with total sympathectomy following high spinal-cord or brain-stem lesions. If adequate ventilation is provided, excellent tissue perfusion with a slow pulse and a low blood pressure may be maintained. Conversely, in severe shock the blood pressure may be raised with vasopressors to normal or hypertensive levels while tissue blood flow is progressively reduced. Measurements of arterial pressure or cardiac output alone do not define the adequacy of tissue perfusion. The status of the microcirculation and, hence, the distribution of blood flow (as well as the routing through to nutritive or nonnutritive channels) are the ultimate determinants of gas exchange at the cellular level.

CARDIAC OUTPUT.—When cardiac output is reduced below the level needed to supply the nutritive demands of the tissues, a state of shock is said to exist. Considered alone, however, the measurement of cardiac output does not always indicate either the presence or the severity of the shock state. The implication often made here is that if the cardiac output is increased sufficiently, the nutritive needs will be supplied. But studies of cirrhotic patients in shock and measurements in septic shock have shown that even though the cardiac output may be within or well above the normal range chemical evidence of severe tissue hypoxia is present. In some cases of sepsis, to be discussed later, the hypermetabolic state raises the nutritive needs above the normal resting level and the accepted norms for resting basal cardiac output can no longer be applied. Oxygen extraction is often reduced, suggesting bypass of nutritive channels, excessive regional perfusion in relation to oxygen demands, or cellular damage limiting oxygen uptake. The latter concept is suggested by in vitro studies using endotoxin which show direct cytotoxic interference with intracellular respiratory intermediaries. It would seem clear therefore that mere increases of cardiac output in these latter two circumstances would not accomplish a reversal of the shock state. Nevertheless, in the majority of cases of shock, cardiac output is reduced. Especially in hypovolemic, cardiogenic, and some of the mixed varieties of shock, the degree of reduction is usually proportional to the severity of the shock. On the other hand, the final outcome in severe shock is often determined by permanent damage to some vital organ such as the kidney, brain, or lung, regardless of any temporary improvement in cardiac output which may have resulted from appropriate therapy. Altered distribution of blood flow and suddenness of fall in cardiac output are as important as the volume of total flow in determining the damaging effects of shock. Gradual reduction in cardiac output, as seen in the patient with advanced mitral stenosis, for example, may produce a total blood flow well within the range seen in patients in shock but without signs of shock. The measurement of cardiac output is of utmost importance in defining the particular pathophysiologic defect in shock and the response to therapy, but it cannot by itself be used as a definition of shock.

TOTAL PERIPHERAL RESISTANCE.—The vasoconstrictor reflexes initiated by many forms of shock-inducing injury are recognized as an appropriate early survival mechanism which conserves blood flow to vital centers. Clearly the degree of vasoconstriction varies from one vascular bed to another, and the values obtained for total peripheral resistance may fail to reflect considerable changes in regional vascular beds; this is strikingly apparent in sepsis. These expressions, derived from measurements of arterial blood pressure and cardiac output, are often accepted as an indicator of over-all vasoconstriction. Most studies reveal raised values for total peripheral resistance in hypovolemic and cardiogenic shock returning toward normal with improvement in the patient's condition. In some forms of septic shock, values significantly lower than the normal level may be found. Shunting through areas of inflammation, the opening up of large numbers of peripheral arterial venous shunts, or generalized vasodilation have been proposed in explanation of this phenomenon. Calculations of total peripheral resistance, based on the measurements of pressure and cardiac output, also fail to provide an absolute measure of shock, but aid in understanding the pattern of hemodynamic response.

CENTRAL VENOUS PRESSURE.—When the amount of blood flowing into a weakened heart exceeds the ability of the heart to pump, central venous pressure rises. Conversely, when the venous return is reduced, right atrial pressure falls. The distinction between myocardial failure and hypovolemia can be made clinically on this basis. The initial measured values may not be definitive and, often, the separation of these two conditions can be made only when the circulatory system is stressed by loading. Venous pressure is also modified by the sympathetic reflex, which increases venous tone and raises venous pressure. The hypovolemic patient responds to volume load with improvement in arterial pressure and cardiac output while the central venous pressure remains within the normal range. Expansion of blood volume in the face of impaired myocardial function results in a rapid rise in central venous pressure. Repeated measurement of arterial blood pressure, cardiac output, and central venous pressure under different conditions provides an invaluable guide in defining the nature and extent of cardiovascular involvement in any particular case and in measuring the response to therapy. Cannulation of the left atrium or left ventricle yields more precise information concerning left ventricular function.

BLOOD VOLUME.—The original studies of Keith, carried out in World War I, and using vital red as an indicator, demonstrated the hypovolemia associated with trauma. Subsequently, the losses of plasma and red cells were shown in burns. While it has often been claimed that rapid loss of over 20% of blood volume would produce shock, more gradual losses of greater quantities than this seem to be tolerated without shock in the adult with normal vital organ reserve and without anemia. The precarious survival of the traumatized animal has been documented by Crile, who showed that a seemingly trivial loss of blood after graded trauma produces abrupt cardiovascular collapse.

The measurement of the circulating blood volume in a resting normal human subject presents little problem when carried out by a variety of techniques available today. In recent years, several semiautomatic electronic devices have been introduced with the intention of simplifying blood volume measurement for rapid clinical use. These devices, sold for bedside use, yield a direct figure for blood volume through measurement of the radioactivity in whole blood without separating plasma from cells. A single measurement is often recommended at the estimated time of tracer equilibrium. Dagher and co-workers, in a critical study of the clinical use of blood volume measurements, emphasized the magnitude of error introduced by counting whole blood with a single tracer at a time of presumed equilibrium. The importance of multiple equilibrium samples cannot be overemphasized when tracer dilution is used to measure blood volume in an acute state such as shock.

In shock, changing dimensions of the intravascular space and variation in cardiac function make the use of standard normal values for blood volume erroneous guides to fluid therapy, in addition to the technical problems associated with determining these values. Many investigators currently measure the adequacy of fluid replacement in shock by functional relationships such as the responses of central venous pressure, cardiac output, and arterial pressure to volume load rather than to absolute measurements of blood volume by indicator dilution techniques.

BIOCHEMICAL DETERMINANTS

One of the fundamental assumptions in the study of shock has been that the problem centers about impaired oxygen delivery or utilization in the mitochondrium. Shock is often assumed to be associated with the development of a tissue oxygen deficit, but quantitative evidence for this idea has been difficult to obtain because the actual oxygen requirements during shock have not been established. While the total oxygen consumption may be within the normal range or even raised, this value may simply reflect altered regional blood flow, giving a net result within the normal range, but failing to point to large hypoxic areas. Crowell and Smith have reported studies on the oxygen consumption of anesthetized dogs subjected to a standard type of hemorrhage. They found that an oxygen debt of less than 100 ml per kg of body weight is compatible with survival, whereas 100% of the animals died when the oxygen deficit reached 150 ml per kilogram.

INDICATORS OF CELLULAR HYPOXIA.—Even though direct measurements of oxygen deficit are not available in human shock, the significance of cellular hypoxia in determining the outcome of the illness is supported both clinically and experimentally. The pioneer study of Cournand and Richards included some measurements of oxygen transport and oxygen consumption in patients in shock from skeletal trauma or external hemorrhage. Average oxygen consumption in this group was not decreased, as compared with a normal value. The group included some patients who were restless and showed symptoms of hyperventilation. They had, as a result, increased their oxygen consumption.

Measurement of mixed venous oxygen content by Cournand and Richards demonstrated a marked widening of the arterial venous oxygen difference brought about by extreme degrees of venous desaturation. The degree of venous blood hemoglobin saturation is often an excellent indicator of reduced tissue perfusion. An exception to this is the high venous blood hemoglobin saturation found in the septic patient. Measurement of the over-all oxygen consumption does not differentiate between the oxygen consumption of large and nonvital tissue masses and that of smaller but more essential organs. The depth of shock and its prognosis is determined best by repeated measurement of blood lactate levels. Levels of excess lactate raised above 2 mM per liter indicate not only a general swing toward anaerobic metabolism but also a severe degree of hepatic dysfunction since the liver is the principal site of lactate metabolism. Weil has used the level of blood lactate to form an accurate prognosis of survival.

In practice the diagnosis of a particular case of shock is made by juxtaposing several factors, including clinical observation, repeated measurements of vital organ function, arterial blood pressure, central venous pressure and, when possible, cardiac output coupled with evidences of cellular hypoxia as shown by metabolic acidosis.

Classification

While advanced shock is associated with failure of several organ systems, the initiating hemodynamic events may be used to form the basis for a simple classification of the common forms of shock:

I. Hypovolemic shock (initially a failure of venous return)
   A. Pure
      1. Hemorrhage
      2. Fluid loss (GI tract, burns, etc.)
      3. Trauma (loss of fluid in and around area of injury)
   B. Complicated (associated sepsis or cardiac failure)
II. Cardiogenic shock
   A. Pure
      1. Failure of left ventricular ejection
         a. Myocardial infarction
         b. Arrhythmias
      2. Failure of left ventricular filling
         a. Tamponade
         b. Massive pulmonary embolism
   B. Complicated (associated anemia, sepsis, or hypovolemia)
III. Septic shock (pathophysiology in man poorly understood)
   A. Pure (without recognizable hypovolemia or heart failure. Hyperdynamic, hypermetabolic, low vascular resistance state)
   B. Complicated
      1. Cardiac failure (cardiac output and vascular resistance variable)
      2. Hypovolemia
IV. Neurogenic shock (generalized interruption of vasomotor control)
   A. Trauma to spinal cord or brain stem
   B. High spinal anesthesia

Classification of shock serves the primary purpose of directing an initial approach to therapy. While the cause of shock is often obvious, the sequential documentation of clinical, hemodynamic, and metabolic measurements provides a running record upon which therapeutic decisions are based.

REFERENCES

HISTORICAL

Archibald, E. W., and McLean, W. S.: Observations upon shock with particular reference to the condition as seen in war surgery, Ann. Surg. 66:281, 1917.
Beecher, H. K. (ed.): *The Physiologic Effects of Wounds* (Washington, D.C.: 1952).

Blalock, A.: Experimental shock: Cause of low blood pressure produced by muscle injury, Arch. Surg. 22:959, 1930.

Blalock, A., and Bradburn, H.: Distribution of blood in shock, Arch. Surg. 20:26, 1930.

Cannon, W. B., and Bayliss, W. M.: Notes on Muscle Injury in Relation to Shock. Special Reports, Medical Research Commission, No. 26, VIII:19, 1919.

Cooper, Sir A.: A Dictionary of Practical Surgery (7th ed., London: Longman, 1838).

Cournand, A., Riley, R. L., Bradley, S. E., Breed, E. S., Noble, R. P., Lauson, H. D., Gregersen, M. I., and Richards, D. W.: Studies of circulation in clinical shock, Surgery 13:964, 1943.

Crile, G. W.: An Experimental Research into Surgical Shock (Philadelphia: J. B. Lippincott Company, 1899).

Dale, H. H., and Richards, A. N.: The vasodilator actions of histamine and other substances, J. Physiol. (London) 52:110, 1918.

Ducastaing, R.: La Vaso-Constriction Peripherique chez les Shockes: Action du Nitrite d'Amyle, Presse méd. 27:782, 1919.

Erlanger, J., and Gasser, H. S.: Studies in secondary traumatic shock. II. Shock due to mechanical limitation of blood flow. III. Circulatory failure due to adrenalin. Am. J. Physiol. 49:151; 345, 1919.

Grant, R. T., and Reeves, E. B.: Clinical observations on air-raid casualties. British Med. J., Aug. 30, 1941, p. 4208, British Med. J., Sept. 6, 1941, p. 329.

Grant, R. T., and Reeves, E. B.: Observations on the General Effects of Injury in Man. Med. Research Council, Special Report Series, No. 277, London: His Majesty's Stationery Office, 1941.

Henderson, Y.: Acapnia and shock. I. Carbon dioxide as a factor in the regulation of the heart rate, Am. J. Physiol. 21:126, 1908.

Johnson, G. S., and Blalock, A.: Experimental shock. XII. A study of the effect of hemorrhage, of trauma to muscles, of trauma to the intestines, of burns and of histamine on the cardiac output and on blood pressure of dogs, Arch. Surg. 23:855, 1931.

Latta, T.: Treatment of malignant cholera, Lancet 2:1831, 1832.

Malcolm, J. D.: Condition of blood vessels during shock, Lancet 2:573, 1905.

Noble, R. L., and Collip, J. B.: A quantitative method for the production of experimental traumatic shock without hemorrhage in unanesthetized animals, Quart. J. Exper. Physiol. 31:187, 1942.

Parsons, E., and Phemister, D. B.: Haemorrhage and "shock" in traumatized limbs. Experimental study, Surg., Gynec. & Obst. 51:196, 1930.

Warren, J. C.: Surgical Pathology and Therapeutics, in Shock (Philadelphia: W. B. Saunders Company, 1895), Chap. XI, p. 279.

Wiggers, C. J.: Physiology of Shock (Cambridge, Mass.: Harvard University Press, 1950).

CLINICAL, HEMODYNAMIC AND BIOCHEMICAL
CONSIDERATIONS IN SHOCK

Ankeney, J. L., Coffin, L. H., Jr., and Littell, A. S.: Experimental evidence that vasoconstriction in hemorrhagic shock does not result in anaerobic metabolism, Ann. Surg. 166:365, 1967.

Broder, G., and Weil, M. H.: Excess lactate. An index of shock reversibility in human patients, Science 143:1457, 1964.

Brody, O. V., and Oncley, J. L.: Effect of Erythrocyte Net Charge on Agglutination and Rouleaux Formation, in Sawyer, P. N. (ed.): Biophysical Mechanisms in Vascular Homeostasis and Intravascular Thrombosis (New York: Appleton-Century-Crofts, Inc., 1965).

Crowell, J. W., and Guyton, A. C.: Cardiac Deterioration in Shock: II. The Irreversible Stage, in Hershey, S. (ed.): Shock—International Anesthesiology Clinics 2:171, No. 2 (Boston: Little, Brown & Company, 1964).

Crowell, J. W., and Guyton, A. C.: Further evidence favouring a cardiac mechanism in irreversible hemorrhagic shock, Am. J. Physiol. 203:248, 1962.

Dagher, F. J., Lyons, J. H., Finlayson, D. C., Shamsai, J., and Moore, F. D.: Blood Volume Measurement: A Critical Study, in Welch, C. E. (ed.): *Advances in Surgery* (Chicago: Year Book Medical Publishers, Inc., 1965), Vol. 1, pp. 69–109.

Haller, J. A., Jr., Ward, M. J., and Cahill, J. L.: Metabolic alterations in shock: The effect of controlled reduction of blood flow on oxidative metabolism and catecholamine response, J. Trauma 7:727, 1967.

Huckabee, W. E.: Relationships of pyruvate and lactate during anaerobic metabolism: III. Effect of breathing low-oxygen gases, J. Clin. Invest. 37:264, 1958.

Kroetz, F. W., Leon, D. F., and Leonard, J. J.: The diagnosis of acute circulatory failure: Shock and syncope, Progr. Cardiovas. Dis. 10:262, 1967.

MacKenzie, G. J., Flenley, D. C., and Taylor, S. H.: Circulatory and respiratory studies in myocardial infarction and cardiogenic shock, Lancet 2:17, 1964.

MacLean, L. D.: Shock and metabolism, Surg., Gynec. & Obst. 127:299, 1968.

Mellander, S., and Lewis, D. H.: Effect of hemorrhagic shock on the reactivity of resistance and capacitance vessels and on capillary filtration transfer in cat skeletal muscle, Circulation Res. 13:105, 1963.

Miller, L. D., Oski, F. A., Diaco, J. F., Sugerman, H. J., Gottlieb, A. J., Davidson, D., and Delivoria-Papadopoulos, M.: The affinity of hemoglobin for oxygen: Its control and in vivo significance, Surgery 68:187, 1970.

Rothe, C. F.: Oxygen deficit in hemorrhagic shock in dogs, Am. J. Physiol. 214:436, 1968.

Sarnoff, S. J., Case, R. B., Warthe, P. E., and Isaacs, J. P.: Insufficient coronary flow and myocardial failure as complicating factor in late hemorrhagic shock, Am. J. Physiol. 176:439, 1954.

Schumer, W.: Lactic acid as a factor in the production of irreversibility in oligemic shock, Nature, London 212:1210, 1966.

Shires, G. T.: Shock and metabolism, Surg., Gynec. & Obst. 124:284, 1967.

Skillman, J. J., Lauler, D. P., Hickler, R. B.: Hemorrhage in normal man. Effect on renin, cortisol, aldosterone, and urine composition, Ann. Surg. 166:865, 1967.

Smith, L. L., and Moore, F. D.: Refractory hypotension in man—Is this irreversible shock? New England J. Med. 267:733, 1962.

Thal, A. P., Wilson, R. F., Kalfuss, L., and Andre, J.: The Role of Metabolic and Humoral Factors in Irreversible Shock, in Mills, L. C., and Moyer, J. H., *Shock and Hypotension* (New York: Grune & Stratton, Inc., 1965), p. 609.

2

The Systemic Response to Shock

THE CAPACITY for self-preservation is nowhere better demonstrated than in shock. Here one sees the evolution of a complex pattern of defense mechanisms designed to negate the effects of the injury (Fig. 2-1). As an example, the cardiovascular system is continuously regulated by a medullary center designed to regulate arterial blood pressure and, to a lesser extent, other circulatory variables within a narrow range. This vasomotor center is continually supplied with information via the 9th and 10th cranial nerves from stretch receptors monitoring pressure in the carotid sinus and aortic arch. A fall in arterial blood pressure within the system normally produces an appropriate response designed to restore the pressure to its former value. The afferent limb of this response is predominantly mediated through the sympathetic nervous system, which reinforces peripheral resistance by arteriolar constriction and cardiac output by increasing the rate and force of cardiac contraction. Meanwhile the effective blood volume is enhanced by increased venomotor tone which squeezes blood from large venous reservoirs into the central circulation (Fig. 2-2). The maximal sympathetic response seen in shock diverts blood flow away from the extremities, bowel, and kidney to the vital areas of heart and brain whose vessels constrict little under intense sympathetic stimulation. While these responses to severe injury are essential for immediate survival, prolonged diversion of blood flow from organs such as liver, kidney, gastrointestinal tract, and muscle masses proves damaging in the long run.

This "selective ischemia" is seen in a highly developed form in the diving mammals in whom, under the threat of hypoxia, blood flow is diverted from nonessential to vital areas. The limited available cardiac output is redistributed from kidney, liver, intestine, and muscle mass to the heart and brain. While differing in some essentials, the circulatory response to hypoxic injury in man bears an over-all similarity to the diving reflex in the seal.

In the microcirculation, hypotension produces a variable effect, depending on the dominance of constrictor influences at each end of the capillary. When capillary hydrostatic pressure falls, there is a net movement of extra-

35

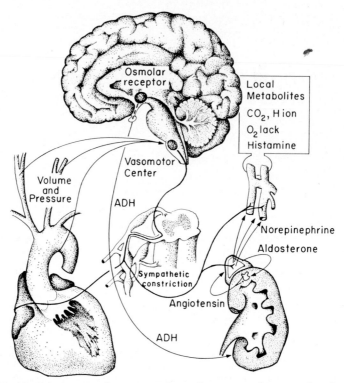

Fig. 2–1.—Homeostatic mechanisms regulating heart rate and contractility, the capacitance of the microcirculation, and plasma volume. (From Thal, Alan P., and Wilson, Robert F.: Shock, in *Current Problems in Surgery* [Chicago: Year Book Medical Publishers, September 1965].)

cellular fluid into the capillary, restoring plasma volume. When capillary hydrostatic pressure increases, plasma is lost from the vascular space and hemoconcentration occurs.

While stabilizing reflexes restore blood pressure in shock by reducing the capacity of the vascular system and increasing the heart rate, other equally powerful homeostatic responses conserve and restore plasma volume. Water and sodium are conserved by the kidney under the influence of antidiuretic hormone (ADH) and aldosterone, respectively. Increased baroceptor firing with hypotension, changes in plasma osmolality, and reduced left atrial filling pressure have been shown to trigger the release of ADH. The juxtaglomerular apparatus stimulated by a number of factors, including a decreased pulse pressure, causes the release of renin, a proteolytic enzyme which forms angiotensin I from plasma protein precursors. Angiotensin I, after being converted to angiotensin II, causes

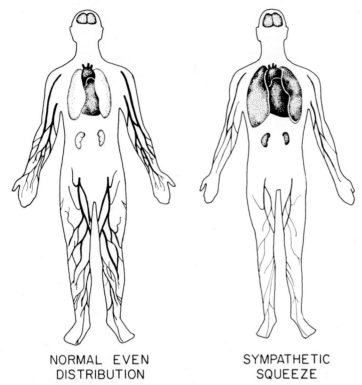

NORMAL EVEN
DISTRIBUTION

SYMPATHETIC
SQUEEZE

Fig. 2–2.—Prolonged vasoconstriction depletes peripheral and splanchnic blood flow, ultimately producing left ventricular failure and pulmonary engorgement.

increased production and release of aldosterone from the adrenal cortex which, in turn, enhances renal retention of sodium and, therefore, water. Additional fluid intake is encouraged by the profound thirst in shock.

Guyton has characterized the control system of the body as a process of negative feedback; that is, the response tends to negate and correct the drift from the norm. A fall in blood pressure, for example, calls for an increase in heart rate and peripheral vasoconstriction. These responses tend to restore the pressure toward normal. Similarly, the response to metabolic acidosis is a ventilatory drive which lowers arterial carbon dioxide tension and tends to restore pH. Governing almost every vital process are similar control systems designed to maintain a near-constant cellular environment.

The initial response of the patient in shock exemplifies the overstressing of these control systems. When a control system fails, a reaction of positive feedback develops. This is illustrated in Figure 2-3, depicting the vicious circle of positive feedback in shock. Under these circumstances, the initi-

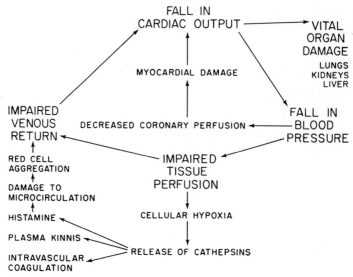

Fig. 2–3.—Positive feedback cycle of shock.

ating stimulus is exaggerated by the response. A fall in blood pressure, for example, reduces coronary blood flow, impairs myocardial function, and results in further reduction in cardiac output, further fall in blood pressure, and further myocardial damage. This positive feedback reaction, which can be endured for only a short period, progresses rapidly to what was once termed irreversible or refractory shock. Ultimately, if a suitable cellular environment is not restored, the injury becomes overwhelming and self-perpetuating; the perimeter defenses are abandoned and the major effective circulation is concentrated in the vital areas of heart, brain, and lungs for a last stand. Unless the vicious cycle of shock (Fig. 2-3) can be reversed rapidly, all treatment may be to no avail because of relentless damage to vital organs. At this stage, pharmacologic manipulations of blood pressure and cardiac output, correction of metabolic acidosis with buffers, and the raising of arterial oxygen tensions give but an illusion of improvement.

The Microcirculation in Shock

Impairment of nutritional blood flow is the ultimate common denominator in all forms of shock. While the capillary circulation is clearly responsive to local metabolic needs and responds promptly to arterial occlusion by reactive hyperemia, when oxygen lack is clearly demonstrable, the requirements of the vital organs take precedence. This lack of oxygen results in a dominating peripheral vasoconstriction and diversion of blood flow from areas not immediately necessary for survival.

The smooth muscle cells regulate the microcirculation by controlling the caliber of peripheral arterioles, precapillary sphincters, and venules. The arteriolar vessels constitute the major resistance to blood flow and the resistance against which the heart must pump. Flow through the nutritional network of capillary vessels is determined by the action of precapillary sphincters. In this way, the surface area for nutrition constantly changes in response to demand. Venules constitute the postcapillary resistance, and the venous system makes up 70% of the reservoir of the vascular space. Postcapillary pressure is of particular importance in determining capillary hydrostatic pressure and, thereby, the efflux and influx of fluid across the capillary endothelium. Contraction of this venous reservoir under sympathetic bombardment can result in a rapid, if short-term, increase in venous return to the heart. The caliber of the venules, therefore, has double importance in regulating both transcapillary fluid exchange and cardiac output.

Local blood flow is controlled by local metabolic requirements under normal conditions, but under a stress condition such as shock, local mechanisms are overridden by the need to maintain central blood pressure. The peripheral vascular resistance rises and the rate of venous return increases. The capillary hydrostatic pressure falls and an influx of interstitial fluid into the vascular space occurs. These two mechanisms—venoconstriction producing an autotransfusion and transcapillary refilling producing a more delayed effect—tend to restore vascular volume and increase cardiac output. These responses serve an adaptive purpose for the support of the central circulation at the expense of peripheral perfusion.

The phenomenon of transcapillary refilling is seen after moderate blood loss (up to 1,500 ml in the adult). In this situation, Moore has measured refilling of approximately 150 ml per hour until plasma volume is restored (Fig. 2-4). In severe shock, postcapillary venous pressure tends to rise and net influx may be reduced or may cease. Large infusions of norepinephrine produce dominant effects on postcapillary venous tone documented by a rising hematocrit. Meanwhile the accumulating tissue metabolites in areas of vasoconstriction produce a powerful stimulus for metabolic vasodilation. According to Zweifach, the small blood vessels react to hemorrhage by becoming highly responsive and show an increase in vasoactivity, causing the blood flow to be confined to direct capillary channels. In the late stages of shock there is a tendency toward decompensation; the microcirculation becomes unresponsive to endogenous pressor amines and the capillary space progressively opens up. Pooling of blood develops in the small venules to the point of stasis. The experimental

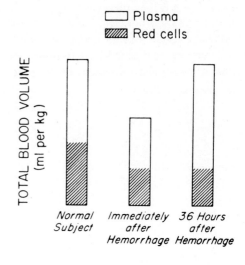

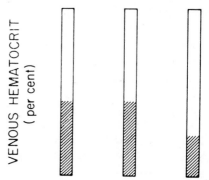

Fig. 2–4.—Restoration of total blood volume by transcapillary refilling 36 hours after hemorrhage. Note the reduced blood volume, but normal hematocrit, in the first few hours after hemorrhage. (From Linman, James W.: in *Principles of Hematology* [New York: The Macmillan Company, 1966], p. 68.)

studies of Mellander and Lewis are pertinent here; using a skeletal muscle bed in cats, they found that postcapillary venous sphincters maintain their state of vasoconstriction long after precapillary sphincters have failed to respond to sympathetic stimulation. This vasoconstriction tends to increase the capillary hydrostatic pressure and decrease the rate of influx of interstitial fluid into the vascular space.

When capillary hydrostatic pressure exceeds plasma colloid osmotic pressure, there is a loss of fluid from the vascular space into the interstitial space. In the experiments of Melander and Lewis, this loss occurred approximately 2 hours after continuous hypotension. Generalizations from this study cannot be made since there is evidence that the circulation of muscle and skin may be under a predominantly vasoconstrictive influence whereas that of the splanchnic viscera or of inflamed areas may be vasodilated. Alpha adrenergic blocking agents, such as phenoxybenzamine, are particularly effective in reducing postcapillary venous resistance and will enhance the movement of fluid into the vascular space. It is clear that both in man and in the experimental animal different vascular beds react with varying degrees of sensitivity to adrenergic vasoconstrictor impulses.

PERIPHERAL SHUNTING

The concept of nonnutritional or shunt flow has gained considerable attention, especially in patients with cirrhosis and septic shock, in which a high cardiac output exists in the face of biochemical evidences of cellular hypoxia. Venous blood from these patients has an oxygen content very near that of arterial blood. In septic shock it is still not clear whether this finding represents diversion of blood from nutritional channels (Fig. 2-5) or results from rapid flow through vasodilated channels or even from cellular damage and impaired oxygen uptake.

Recent studies on experimental sepsis have been revealing in delineating the hyperdynamic circulatory response to sepsis. When a septic leg is developed experimentally in the dog, there is a progressive increase in blood flow and venous blood hemoglobin saturation within the area of sepsis. Blood flow within the septic leg may be doubled or tripled, but the rise in cardiac output is disproportionately large and cannot be accounted

Fig. 2–5.—Arteriovenous communication (shown in bars). This may become a preferential route in septic shock producing the low vascular resistance state. (From Zweifach, B. W., *Functional Behavior of the Microcirculation* [Springfield, Ill.: Charles C Thomas Publisher, 1961], p. 18, Fig. 3, *C*.

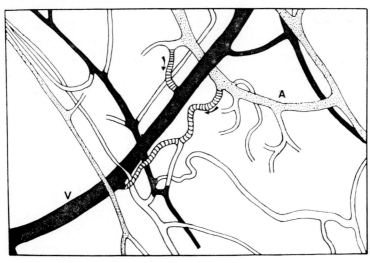

for by the rise in blood flow through the area of sepsis. It appears that a vasodilator substance released from the septic region lowers vascular resistance within the renal and splanchnic beds, increasing flow considerably through these organs. Concurrently the resistance in skin and muscle appears to rise, thereby reducing flow. The system is labile and responds to dominant influences; a powerful sympathetic response to an additional injury, such as blood loss, produces an over-all rise in resistance and a drop in flow even in the area of sepsis.

RED CELL AGGREGATION AND VISCOSITY FACTORS

Chiefly as a result of Kniseley's work, a great deal of interest has centered upon the possibility that red cell aggregation impedes the microcirculation. The question still being debated is whether the red cell aggregation causes or results from the low-flow states. Aggregation of red cells has been noted in a number of normal and diseased states in man and in the experimental animal. Under most circumstances, the aggregation appears to be reversible, but in some disease states it is thought to develop as an irreversible aggregation. Some investigators feel that the suspension stability of the red cell is maintained by the action of the negative surface charge in repelling adjacent cells. Bernstein, by measuring electrophoretic mobility of red cells, has indicated that the net negative surface charge may be increased by agents such as low-molecular-weight dextran. This observation has been fundamental in supporting the extensive use of the substance, but recent studies by Brody and Oncley have questioned the importance of electronegativity of red cell surface in maintaining suspension stability. Grendahl, who measured the force required to separate aggregated red cells, concludes that the energy required for separation was greater than can be accounted for by ionic charge forces.

On the other hand, fibrinogen coating of the red cell surface appears to be an important factor in promoting aggregation. Replogle has differentiated the easily broken-apart aggregate seen when normal red cells are coated with fibrinogen from the agglutination which occurs when sensitized red cells are suspended in specific antibody. These latter masses of erythrocytes cannot be separated readily. Merril, Replogle, and Wells emphasized the non-Newtonian behavior of blood (Fig. 2-6) by measuring viscosity under various conditions. Plasma has Newtonian characteristics shown by a viscosity that does not alter with change in velocity of flow. The term *shear rate*, or velocity gradient, is the measure applied to these forces. When flow stops at zero shear rate, a certain force which has been called "the yield stress" must be applied to the blood to cause it to yield and begin to flow. Washed red cells suspended in saline or defibrinated

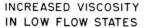

INCREASED VISCOSITY
IN LOW FLOW STATES

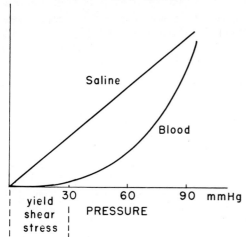

Fig. 2–6.—A plot demonstrating the non-Newtonian characteristics of blood in low-flow states.

blood result in a solution which becomes nearly Newtonian. In these solutions the yield shear stress is small.

When fibrinogen is added to saline suspensions of red cells, the non-Newtonian characteristics are again observed and the yield shear stress is increased. This is thought to represent the effect of fibrinogen acting as a bonding material between red cells. In low-flow states, such as shock, the propensity for aggregation is increased. The same is true after extensive surface burns, and in cyanotic heart disease, where the hematocrit is high. After successful treatment of low-flow states, the velocity of flow through the capillary bed increases, the erythrocyte aggregates are broken apart and, at high shear rates, the blood viscosity is lowered. Preliminary studies suggest that in low-flow states, and particularly following a prolonged period of shock, the alteration in the red cell surface leads to coating with gamma globulin similar to the coating seen when sensitized red cells are exposed to specific antibody.

Studies of the microcirculation in low-flow states in man have been restricted to a few vascular beds only, such as those of the conjunctiva or skin. The most elegant studies now available are those of Branermark, who implanted transparent chambers into the skin of human volunteers under circumstances in which flow could be regulated by compression of a skin-tube pedicle. Under normal conditions, there is no tendency for erythrocytes to adhere. When blood flow was reduced by compression of the pedicle, however, erythrocyte aggregation was seen in rouleaux formation. When flow was reestablished, these rouleaux were quickly broken apart and washed away. Even when flow had been reduced for 3 hours there was aggregation, but no tendency for agglutination. Under conditions of elevated hematocrit, together with low flow, red cell aggregates appeared to plug capillaries and venules. Again, restoration of flow readily initiated breakup of the erythrocyte mass. Weighing the evidence regarding the phenomenon of red cell agglutination in low-flow states, Replogle concludes that intravascular aggregation should, at the moment, be viewed as the result of diminished flow rather than as its cause.

Release of Humoral Agents Affecting the Microcirculation

In addition to the local blood and fluid losses which occur in most forms of shock, diffusible products emanate from damaged tissue and may have profound effects on the circulation locally and systemically. It should be recognized that edema and fluid loss into an inflamed or injured area result in large measure from the local action of humoral agents such as histamine, serotonin, and vasoactive polypeptides. Some of the potentially toxic agents that have been identified in a human or in an experimental animal in shock will be discussed.

CATECHOLAMINES.—Release of catecholamines is part of the vital primary reaction to injury which enables the animal to maintain blood flow to the heart and brain. Erlanger and Gasser postulated that tissues were asphyxiated by prolonged vasoconstriction. This work has been repeatedly confirmed; 5 mg per kilogram of body weight of norepinephrine given for 60 minutes to dogs produces an initial hypertension and rise in cardiac output which is then followed by a fall in cardiac output and shock. The autopsy findings in these animals closely resemble those seen in endotoxin shock.

The electron microscope and the use of radioisotopes have revealed norepinephrine storage in "granulated vesicles" in postganglionic sympathetic nerve endings. This stored norepinephrine can be released by reserpine, tyramine, amphetamine, cocaine, and other drugs. Prolonged use of these drugs may so deplete the nerve endings of their catecholamine content that shock may result from minimal stress. Many so-called sympathomimetic drugs were thought to act directly on vascular smooth muscle, but it now seems clear that several of these agents liberate norepinephrine from "granulated vesicles" in the postsynaptic sympathetic nerve ending. This liberated catecholamine then stimulates the effector organ. A current concept of the site of action of these agents at the nerve terminal is shown in Figure 2-7.

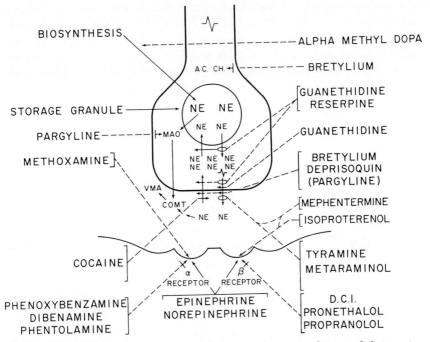

Fig. 2–7.—Diagrammatic concept of biosynthesis of norepinephrine and drug action at the adrenergic nerve ending. (Modified and reproduced with permission of Dr. William B. Abrams.)

The best-known hemodynamic effects of the catecholamines are related to inotropic and chronotropic stimulation of the heart, constriction of arterioles in skin, kidney, and viscera, dilatation of arteries in striated muscle and the myocardium, and constriction in most veins. These effects vary considerably, depending upon the metabolic state of the experimental animal, blood volume, anesthesia, and the dose and type of adrenergic drug given.

Evidence for the participation of catecholamines in the genesis of and response to shock are many, and increased catecholamine levels have been regularly measured in the plasma in many forms of shock. Moreover the effects of bacterial endotoxin are enhanced locally and systemically with epinephrine or norepinephrine.

HISTAMINE.—The discovery by Dale in 1912 that histamine is a vasodilator substance which increases tissue permeability and produces severe hypotension when given in large doses to cats seemed to provide a biochemical basis for many of the microvascular changes in shock. Further studies by Sir Thomas Lewis indicated that in areas of skin injury an

H-substance similar to histamine was released. Interest in this substance has been rekindled by Schayer, who suggests that a balance between histamine and catecholamines exerts the main control over circulatory homeostasis and that histamine is the main regulator of the microcirculation. His work, showing increased synthesis of histamine-decarboxylase in shock tissues, implies that the local synthesis of histamine ("induced histamine") rather than the "preformed histamine" in mast cells is the important physiologic mechanism controlling the microcirculation. This increased synthesis of histamine during shock may then produce small-vessel damage. On the basis of pressure measurements of small vessels, Haddy and Visscher felt that the increased capillary permeability brought about by histamine results from postcapillary venular spasm rather than from a direct toxic effect on endothelial cells. The role of this substance remains to be elucidated in shock, but it seems probable that it is released in concert with other agents affecting the microcirculation.

SEROTONIN.—Serotonin (5-hydroxytryptamine) is present throughout the body, but has been found in largest concentration in the brain, gastrointestinal tract, platelets, and mast cells. This vasoactive agent is released during various forms of experimental and clinical shock and during prolonged pump oxygenation when there is continued trauma to the solid elements of blood. Its effects on vascular smooth muscle are highly variable and can best be described as amphibaric in that it may either raise or lower pressure, depending on the circumstances. The action on vessel tone is often opposite to that already present. One of the most noticeable effects of serotonin is on the pulmonary vasculature, where it greatly increases pulmonary vascular resistance. The possibility has been raised by Daicoff that it produces pulmonary venular spasm and pulmonary edema.

VASOACTIVE POLYPEPTIDES.—*Bradykinin.*—Bradykinin is a vasoactive nonapeptide released by the action of a protease such as trypsin or kallikrein on its inactive precursor, bradykininogen. Experiments by Fox suggest that bradykinin may be the hormone that regulates the caliber of the small vessels. In clinical experiments, bradykinin was shown to dilate the small vessels of skin and muscles in doses comparable to those of histamine and was a more universal vasodilator. Upon the coronary vessels and pial vessels it was found to be a very potent vasodilator. Doses on the order of a nanogram (10^{-9} gm) produce a detectable increase in coronary flow of the isolated guinea pig heart.

Bradykinin release has now been documented in several forms of experimental and clinical shock. In hemorrhagic shock, Diniz and Carvalho found that bradykininogen levels rose initially and then declined rapidly to levels below control. Nies and associates, working in Melmon's laboratory, have identified circulating kinins in rhesus monkeys given endotoxin.

In anaphylactic shock, Beraldo found that bradykininogen levels decreased as the bradykinin activity of plasma increased. It was also noted that the local Shwartzman and Thomas reactions were potentiated by bradykinin. Trasylol, trypsin kallikrein inhibitor (TKI), stops the formation of bradykinin from bradykininogen and has been used in the management of human pancreatitis and septic shock. Its value is as yet unestablished. The extremely rapid inactivation of bradykinin in blood makes it likely that its actions are limited to the site of formation, where it produces local vasodilation and increased capillary permeability.

Kallidin II.—Kallidin II closely resembles bradykinin in its formation, structure, and function. This decapeptide is formed by the action of kallikrein upon kallidinogen, a substrate in the alpha-$_2$-globulin fraction of plasma. Attention has been directed to these substances since 1950 when Werle published his classic work on kallikrein, the hypotensive proteolytic material from the pancreas. Although previous work indicated that intravenous infusion of urinary kallikrein could produce shock, Webster and Clark found that a more purified form failed to kill dogs in amounts nine times that previously reported. After further investigation, they suggested that a possible synergistic effect and relationship existed between endotoxin, kallikrein, and plasmin.

Angiotensin II.—This vasoactive octapeptide is formed by the action of the protease renin on angiotensinogen. Its vascular effects are generally opposite to those of bradykinin. Clinically angiotensin II has been found to raise blood pressure by arterial vasoconstriction. In patients treated with this drug, there has been an increased total peripheral resistance, central venous pressure, and arterial blood pressure with a decrease in cardiac output.

Toxic Phenomena in Shock

The noxious effects of blood from damaged tissues.—Blood or lymph draining from damaged tissues produces an adverse effect on the circulation as a whole. An example of this is seen in animal experiments when a completely occluding tourniquet placed around the leg produces arterial ischemia for several hours. Release of this tourniquet is followed by hypotension which can be explained largely by loss of fluid into the leg. If blood and lymph draining from this damaged tissue is collected, vasodilator substances may be identified, including histamine, polypeptides released by proteases from damaged cells, and adenosine. Under certain circumstances the products released by cellular damage appear to play a major role in initiating and perpetuating the damage to the cardiovascular system, but this role at the moment is unclear. In man the most important effects brought about by muscle-crushing injury or tourniquet injury are fluid loss into the injured limb coupled with release of myoglobin and potassium. High circulating levels of both myoglobin and potassium produce acute renal failure and impaired myocardial function respectively.

THE EFFECTS OF BACTERIAL TOXINS.—Endotoxin, a lipopolysaccharide derived from the disintegration of gram-negative bacterial cell wall has many varied effects in different species of animals and in humans, depending on the amount used and on the species studied. In general the substance produces severe metabolic damage with hypotension, leading ultimately to death. In dogs, severe congestion and engorgement of the liver with hemorrhagic necrosis of the bowel are conspicuous, but this lesion is extremely rare in septic shock in man. Acting through the release of tissue mediators, bacterial endotoxins produce an extraordinary hypersensitivity of the muscular venules and small veins and a tendency to extensive capillary damage as seen in the transilluminated preparation.

Endotoxin itself has no effect on isolated smooth muscle preparations, but when incubated with blood or homogenized tissue, it releases histamine and vasoactive polypeptides. The generalized Shwartzman reaction described in 1929 demonstrated that when two sublethal doses of endotoxin were given intravenously (approximately 18 hours apart) to a rabbit, intravascular platelet and fibrin thrombi formed with the production of symmetrical renal cortical necrosis. The local Shwartzman reaction occurs when the first dose is given subcutaneously and the second intravenously, producing a similar form of hemorrhagic necrosis in the skin.

Blockade of the reticuloendothelial system with particulate material, the addition of steroids, or pregnancy produces the Shwartzman reaction with only one injection of endotoxin. From the experimental point of view, endotoxin is fascinating, and with suitable manipulation it can be made to potentiate or inhibit the function of the reticuloendothelial system or the effects of hemorrhage, catecholamines, etc. The release of endotoxin in patients previously exposed to this substance may result in severe intravascular thrombosis, thrombocytopenia, and hemorrhagic phenomena. Meningococcemia appears to be a phenomenon of this type. Recent work, previously discussed, points up serious differences between the experimental endotoxin model and clinical sepsis.

Bacterial exotoxin, in particular that of pathogenic staphylococci, is more commonly associated with local tissue necrosis. The staphylococcus, alpha hemolysin, which has the property of producing severe spasm in small blood vessels leading to tissue necrosis, is a lipoprotein. Unlike endotoxin, alpha hemolysin produces a severe constriction when applied to vascular smooth muscles. It is an extremely potent liberator of serotonin and histamine. Shock associated with gram-positive bacteremia is far less common than with gram-negative microorganisms.

Coagulation

Hemorrhagic shock is followed by a marked shortening of the coagulation time and an increased tendency to thrombosis. In virtually every clinical or experimental situation in which disseminated intravascular coagulation (DIC) occurs, some degree of low tissue perfusion and hypotension has been found. Naturally the question of cause and effect has arisen. This question remains unanswered, but the importance of the clotting defect in shock should not be underestimated.

Under normal circumstances blood remains fluid in the vascular system unless there is injury to blood vessels, at which time it is able to clot rapidly to prevent excessive hemorrhage. This function is only part of the complex hemostatic mechanism which depends on the reactivity of blood vessels and platelets as well as on the ability of the blood to form stable clots speedily. The relative importance of these factors and the exact sequence of events are variable, but eventually the openings in damaged vessels must be closed so that blood can no longer escape from them. Except in very small venules and capillaries where adhesion of endothelial surfaces and local aggregation of platelets alone is sufficient, hemostasis is accomplished by the formation of clots within the lumens of the vessels.

The mechanism by which blood remains fluid and does not clot in the intact circulation is similarly complex and not nearly as well understood as the hemostatic one. Some contributing factors are the "nonwettable" and fibrinolytic surface of the vascular endothelium, the slowness of clotting via the intrinsic pathway, the avidity of the reticuloendothelial system for circulating active coagulant substances, and the physiologic anticoagulant activities of plasma. Whatever the exact roles of these factors, under pathologic conditions the normal fluidity of the blood may be lost and DIC may result in the deposit of clots in arterioles, capillaries, and venules without any apparent initiating trauma to these vessels. Thus the hemostatic mechanism which is so necessary to preservation of life may actually become life threatening. Improved understanding of normal hemostasis and careful study of individual cases have made it possible to understand many aspects of disseminated clotting and its effect on the body as a whole.

THE HEMOSTATIC MECHANISM

Study of blood clotting has been greatly aided by the general acceptance of an International Nomenclature for the recognized coagulation factors.

These have been assigned Roman numerals and now number thirteen; besides these factors, many less-well-defined substances are involved in the formation and destruction of clots and will be referred to by name. The following is a list of the numbered factors and their equivalents.

Factor I	Fibrinogen
Factor II	Prothrombin
Factor III	Thromboplastin (tissue)
Factor IV	Calcium
Factor V	Labile factor, proaccelerin, accelerator globulin (AcG)
Factor VI	(No longer used—accelerin)
Factor VII	Stable factor, proconvertin, serum prothrombin conversion accelerator (SPCA), autoprothrombin I
Factor VIII	Antihemophilic factor (AHF), antihemophilic globulin (AHG), thromboplastinogen, platelet cofactor I
Factor IX	Plasma thromboplastin component (PTC), Christmas factor, platelet cofactor II, autoprothrombin II
Factor X	Stuart-Prower factor
Factor XI	Plasma thromboplastin antecedent (PTA)
Factor XII	Hageman factor
Factor XIII	Fibrin stabilizing factor

Almost immediately after injury to the wall of a small blood vessel, platelets adhere to the exposed collagen and changes begin to occur, resulting in the aggregation of platelets; within 30 seconds small fibrin loci form. Fibrinogen is present in plasma and absorbed onto the surfaces of platelets so that the newly formed fibrin is closely associated with the platelets. The platelet aggregates then begin to disintegrate, liberating vasoconstrictor and clot-promoting (phospholipid) substances. Fibrin formation continues and fibrin masses become confluent with the platelet aggregates, forming a plug which is firm enough to stop the flow of blood temporarily. Tissue thromboplastin (factor III) is responsible for the initial rapid formation of these small amounts of fibrin. This mechanism is often referred to as the *extrinsic pathway* (Fig. 2-8). "Extrinsic" is used to describe this process because the coagulant material which initiates clotting in this situation is released into the blood stream from tissues and is not ordinarily present in the circulating blood. The *intrinsic pathway* (Fig. 2-9), on the other hand, is the sequential activation of the coagulation proteins which normally circulate in inactive form in the blood. The fibrin which forms is the same in both cases.

When the column of circulating blood is stopped or slowed behind the platelet plug, the slower changes of intrinsic clotting begin to occur and, eventually, a whole-blood clot forms, usually extending as far backward from the platelet plug as the nearest connecting vessel. This intrinsic pathway involves the sequential interaction of platelet phospholipid and at

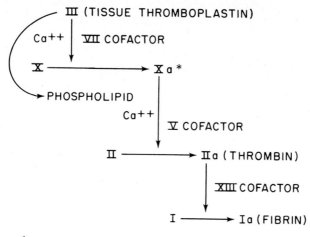

*Activated form

Fig. 2–8.—Extrinsic pathway.

least nine coagulation proteins, and it is not perfectly understood; however, it probably progresses in the manner shown in Figure 2-9, taking several minutes to reach completion. The final step is the formation of the fibrin network which contains red blood cells and platelet aggregates in its meshes.

The initial stages of this process are the most time-consuming ones, and moderate deficiencies of factors XII, XI, IX, and VIII are more likely to prolong the over-all coagulation time than those of the later-acting factors, V, X, II, XIII, and I. Either a severe deficiency of any one factor or multiple deficiencies of more than one factor will significantly delay clotting. The final conversion of factor I (fibrinogen) to fibrin is accomplished by the proteolytic splitting off of fibrinopeptides A and B and the subsequent polymerization of the fibrin monomers that are left, thus forming the supportive framework of the clot. This fibrin clot and certain other less-well-defined substances act as antithrombins to prevent the accumulation of too much thrombin (factor IIa), which is always produced in excess.

Fortunately the formation of fibrin is not a permanent matter, and the body has many ways of disposing of unneeded fibrin. One method is the slow enzymatic digestion, which includes not only proteolytic enzymes from tissues and leukocytes, but also a potent plasma protease called plasmin. Plasmin exists in the normal plasma in the form of an inactive precursor, plasminogen, which can be activated in a variety of ways: by anoxia, surface contact, tissue extracts, chloroform, streptokinase, and

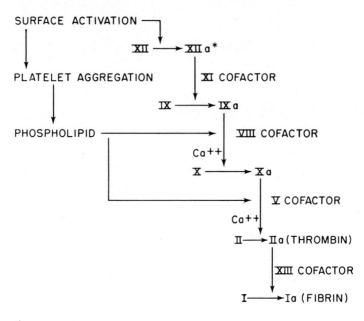

*Activated form

Fig. 2–9.—Intrinsic pathway.

urokinase. This plasminogen-plasmin system is integrally related to and in many ways very similar to the blood-clotting system (Fig. 2-10).

Usually plasminogen is closely associated with fibrinogen and is deposited in the clot with the fibrin during clotting. When activating substances from tissues, blood vessels, or plasma penetrate the clot, localized secondary fibrinolysis occurs. Usually this is a relatively slow process, allowing the clot to remain as a hemostatic plug until other processes, such as organization, can provide permanent repair. If a clot is lysed too rapidly, there may be a recurrence of local bleeding after the original adequate hemostasis. With such local fibrinolysis, there is no evidence of an increase in circulating plasmin.

The lysis of fibrin clots by plasmin results in the formation of fibrin split products (FSP). These are partially digested fragments that can react with antifibrinogen sera but are incoagulable with thrombin. Under normal conditions they are found in serum in very minute quantities. Primary systemic fibrinolysis (which apparently occurs rarely, if at all) and fibrinolysis secondary to DIC may produce large quantities of these products, which have been shown to act as anticoagulants. They impair aggregation, adhesiveness, and the release reaction of platelets and interfere

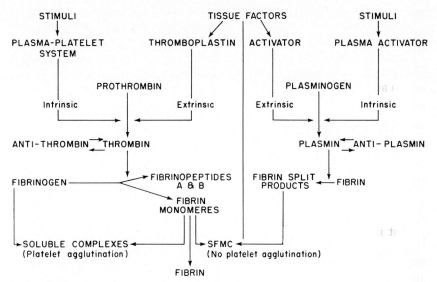

Fig. 2–10.—Comparison of the plasminogen-plasmin system to the blood-clotting system.

with plasma thromboplastin formation, the thrombin-fibrinogen reaction, and fibrin polymerization. Small amounts of these split products may form inactive complexes with fibrin monomers called *soluble fibrin monomer complexes* (SFMC). The presence of both split products and some of these complexes in normal persons indicates that there is some intravascular clotting with secondary lysis occurring all the time.

Plasmin, being a nonspecific proteolytic enzyme, is also capable of digesting fibrinogen and other coagulation proteins when it circulates freely with them in the plasma. Normally, however, when increased amounts of plasmin are formed, they are rapidly inactivated by antiplasmin. Rare cases of primary systemic fibrinolysis have been described in which excessive plasmin could be demonstrated with rapid lysis of clots formed in vitro. The opposite situation occurs in liver disease when there is increased lytic activity because of a decrease in antiplasmin. In both situations, increased lytic activity and increased levels of fibrin split products can be demonstrated, usually with decreases in plasminogen. Figure 2-11 compares the situation in the clot and in the circulating plasma.

PATHOPHYSIOLOGY

Only by understanding the hemostatic mechanism and what is essential to produce clotting can one postulate a sequence of events most likely to occur in DIC and predict the clinical situations in which it will be found. A variety of initiating stimuli can act in different ways and at different stages in the clotting process. Primarily these stimuli include damage to endothelial surfaces, changes in platelets which increase their tendency to adhesiveness and aggregation, and the infusion of tissue thromboplastin into the circulating blood. Platelet aggregation may be initiated by contact with injured vascular endothelium or by interaction with certain agents in the circulating blood. How substances such as bacterial endotoxin, antigen-antibody complexes, viruses, and thrombin bring about these changes in platelets is not well understood, but may involve release of adenosine diphosphate (ADP) or immune adherence. Some stimuli may act in more than one manner, and in many cases more than one stimulus may be active at a given time. Possible initiating stimuli and their sites of action are shown in Figure 2-12.

Even though the type of stimulus varies, the end result is essentially the same—the formation of thrombin (IIa) with the deposition of microthrombi of different combinations of agglutinated platelets, fibrin, and red and white blood cells in the microcirculation, resulting in occlusion of these small vessels (Figs. 2-13 to 2-15). In low-perfusion shock, slowing of blood flow, tissue acidosis, and a temporary stimulus to increased and more-rapid clotting enhances intravascular coagulation. Local fibrinolysis almost invariably accompanies the clotting but, in some patients, activation is insufficient and thrombosis with infarction and necrosis of tissue occurs. In some cases, the fibrinolytic system is rapidly and generally activated so that fibrinolysis overshadows the initiating clotting process. Also, a variety of vasoactive substances participate in the development of the

Fig. 2–11.—Comparison of the activity of the plasminogen-plasmin system in plasma and in the clot. (From Sirridge, Marjorie: *Laboratory Evaluation of Hemostasis.* Used by permission of Lea & Febiger.)

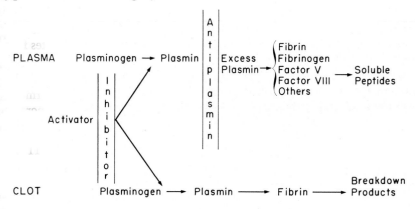

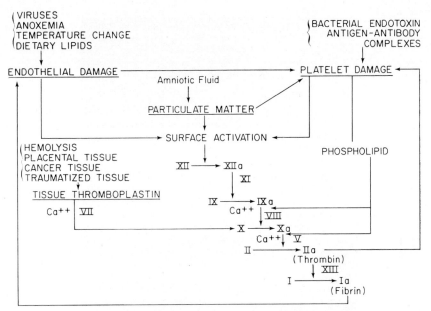

Fig. 2–12.—Possible sites of action of initiating stimuli in disseminated intravascular coagulation.

whole picture. The reticuloendothelial system normally serves as a protective mechanism by phagocytizing both coagulant substances and fibrin aggregates.

With massive coagulation, a patient may die rapidly in irreversible shock. Minor clotting episodes usually result only in transient platelet agglutination with a slight deposition of fibrin and mild, reversible shock. With somewhat more severe stimuli, the patient may survive shock only to develop a bleeding diathesis due to the consumption of platelets, fibrinogen, and other clotting factors (V, VIII, and X most often) during the intravascular coagulation. This is the so-called consumption coagulopathy. Should a patient survive both shock and hemorrhage, he may develop symptoms referable to thrombosis and tissue necrosis.

With any degree of DIC, hemorrhage usually occurs. It is most often manifested by bleeding where surgical or obstetric trauma has left an open wound, but it may occur from all mucous membranes in the severely affected patient. Bleeding from the stomach, the duodenum, and the esophagus is an especially common complication in surgical shock. The bleeding problem produced by consumption of the coagulation proteins is further aggravated by the anticoagulant activity of the fibrin split products that form and may not be cleared from the circulation for 6 to 9 hours.

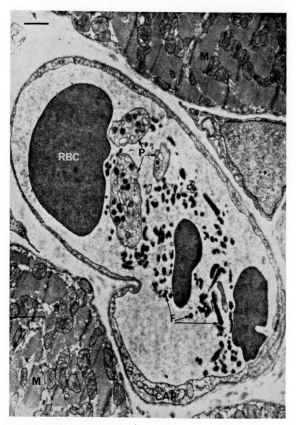

Fig. 2–13.—Endotoxin shock; myocardial capillary in rhesus monkey. Fibrin strands appear to be floating free in the plasma, clearly demonstrating that intravascular clotting is triggered in this type of shock. Reduced from ×10,600 (line represents 1 μ). (F = fibrin, CAP = capillary endothelium, RBC = red blood cell, P = platelet, M = myocardium.) (From McKay, Donald G.: Intravascular coagulation, J. Trauma 9:646, 1969. Used by permission of The Williams & Wilkins Company.)

Disseminated intravascular coagulation is an intermediary mechanism of disease. Behind every clotting episode lies a causative factor which initiates the process. Table 2-1 includes the substances used experimentally to produce disseminated clotting and the clinical syndromes in which this process has been shown to occur. Although these syndromes have in common an association with diffuse intravascular clotting, their many dissimilarities in manifestations may be explained, at least in part, by the following considerations.

1. The nature of the clot-promoting stimulus varies both in the speed of

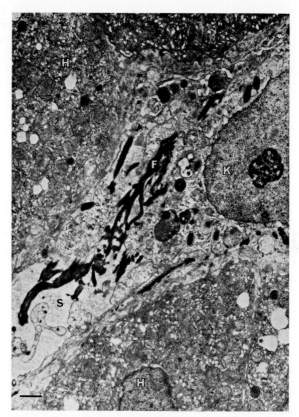

Fig. 2–14.—Endotoxin shock; liver sinusoid in rhesus monkey. Intravascular fibrin strands are attached to the surface of a Kupffer cell. Reduced from ×9,600 (line represents 1 μ). (F = fibrin, H = hepatic cell, S = sinusoidal lumen, K = Kupffer cell.) (From McKay, Donald G.: Intravascular coagulation, J. Trauma 9:646, 1969. Used by permission of The Williams & Wilkins Company.)

response it elicits and in the amount of material required to produce significant clotting. Bacterial endotoxin, for example, requires at least an hour to produce clotting even though only minute amounts are effective.

2. Dosage and speed of administration are important in determining the eventual outcome. With very low dosages given slowly, no functional or anatomic changes may be detected; with intermediate dosage, usually disseminated clotting and shock occur; with large doses, death in profound shock with the absence of demonstrable thrombosis is most often found.

3. Portal of entry and condition of the vascular bed during the clotting episode determines primarily the site of localization of thrombi. Illustra-

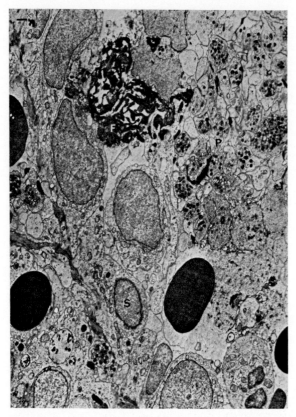

Fig. 2–15.—Endotoxin shock; spleen of rhesus monkey. The sinusoid contains a large clump of platelets in various stages of preservation and a twisted skein of fibrin. Reduced from ×4,400 (line represents 1 µ). (F = fibrin, P = platelets, S = sinusoidal lining cells.) (From McKay, Donald G.: Intravascular coagulation, J. Trauma 9:646, 1969. Used by permission of The Williams & Wilkins Company.)

tive of this is the tendency to thrombosis in the gastrointestinal mucosa and kidney in patients who have undergone surgical trauma and have developed stasis of blood in the splanchnic circulation.

4. "Blockade" of the reticuloendothelial system by substances such as fibrin aggregates prevents the normal phagocytosis of excess coagulant materials with resulting increased tendency to thrombosis and infarction (Shwartzman reaction).

5. The importance of fibrinolysis is shown by the persistence of thrombi in patients who have received a fibrinolytic inhibitor such as ε-aminocaproic acid (EACA) during a clotting episode.

TABLE 2-1.—DISSEMINATED INTRAVASCULAR COAGULATION

EXPERIMENTALLY PRODUCED	CLINICAL SYNDROMES
Thrombin intravenously	Premature separation of placenta
Tissue thromboplastin intravenously	Dead fetus syndrome
Snake venoms	Amniotic fluid embolism
Hemolyzed blood intravenously	Septic abortion
Dextran intravenously	Incompatible blood transfusion
Trypsin intravenously	Bacterial endotoxin
	(gram-negative bacteremia)
Bacterial endotoxin intravenously	Viremia
	(exanthematous and arbovirus diseases)
Amniotic fluid intravenously	Acute hemolytic anemias
	Pseudomembranous enterocolitis
	Shwartzman reaction
	Purpura fulminans
	Extracorporeal circulation
	Tissue injury with shock
	Leukemia
	Disseminated malignancy

6. Concentrations of clotting factors prior to an episode may determine the effects of the clot-promoting agent. Disseminated coagulation is more severe and more common in pregnancy when levels of platelets, fibrinogen, and other clotting factors are significantly increased.

7. The duration of any clotting episode is dependent upon whether or not there is a continuing source for the stimulating agent. When this syndrome occurs during parturition, usually it is acute and terminated with delivery. In the dead-fetus syndrome and in disseminated malignancy, however, there is a continuing slow infusion of small amounts of thromboplastic material which results in a subacute process of milder symptomatology.

IDENTIFICATION OF CLOTTING DEFECTS

Fortunately, the changes in the coagulation system that occur with DIC can be measured by a variety of laboratory tests. Blood for such testing should be drawn as soon as the condition is suspected and certainly before large amounts of intravenous fluids, blood, and drugs have been given. Careful evaluation of the status of the clotting mechanism can give valuable information concerning the diagnosis and the proper therapy. In acute situations, the following group of tests will most likely be helpful and the majority of tests can be completed in approximately 30 minutes by a single technologist. If possible, 20 ml of blood is drawn: 5 ml in EDTA, 10 ml in sodium oxalate or sodium citrate anticoagulant, and 5 ml without anticoagulant.

1. *Fibrinogen titer.* This test is done by adding thrombin to serial dilutions of plasma and will quickly estimate the level of clottable fibrinogen. It will be moderately to severely decreased in DIC.

2. *Platelet estimation or count.* Platelets tend to be decreased in about the same proportion as fibrinogen. Estimation of the numbers on a blood smear is not always satisfactory, and a count should be done if platelets appear to be less than normal.

3. *Observation of a tube of whole blood for clotting and lysis.* In DIC whole blood tends to clot in normal or near-normal time, and the clot retracts rapidly so that it is characteristically very small and fragile with increased red cell fallout. It may not even be visible unless the blood is poured into a petri dish. Either a Diluted Whole Blood Clot Lysis or Euglobulin Clot Lysis should also be set up, as these tests are much more sensitive to minor increases in fibrinolytic activity.

4. *Prothrombin time.* This test measures the time required for clotting by the extrinsic pathway and is done by adding tissue thromboplastin and Ca^{++} to plasma. This is a nonspecific test, but in DIC it is usually slightly prolonged, due to decreases in fibrinogen and factors V, X and, possibly, II. Fibrin split products also cause prolongation. If this test is completely normal, it is against the diagnosis of significant DIC, particularly of the acute type.

5. *Activated partial thromboplastin time (APTT).* This test measures the time required for clotting by the intrinsic pathway and is done by adding a surface activator, a platelet substitute, and Ca^{++} to plasma. This is also nonspecific but detects decreases in factor VIII in addition to the other factors measured in the prothrombin time test. It tends to show more marked prolongation than the prothrombin time and is also influenced by fibrin split products. If the test is prolonged, it should be repeated with a mixture of the patient's plasma and an equal volume of normal plasma. Correction would indicate that the abnormal result was due to a deficiency of clotting factors rather than to the anticoagulant effect of fibrin split products. It would also suggest that the patient's situation could be improved by giving blood or plasma.

6. *Thrombin time.* This test measures the time required for the clotting of plasma after adding extrinsic thrombin. It is influenced by the level of fibrinogen and fibrin split products. If the fibrinogen level is normal, a Serial Thrombin Time may be useful to detect increased plasma fibrinolytic activity.

7. *Study of the serum for fibrin split products (FSP).* These products are detected qualitatively in serum with the Fi test by their reaction with an Antifibrinogen Serum in the presence of latex particles to produce agglutination. Semiquantitation may be achieved by using serial dilutions of

serum. Quantitation requires some type of immunoassay such as the Tanned Red Cell Hemagglutination Inhibition Immunoassay.

Other tests that may be helpful if time permits and if such procedures are available include:

1. *Plasminogen level.* This should be significantly decreased in all cases of primary or secondary fibrinolysis, but it requires considerable time to perform and would seldom be useful in an emergency situation.

2. *Chemical determination of fibrinogen.* This is more accurate than the Fibrinogen Titer but is also time consuming.

3. Special tests to detect abnormal products of thrombin and plasmin action are:

   a. Refrigeration of plasma overnight to detect cryofibrinogen.

   b. Protamine sulfate precipitation to detect soluble fibrin monomer complexes.

   c. Ethanol gel formation to detect fibrin monomers.

4. Examination of the blood smear for red cell fragmentation produced by forcing the cells through fibrin meshes in the microcirculation.

5. *Tests for platelet adhesiveness and aggregation.* The adherence of platelets to glass surfaces can be measured by comparing the standard platelet count of a patient to one done after his blood has been passed through a column of glass beads. Platelet aggregation is usually measured by determining the decrease in optical density of platelet-rich plasma after ADP has been added since more light passes through a suspension of aggregated platelets than through a cloudy suspension of single platelets. Both of these properties may be changed by drugs, clot-promoting stimuli, and episodes of intravascular clotting. Thrombin causes increased aggregation of platelets, whereas fibrin split products have the opposite effect.

See Table 2-2 for laboratory findings in three possible clinical situations. Defibrination with fibrinolysis occurs most often.

TABLE 2-2.—POSSIBLE CLINICAL SITUATIONS

	DEFIBRINATION ONLY	DEFIBRINATION AND FIBRINOLYSIS	FIBRINOLYSIS ONLY
Fibrinogen	Low	Low	Normal or low
Platelets	Low	Low	Normal
Prothrombin time	Slightly increased	Increased	Normal or increased
APTT	Slightly increased	Increased	Normal or increased
Thrombin time	Increased	Increased	Increased
Clot lysis	Normal	Normal or increased	Increased
Fibrin split products	None	Present	Present
Plasminogen	Normal	Decreased	Decreased
Possible specific therapy	Heparin	Heparin and EACA	EACA

THERAPY IN DEFIBRINATION SYNDROMES

The need for therapy in defibrination depends upon the severity and duration of the clotting. If the episode is minor, no therapy should be instituted. If the patient is in clinical shock and massive hemorrhage is accompanied by a consumption coagulopathy, the most immediate need is the restoration of tissue perfusion, preferably by the administration of whole blood. It is important to repeat that blood for the coagulation studies should be drawn before therapy is started. Transfused blood not only replaces the blood being lost in hemorrhage, but may replace to some extent the coagulation factors that have been consumed during the clotting episode. Only very fresh blood (less than 24 hours old) will contain platelets, and there is also significant loss of the labile coagulation factors (V and VIII) with storage of blood. Frequently, transfusions are all that will be needed. Fibrinogen should never be given unless blood loss is severe, because it furnishes further substrate for the clotting process if the stimulus is still present, and also, it carries the large danger of producing homologous serum jaundice. But if the patient has open wounds in which local control of bleeding is difficult, fibrinogen may be helpful when the plasma fibrinogen level is low.

If there is good evidence that the stimulus to clotting is still operating, and judgment of this will depend to a large extent on careful clinical observation and determination of the cause of the condition, intravenous heparin is the treatment of choice. Though it may seem paradoxical to treat hemorrhage with an anticoagulant, there is good evidence both in experimental and clinical situations that heparin inhibits the clotting reaction sufficiently to allow the gradual return to normal of depleted coagulation factors. It acts immediately when given intravenously, but the effect lasts only 4–6 hours, so it must be repeated at regular intervals or given by continuous intravenous drip. The dosage should be sufficient to double the clotting time (usually 50–100 units/kilo every 6 hours), and it should be given as long as the stimulus to clotting is present. Fortunately for the obstetrician, heparin does not cross the placenta. In many acute defibrination syndromes, the stimulus to clotting is frequently over by the time the situation becomes clinically manifest, and the main need is to establish and maintain blood pressure and tissue perfusion and to replace the blood being lost.

Antifibrinolytic agents act by inhibiting the fibrinolytic enzyme system, and this causes the preservation of thrombi beyond the time they would ordinarily be lysed. Obviously, these agents should not be used while intravascular clotting is occurring. The four possible situations in which antifibrinolytic agents may be helpful are (1) when a patient is bleeding due to the rare syndrome of isolated primary systemic fibrinolysis; (2) when hemorrhage is due to the activation of the fibrinolytic system secondary to disseminated intravascular clotting in a patient in whom clotting has stopped and fibrinolysis has persisted; (3) when hemorrhage is associated with a decrease in antifibrinolytic activity, as occurs in liver disease; and (4) to preserve thrombi and thus control local bleeding in a patient with no systemic clotting disorder, as in prostatic surgery.

Epsilon-aminocaproic acid is a synthetic amino acid which inhibits the conversion of plasminogen to plasmin and thus acts as an antifibrinolytic agent. It is active when it circulates at appropriate levels, is rapidly excreted by the kidneys, and may be given intravenously or orally. The initial or priming dose is 5 gm followed by 1–1¼ gm doses at hourly intervals. The drug should never be given if there is even a suspicion that intravascular clotting is still going on, because of the danger of thrombosis leading to ischemic necrosis. Even in patients undergoing prostatectomy without evidence of systemic clotting there has been an increased incidence of thromboembolism when the drug is used prophylactically. When heparin was used with EACA in similar patients, this danger was greatly reduced, suggesting that the combination of these two drugs may represent an effective way of treating patients with continuing clotting and exaggerated lysis. If increased clot lysis cannot be demonstrated in vitro as the primary abnormality, there is no indication for the isolated therapeutic use of this drug.

CASE HISTORIES

CASE 1.—POSTPARTUM DISSEMINATED INTRAVASCULAR COAGULATION

A 29-year-old female (gravida 6, para 3) was admitted at term on 7/17/69 with ruptured membranes. Pitocin induction of labor was attempted on 7/18/69, and at 10:05 P.M. the patient had a precipitous delivery after the cervix had dilated from 3 to 10 cm in the 20 minute period prior to this. By 11:00 P.M. vaginal blood flow was excessive and IV fluids were started, but at that time BP was still 110/70 with a pulse rate of 110. By 12:00 midnight the BP was 60/30 and the temperature was 103°. Whole blood and IV fluids were given, and the blood pressure was maintained at 80/50 despite continued heavy vaginal flow. An attempt was made during this time to suture the cervix, which had been torn during delivery, but there was little decrease in bleeding. By 7:00 A.M., the patient was anuric and the hemoglobin had dropped to 9.8 gm. Clotting and bleeding times were reportedly normal, but the fibrinogen was 96 mg%, platelets were 91,000, ProTime 18 sec., and APTT 108 sec. A mixture of the patient's plasma with normal plasma corrected the prolonged APTT to normal. The clot was small and fragile with no evidence of lysis. Fresh blood was given with a gradual decrease in bleeding. By 11:00 P.M. the urine output was normal, ProTime was 16 sec., and APTT was 50 sec., but the thrombocytopenia persisted for 3 days. Studies for FSP and plasminogen were not done.

This patient represents a typical case of disseminated intravascular clotting with shock and hemorrhage. Most likely the stimulus for clotting was the release of tissue products from the placental site into the maternal circulation during the precipitous delivery. Presumably this acted like an intravenous infusion of thromboplasmin. Because the stimulus was temporary, it was possible to maintain the patient in satisfactory condition with blood and IV fluids without the use of a clot-preventing drug such as heparin. The severe injury to the cervix contributed to the heavy bleeding, but a mild consumption coagulopathy had obviously developed.

CASE 2.—EXAGGERATED FIBRINOLYSIS FOLLOWING DISSEMINATED INTRAVASCULAR COAGULATION

An 18-year-old male was admitted to the hospital 15 minutes after being shot in the abdomen. On admission, his BP was 68/48, Hb 12.7, and Hemat. 37. Within the next 1½ hours he received 6,000 ml of lactated Ringer's solution and 2 units of blood. He was then taken to surgery, and during the next 4 hours received 8,000 ml fluid, 5,000 of which was whole blood, in order to maintain blood pressure at 80 to 100 systolic. The estimated blood loss during surgery was 7,000 ml. There was free blood in the peritoneal cavity in addition to a large retroperitoneal hematoma. Lacerations of bowel and stomach were repaired. Bleeding seemed to be controlled until just prior to closing when there was some oozing around the spleen. The spleen was then removed. About 1½ hours after surgery, bloody drainage was noted from multiple drain sites; BP was 50/0. The patient had received 1,500 ml more blood after surgery and an additional 1,500 ml before he died about 3 hours later. Coagulation studies done during this period of postoperative bleeding were as follows:

ProTime 23 sec. (control 13 sec.)
APTT 3 min. (control 45 sec.) 1/1 mixture with control 94 sec.
Thrombin time 14 sec. (control 12 sec.)
Fibrinogen titer 200 mg%
Whole blood clot formed in 8 minutes, but was lysed in 5 minutes after
    forming
Fibrin split products—positive in serum in a 1-256 dilution (Fi test)
Platelet estimated to be 50,000–100,000

This case is an example of the situation in which hemorrhage is due to the activation of the fibrinolytic system secondary to disseminated intravascular clotting in a patient in whom clotting had stopped and fibrinolysis had persisted. The transfused blood had apparently been adequate to replace fibrinogen, but not platelets and other labile coagulation factors. The clotting defect was aggravated by the anticoagulant effect of the fibrin split products. Fresh blood and ε-aminocaproic acid should have benefited this patient.

CASE 3.—ABRUPTIO PLACENTA WITH DISSEMINATED INTRAVASCULAR CLOTTING

A 24-year-old female (gravida I, para 0), who was 8 months pregnant, had the sudden onset of acute abdominal pain with vaginal bleeding and faintness at 9 A.M. on 1/8/70. She arrived at the hospital at 9:30 A.M. with heavy vaginal bleeding and a BP of 90/60 with marked peripheral vasoconstriction. No fetal heart tones were heard. Between 9:30 and 11:30, when the clotting studies were reported, she received 2,000 ml of 5% glucose in lactated Ringer's which maintained her BP at about 100/60. As soon as it became evident that the blood was almost completely lacking in clottable fibrinogen, heparin (7,500 units) was given IV and two units of blood were administered very rapidly. Vaginal bleeding diminished and the BP rose to 120/70 with much less peripheral vasoconstriction. In 1½ hours repeat coagulation studies showed formation of small visible clots which did not lyse. After two more units of blood had been administered the clinical condition was even better and the fibrinogen titer was 1:16 (app. 50 mg%) with other studies, as shown in Table 2-3. The cervix was very firm and undilated, and rupture of the membranes had not resulted in any significant uterine contractions. The patient was then taken to surgery where a cesarean section was performed with about 500 ml of measurable blood loss. Two units of blood were given during the procedure because a blood volume done just prior to surgery had revealed a circulating blood volume of only 3.7 liters (expected 4.4). The patient tolerated the procedure well and the fibrinogen titer was 1:64 (100–200 mg%) 2 hours after surgery and up to 1:256 (>400 mg%) 36 hours later. Postoperative course was uneventful except for some increased vaginal bleeding probably due to moderate thrombocytopenia.

In this case of disseminated intravascular clotting, thromboplastic material from the separated placental site entered the maternal circulation to initiate clotting. Obviously the resulting shock state contributed to this. Rapid fibrinolysis of the microclots had already taken place before the

TABLE 2-3.—CASE OF ABRUPTIO PLACENTA WITH DISSEMINATED INTRAVASCULAR CLOTTING

| DATE | 1/8/70* | 1/8/70 | 1/8/70** | 1/8/70 | 1/9/70 | 1/10/70 |
TIME	11:30 AM	1:30 PM	3:30 PM	8:00 PM	8:00 AM	8:00 AM
Platelets mm³	136,000	100,000	85,000		75,000	68,000
Fibrinogen titer	0	1:8	1:16	1:64	1:64	1:256
Clot lysis	No clot	No lysis	No lysis		No lysis	
ProTime seconds	35 (12)	20.5 (11)	15 (11)	13.8 (11)	12.5 (12)	
APTT seconds	No clot	146 (40)	51 (40)	43 (39)	34 (38)	
Thrombin time seconds	No clot		47 (17)		12 (15)	
Fibrin split products	1:128	Plasminogen 1%			Absent	
Hemoglobin Gm%	11	10	12	12	10	9
Blood given units	2	2	2			

*Heparin 7,500 units given   **Cesarean section   ( ) Control values blood was drawn for the initial coagulation studies and fibrin split products were present in that serum specimen in high titer (1:128). Since the source of thromboplastic material was still present, it was necessary to give intravenous heparin to prevent further clotting. With the fibrinogen and other coagulation proteins in transfused blood and those the patient was able to manufacture, it was possible to improve the hemostatic situation sufficiently to allow the patient to undergo a cesarean section. Despite the low level of fibrinogen and platelets, there was no serious bleeding during or after surgery.

Metabolic Response to Severe Trauma and Sepsis

Shock frequently occurs in patients who have been subjected to major trauma or who are septic and chronically ill. When an operation has to be performed under such tenuous circumstances, relatively minor trauma, minor blood and fluid loss, or operative manipulation of a septic area may tip the balance and result in rapid deterioration. These patients respond with increases in adrenocorticoid output and are in a state of negative nitrogen balance. Especially after major burns or severe sepsis, energy demands are at a maximum. The urinary corticoid levels reach three times their normal level. There is an increase in aldosterone and antidiuretic activity. Moreover, the febrile patient has increased vaporizational losses of heat and water and cannot achieve positive nitrogen balance until sepsis has been controlled. Since the rate of metabolism increases in proportion to the degree of fever, corresponding demands are placed upon pulmonary ventilation. In order to cope with the increased needs for oxygen intake and carbon dioxide elimination, hyperventilation is an almost uniform occurrence after trauma or with sepsis.

To demonstrate that the respiratory center is sensitive to small changes in blood temperature, Kahn infused warm blood into the carotid artery and produced a considerable increase in respiratory rate before there was any rise in rectal temperature. The effect of hyperthermia appears to override the control of depth and rate of inhalation by levels of P_{CO_2}, since a rise in temperature continues to produce hyperventilation in spite of low P_{CO_2} levels. The basis for the hypermetabolism which follows trauma is not completely clear but is, in part, accounted for by the measurable increase in the production of catecholamines. There is also a large increase in protein catabolism. The breakdown of tissue protein causes an increase in metabolic rate as a result of the increase in amino acid oxidation and the specific dynamic action of protein. After burn trauma, there is an additional factor, namely, the unrestricted passage of water molecules through the burn eschar. This may amount to several liters per day and result in an enormous heat loss, causing additional metabolic demands for heat production to maintain the temperature setting. Sepsis is also associated with increased energy expenditure, but not to the same degree as in burns, when maximal energy demands are placed upon the body metabolism.

TEMPERATURE REGULATION

The body temperature in mammals is the result of a balance between heat production and heat loss. A homeothermic animal has a complex regulatory system for maintaining a steady temperature involving a central hypothalamic control center linked very closely with the activity of the thyroid gland, the adrenal glands, and the circulatory system. Roe, Hammell, and Hardy have noted the similarities of the mammalian temperature-regulating mechanism to the feedback control systems developed for engineering application. The main sensory area of the heat-regulating system appears to be in the hypothalamus, which responds to changes in environmental blood temperature. The human thermostat is normally set in the vicinity of 37°C; any deviation from this level results in negative feedback response tending to maintain the steady state. In pyrexia, the setting of the thermostat is reestablished at a higher level.

HEAT PRODUCTION

The amount of fuel burned by the body for heat production is most conveniently measured by the amount of oxygen consumed per minute. The oxygen consumption of the average adult male is from 200 to 250 ml in the resting state. This reflects the oxygen needs for muscle contraction, glandular activity, and respiratory effort. About 25% of the total body heat production at rest is thought to come from muscular activity. Increased heat production by the body is largely a function of increased muscular activity, and this is the mechanism for rapid production of heat under circumstances of excessive heat loss. Shivering may increase the heat production approximately threefold. The calorigenic effects of catecholamines are brought about by increase in the rate of mitochondrial oxidation. Thyroxin increases heat production by its action as an uncoupling agent, resulting in partial dissociation of the multiple steps of the electron transport system yielding heat rather than energy stored as adenosine triphosphate.

HEAT LOSS IN SHOCK

Heat loss occurs from four principal routes: (1) radiation; (2) evaporation; (3) convection; and (4) conduction. The first two are under physiologic control. Radiative heat loss occurs from approximately 78% of total body surface. Recent studies indicate that approximately 60% of total heat loss from the body is by radiation. Evaporative heat loss is the most labile of all the methods employed to rid the body of the excess heat. The loss of water from the skin and respiratory tract approximates 750 ml per day and accounts for approximately 25% of the total heat loss from the body. Since this evaporation is an energy-consuming process, every milliliter of water evaporated requires 0.58 kcal of heat. Heat loss by conduction and convection accounts for a relatively small proportion of the total loss.

In septic shock, metabolic demands are raised in proportion to the degree of pyrexia. Variations in skin temperature determine the degree of heat conservation by vasoconstriction or heat loss from vasodilation. In other forms of shock, heat is conserved by cutaneous vasoconstriction, but in terminal shock, core temperature falls in spite of this. Failure of heat conservation is seen with the hypotension that follows high spinal cord section and renders the patient poikilothermic for about 7 days. During this time, the core temperature drifts according to the ambient temperature. This serious heat loss may be mitigated by judicious titration with alphamimetic adrenergic drugs. Because of the need for close observation, shock patients are frequently nursed with little or no covering—again leading to heat loss and an increase in metabolic demand.

REFERENCES

Systemic Response to Injury

Britton, K. E.: Renin and angiotensin, Lancet 2:335, 1968.
Davis, J. O., Carpenter, C. C. J., and Ayers, C. R.: Relation of renin and angiotensin II to the control of aldosterone secretion, Circulation Res. 11:171, 1962.
Guyton, A. C.: Regulation of cardiac output, Anesthesiology 29:314, 1968.
Korner, P. I.: Circulatory adaptations in hypoxia, Physiol. Rev. 39:687, 1959.
Moore, F. D.: Terminal mechanisms in human injury, Am. J. Surg. 110:317, 1965.
Rothe, C. F., Schwendenmann, F. C., and Selkurt, E. E.: Neurogenic control of skeletal muscle vascular resistance in hemorrhagic shock, Am. J. Physiol. 204:925, 1963.
Scholander, P. F.: The master switch of life, Scient. Am. 209:92, 1963.
Skillman, J. J., Lauler, D. P., Hickler, R. B., Lyons, J. H., Olson, J. E., Ball, M. R., and Moore, F. D.: Hemorrhage in normal man: Effect on renin, cortisol, aldosterone, and urine composition, Ann. Surg. 166:865, 1967.
Verney, E. B.: Water diuresis, Irish J. M. Sc. 345:377, 1954.

Microcirculation

Amundsen, E.: Possible roles of plasma kinins in shock states, T. Norsk Laegforen 86: 633, 1966.
Anas, P., Neely, W. A., and Hardy, J. D.: Interstitial fluid pressure changes in endotoxin shock, Surgery 63:938, 1968.
Back, N., Jainchill, M., Wilkens, J. H., and Ambrus, J. L.: Effect of inhibitors of plas-

min, kallikrein and kinin on mortality from scalding in mice, Medical Pharmacol. Exp. no. 6, 15:597, 1966.

Beraldo, W. T.: Formation of bradykinin in anaphylactic and peptone shock, Am. J. Physiol. 163:283, 1950.

Bernstein, E. F., Emmings, F. G., Mackey, G. C., Castaneda, A., and Varco, R. L.: Effect of low molecular weight dextran on red blood cell charge during extracorporeal circulation, Tr. Am. Soc. Art. Int. Organs 8:23, 1962.

Border, J. R., Gallo, E., and Schenk, W.: Systemic arteriovenous shunts in patients under severe stress: A common cause of high output cardiac failure? Surgery 60:225, 1966.

Brake, C. M., Emerson, T. E., Wittmers, L. E., and Hinshaw, L. B.: Alterations of vascular responses to endotoxin by adrenergic blockade, Am. J. Physiol. 207:149, 1964.

Branemark, P. I., Aspergren, K., and Breine, U.: Microcirculation studies in man by high resolution vital microscopy, Angiology 15:329, 1964.

Branemark, P. I.: Rheological Aspects of Low Flow States, in Shepro, D., and Fulton, G. P. (eds.): Microcirculation as Related to Shock (New York: Academic Press, 1968).

Braude, A. I.: Bacterial endotoxins, Scient. Am. 210:36, 1964.

Brody, O. V., and Oncley, J. L.: Effect of Erythrocyte Net Charge on Agglutination and Rouleaux Formation, in Sawyer, P. N. (ed.): Biophysical Mechanisms in Vascular Homeostasis and Intravascular Thrombosis (New York: Appleton-Century-Crofts, Inc., 1965).

Chien, S., Chang, C., Dellenback, R. J., Usami, S., and Gregersen, M. I.: Hemodynamic changes in endotoxin shock, Am. J. Physiol. 210:140, 1966.

Chien, S., Sinclair, D. G., Dellenback, R. J., Chang, C., Peric, B., Usami, S., and Gregersen, M. I.: Effect of endotoxin on capillary permeability to macromolecules, Am. J. Physiol. 207:518, 1964.

Chien, S., Shunichi, U., Taylor, H. M., Lundberg, J. L., and Gregersen, M. I.: Effects of hematocrit and plasma proteins on human blood rheology at low shear rates, J. Appl. Physiol. 21:81, 1966.

Corrado, A. P., Reis, M. L., Carvalho, I. F., and Diniz, C. R.: Bradykininogen and bradykinin in the cardiovascular shock produced by proteolytic enzymes, Biochem. Pharmacol. 15:959, 1966.

Crowell, J. W., Bounds, S. H., and Johnson, W. W.: Effect of varying the hematocrit ratio on the susceptibility to hemorrhagic shock, Am. J. Physiol. 192:171, 1958.

Dale, H. H., and Richards, A. N.: Vasodilator actions of histamine and other substances, J. Physiol. 52:110, 1918.

Diniz, C. R., and Carvalho, I. F.: A micromethod for determination of bradykininogen under several conditions, Ann. New York Acad. Sc., 104:77, 1963.

Erdos, E. G.: Hypotensive peptides: Bradykinin, kallidin, and eledoisin, Advances Pharmacol. 4:1, 1966.

Fairchild, H. M., Ross, J. M., and Guyton, A. C.: Identity of oxygen lack hyperemia and reactive hyperemia, Am. J. Physiol. 210:490, 1966.

Fine, J., and Minton, R.: Mechanism of action of bacterial endotoxin, Nature (London) 210:97, 1966.

Fine, J., Frank, E. D., Ravin, H. A., Rutenburg, S. H., and Schweinburg, F. B.: The Bacterial Factor in Traumatic Shock, in Stoner, H. B., and Threlfall, C. J. (eds.): The Biochemical Response To Injury (Springfield, Ill.: Charles C Thomas, Publisher, 1960).

Fischer, M. J., and McArtor, R. E.: Staphylococcal septicemia. A study of 100 cases, Ohio Med. J. 63:1325, 1967.

Fox, R. H., Goldsmith, R., Kidd, D. J., and Lewis, G. P.: Bradykinin as a vasodilator in man, J. Physiol. 157:589, 1961.

Gelin, L. E.: Disturbance of the flow properties of blood and its counteraction in surgery, Acta Chir. Scand. 122:287, 1961.

Grendahl, M. J., Olson, C. R., and Evans, R. L.: Intercellular forces and separation energy of red cells sludged by contrast medium, Proc. Soc. Exper. Biol. & Med. 118: 1124, 1965.

Janoff, A., and Aeligs, D.: Vascular injury and lysis of basement membrane in vitro by neutral protease of human leukocytes, Science 161:702, 1968.

Katz, W., Silverstein, M., Kobold, E. E., and Thal, A. P.: Trypsin release, kinin production and shock, Arch. Surg. 89:322, 1964.

Kellermeyer, R. W., and Grahan, R. C., Jr.: Kinins—possible physiologic and pathologic roles in man, New England J. Med. 279:754, 1968.

Kitamura, S., Shelton, J., and Thal, A. P.: Isolation and characterization of Staphylococcus alpha-hemolysin, Ann. Surg. 160:926, 1964.

Knisley, M. H.: Intravascular erythrocyte aggregation (blood sludge), Handbook of Physiology, Sec. 2, Vol. III: Circulation (Washington, D.C.: American Physiological Society, 1965), p. 2257.

Kobold, E. E., Lowell, R., Katz, W., and Thal, A. P.: Chemical mediators released by endotoxin, Surg., Gynec. & Obst. 118:807, 1964.

Linman, J. W.: Physiologic and pathophysiologic effects of anemia, New England J. Med. 279:812, 1968.

Lister, J.: Factors influencing homeostatic responses to hemorrhage, Surgery 60:43, 1966.

Nicoll, P. A., and Frayser, R.: Physiological considerations of the microcirculation as related to shock, Cardiovas. Dis. 9:558, 1967.

Niles, A. S., Forsyth, R. P., Williams, H. E., and Melmon, K. L.: Contribution of kinins to endotoxin shock in unanesthetized rhesus monkeys, Circulation Res. 22:155, 1968.

Page, I. H.: Serotonin (5-hydroxytrytamine), Phys. Rev. 34:571, 1954.

Replogle, R. L., and Merrill, E. W.: Hemodilution: Rheologic, hemodynamic and metabolic consequences in shock, Surg. Forum 18:157, 1967.

Replogle, R. L., Meiselman, H. J., and Merrill, E. W.: Clinical implications of blood rheology studies, Circulation 36:148, 1967.

Rittenbury, M. S., and Egdahl, R. H.: The effect of total pancreatectomy on experimental hemorrhagic pancreatitis, Fed. Proc. 19:504, 1960.

Rosenberg, J. C., Lillehei, R. C., Moran, W. H., and Zimmerman, B.: Effect of endotoxin on plasma catecholamines and serum serotonin, Proc. Soc. Exper. Biol. & Med. 102:335, 1959.

Schayer, R. W.: Relationship of stress-induced histidine decarboxylase activity in histamine synthesis to circulatory homeostasis and shock, Science 131:226, 1960.

Shwartzman, G.: Phenomenon of local tissue reactivity and its immunological, pathological and clinical significance (New York: Med. Div., Harper & Row, 1937).

Smith, H. W.: Lectures on the kidney, University Extension Division, University of Kansas, Lawrence, Kansas, 1943.

Spector, W. G., Walters, M. N., and Willoughby, D. A.: Venular and capillary permeability in thermal injury, J. Path. & Bact. 90:635, 1965.

Spink, W. W., and Starzecki, B.: Experimental canine endotoxin shock: Failure to correlate outcome with persistent endotoxemia, Proc. Soc. Exper. Biol. & Med. 126:574, 1967.

Thal, A. P.: Surgical Physiology of the Exocrine Pancreas, in Davis, J. H., Current Concepts of Surgery (New York: McGraw-Hill Book Company, 1965).

Thal, A. P., and Egner, W. E.: Mechanism of shock produced by means of staphylococcal toxin, Arch. Path. 61:488, 1956.

Thal, A. P., and Egner, W. E.: The site of action of Staphylococcus alpha toxin, J. Exper. Med. 113:69, 1961.

Thal, A. P., Kobold, E. E., and Hollenberg, M. J.: Release of vasoactive substances in acute pancreatitis, Am. J. Surg. 105:708, 1963.

Thal, A. P., and Sardesai, V. M.: Shock and the circulating peptides, Am. J. Surg. 110: 308, 1965.

Thal, A. P., Wilson, R. F., Kalfuss, L., and Andre, J.: The Role of Metabolic and Humoral Factors in Irreversible Shock, in Mills, L. C., and Moyer, J. H. (eds.): *Shock and Hypotension* (New York: Grune & Stratton, Inc., 1956).

Webster, M. E., and Clark, W. R.: Significance of kallikrein-kallidineogen-kallidin system in shock, Am. J. Physiol. 197:406, 1959.

Werle, E.: *Kallikrein, Kallidin and Related Substances: Polypeptides which Affect Smooth Muscles and Blood Vessels* (New York: Pergamon Press, 1960).

Zweifach, B. W., Nagler, A. L., and Thomas, L.: The role of epinephrine in the reactions produced by the endotoxin of gram-negative bacteria. II. The changes produced by endotoxin in the vascular reactivity to epinephrine, in the rat mesoappendix and the isolated, perfused rabbit ear, J. Exper. Med. 104:881, 1965.

TRAUMA AND SEPSIS

Beeson, P. B.: Temperature-elevating effect of a substance obtained from polymorphonuclear leukocytes, J. Clin. Invest. 27:524, 1948.

Bennett, I. L., Jr., Petersdorf, R. G., and Keene, W. R.: Pathogenesis of fever: Evidence for direct cerebral action of bacterial endotoxins, Tr. A. Am. Physicians 70:64, 1957.

Benzinger, T. H., Kitzinger, C., and Pratt, A. W.: The Human Thermostat, in Hardy, J. D. (ed.): *Temperature: Its Measurement and Control in Science and Industry* (New York: Reinhold Publishing Corporation, 1963), Vol. III, Part 3, p. 637.

Cooper, K. E.: Mechanisms of action of pyrogens, Fed. Proc. 22:721, 1963.

Goldberg, M. J., and Roe, C. F.: Temperature changes during anesthesia, Arch. Surg. 93:365, 1966.

Gump, F. E., Kinney, J. M., Long, C. L., and Gelber, R.: Measurement of water balance—A guide to surgical care, Surgery 64:164, 1968.

Hammel, H. T.: Neurons and Temperature Regulation, in Yamamoto, W. S., and Brobeck, J. R. (eds.): *Physiological Controls and Regulation* (Philadelphia: W. B. Saunders Company, 1965), p. 71.

Hardy, J. D.: The "Set-Point" Concept in Physiological Temperature Regulation, in Yamamoto, W. S., and Brobeck, J. R. (eds.): *Physiological Controls and Regulation* (Philadelphia: W. B. Saunders Company, 1965), p. 98.

Roe, C. F.: Fever and energy metabolism in surgical disease, Monogr. Surg. Sc. 3:85, 1966.

Roe, C. F., Goldberg, M. J., Blair, C. S., and Kinney, J. M.: The influence of body temperature on early postoperative oxygen consumption, Surgery 120:85, 1966.

Simeone, F. A.: Hemorrhagic shock: Metabolic effects, Science 141:536, 1963.

Simeone, F. A.: Shock, trauma and the surgeon, Ann. Surg. 158:759, 1963.

3

The Pathophysiology of Shock

Lung

ULTRASTRUCTURE OF THE LUNG

THE ELECTRON MICROSCOPIC STUDIES of Lowe and others have demonstrated that alveoli are made up of a continuous lining of epithelial cells, two types of which have been identified. The type I cells are extremely thin, measuring approximately 0.1–0.7 microns. They are continuous with the epithelium of the bronchioles and are occasionally interrupted by the pores of Kohn. These cells line the outer surface of the pulmonary capillaries and endocapillary tissue (Fig. 3-1).

Type I cells constitute the main lining of the alveolar surface, and their extreme thinness is important in permitting rapid diffusion of gases between blood and air. They have no phagocytic activity and, where they contact the capillary, the basement membrane appears to be a single layer. These cells have been variously described as membranous pneumocytes, surface epithelial cells, and small alveolar cells. The type II cell, often called the granular pneumocyte, or great alveolar cell (Fig. 3-1), is periodically scattered over the surface of the alveolar wall, interrupting the continuity of the type I cells. It appears that the type II cell has phagocytic properties and is capable of moving over the alveolar surface. Some consider it as identical with the pulmonary macrophage or "heart-failure cell." Unlike the thin, relatively structureless type I cell, the type II cell is plump and contains an eccentric nucleus, mitochondria, Golgi apparatus, granular endoplasmic reticulum, and so-called inclusion or lamellar bodies (Fig. 3-1).

Electron microscopy has also demonstrated that the alveolar walls are lined by an acellular lipid material (Fig. 3-1) commonly known as surfactant, which is scanty or absent in atelectasis, respiratory distress syndrome, and possibly in the shock lung. Strong evidence now indicates that the inclusion or lamellar bodies of the type II cell contain lipids that are extruded into the alveolar space and constitute the source of surfactant.

The importance of this substance in maintaining alveolar patency will be discussed later. The ultrastructural changes in the respiratory distress syndrome, which so often accompanies shock or severe trauma, are described in Figure 3-2, A–C.

NORMAL PHYSIOLOGY OF THE LUNG

Intrapulmonic pressure is less than atmospheric pressure during inspiration and greater than atmospheric pressure during expiration (Fig. 3-3). These intrapulmonic pressure changes occur passively in response to active changes in the volume of the thoracic cavity. With an open glottis during quiet breathing, intrathoracic pressure is less than atmospheric and less than intrapulmonic throughout the respiratory cycle. The basis for this phenomenon is as follows: In the newborn infant, before the first breath, the solid, noninflated lungs fill the chest and intrathoracic pressure approximates atmospheric pressure. With growth, the size of the thoracic cavity exceeds that of the lungs, and the elastic lung becomes expanded and stretched to fill the thoracic cavity. The subatmospheric intrathoracic pressure is present because the stretched elastic lung tends to assume a lower potential energy state. The difference between intrathoracic pressure and atmospheric pressure is a rough index of the potential energy stored in the stretched elastic lung.

Intrathoracic pressure seldom exceeds atmospheric pressure during expiration, except in asthmatic conditions and during extreme, forced expiratory efforts. With the glottis closed, however, intrathoracic pressure can frequently exceed 100 mm Hg with coughing, defecation, guarding of the acute abdomen, crying in the newborn, and extreme muscular efforts. Negative intrathoracic pressure plays an important role in aiding venous return to the heart. With maintained positive intrathoracic pressure, this aid to cardiac filling is lost. No significant problem arises in terms of cardiac function with transient positive intrathoracic pressures as long as blood volume is normal and the sympathetic nervous system is intact. With blood volume deficits or depressed sympathetic activity, however, intermittent positive-pressure ventilation with large tidal volumes and high peak airway pressures may cause a precipitous drop in systemic blood pressure and cardiac output by raising mean intrathoracic pressure. Venous return to the heart is reduced, pulmonary vascular resistance is increased, and ventricular filling is impaired. This is a particular hazard when continuous positive-pressure ventilation is employed in shock patients. Central venous pressure measurements may be raised considerably by assisted ventilation at high peak airway pressures. This aberration must

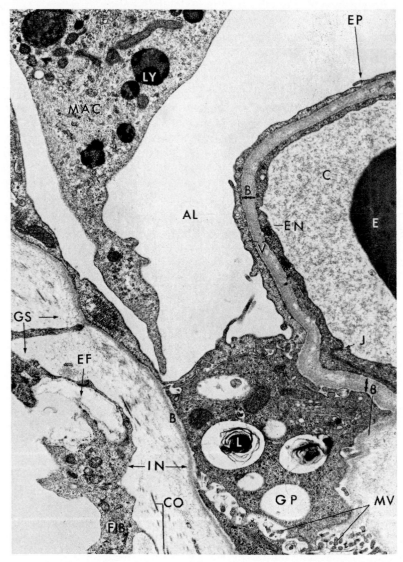

Fig. 3–1.—Ultrastructure of the normal lung. Electron micrograph of normal human lung showing all vital ultrastructural components of the alveolus and interalveolar septum. The alveolus (*AL*) is lined by long, thin squamous epithelium (*EP*)—type I— which is separated from the endothelium (*EN*) of a septal capillary (*C*) by a common basement membrane (*B*). The capillary lumen (*C*) contains finely granular gray plasma protein and an erythrocyte (*E*). Both endothelial and epithelial cells contain pinocytotic vesicles (*V*). An interendothelial junction is noted at *J*. A granular pneumocyte (*GP*)— so-called great alveolar cell—shows typical lamellar bodies (*L*) containing the black phos-

be taken into account and not be mistaken for evidence of failure of the right side of the heart, but properly attributed simply to impedance of venous return to the heart.

LUNG VOLUMES

Total lung capacity has been partitioned into a number of subdivisions (Fig. 3-4). Some of these volumes are measured routinely in pulmonary function laboratories. They describe the size and capacity of the lungs, but they give no information about the rate of ventilation of the lungs or of gas exchange between alveolar air and blood. Rate of ventilation of the lungs (minute volume) is the product of tidal volume (V_T) and respiratory rate (f). Thus, a minute volume of 6 liters could be provided by a tidal volume of 600 ml, and a respiratory rate of 10; a tidal volume of 400 ml and a respiratory rate of 15; a tidal volume of 300 ml and a respiratory rate of 20; and so on. These combinations are not equally effective in producing ventilation of the lungs, however, because only part of each tidal volume reaches the alveoli and participates in gas exchange with the blood.

The part of each tidal volume that does not take part in gas exchange is known as dead space. Dead space is the volume of the respiratory tract from oral or nasal pharynx down to the respiratory bronchioles since the air in these passages does not participate in gas exchange with pulmonary capillary blood. This volume is known as anatomic dead space and averages about 150 ml in adults. In addition to the anatomic dead space, the volume of gas that ventilates any unperfused alveoli or the ventilation of any alveoli in excess of that necessary to oxygenate the blood perfusing those alveoli adds to the dead space. The sum of these dead spaces is physiologic or total dead space. In conditions in which uneven ventilation and uneven perfusion of the lungs are present, physiologic (or functional) dead space may be much larger than anatomic dead space.

The importance of considering dead space in evaluating the respiratory status of a patient is emphasized by referring again to the combinations of

pholipid material which is eventually extruded into the alveolus as surfactant. This epithelial cell (type II) rests on basement membrane (B) and extends out characteristic microvilli (MV) which appear seemingly unattached in this cross-sectional view. A pulmonary macrophage (MAC) with its prominent hydrolytic enzyme-containing lysosomes (LY) is seen with a protruded (ameboid) cytoplasmic process. The interstitial space or interstitium (IN) of a larger septum contains an inactive fibroblast or fibrocyte (FIB), collagen fibrils (CO), elastic fibers (EF) and amorphous lightly stained connective tissue ground substance (GS), which is somewhat increased in this elderly man. (Reduced from ×19,200.) (Courtesy of Dr. Carl Teplitz.)

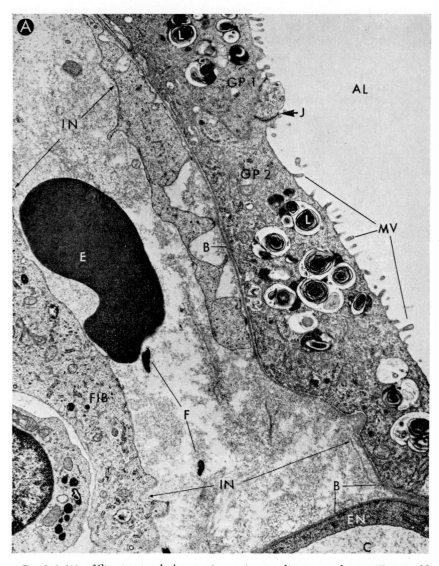

Fig. 3–2 (A).—Ultrastructural changes in respiratory distress syndrome. 59-year-old woman dying from pulmonary insufficiency, following a 95% total body surface burn. Patient was severely hypoxemic despite continued, prolonged use of 70% oxygen therapy. Pulmonary parenchyma instantly fixed at the time of death by intratracheal perfusion of electron microscopy fixative. The gross and light microscopical findings were characteristic of patients dying with post-traumatic pulmonary insufficiency while on high concentrations of oxygen. Hyperplasia of granular pneumocytes is present; i.e., the thin, elongated type I epithelial cells have undergone transformation into type II

tidal volume and respiratory rate that will produce a minute volume of 6 liters. If we assume that the normal adult has a dead space of 150 ml, then the effective or alveolar minute volume is 4.5 liters with a respiratory rate of 10; 3.75 liters with a respiratory rate of 15; 3 liters with a rate of 20; and the effective ventilation approaches 0 at a respiratory rate of 40.

Dead space may be calculated by the following equation:

$$V_D = V_T \frac{P_{A_{CO_2}} - P_{E_{CO_2}}}{P_{A_{CO_2}}}$$

in which $P_{A_{CO_2}}$ is the CO_2 tension of alveolar air and $P_{E_{CO_2}}$ is the partial pressure of CO_2 in mixed expired air. This equation is derived in Chapter 5.

COMPLIANCE

Pulmonary tissue often becomes less distensible, "stiff" in chronic disease states and in acute conditions such as shock, pulmonary edema, or fat embolism. A common and simple measure of distensibility of the lung is compliance, $\frac{\Delta V}{\Delta P}$, where ΔP is the total change in pressure required to elicit a change in volume (ΔV). Compliance is measured under static conditions. Patients are simply required to inspire varying tidal volumes (600–2,000 ml) and to hold the breath for 1–2 seconds while the change in intrathoracic pressure is recorded via an esophageal catheter. The change in esophageal pressure is plotted against the change in lung volumes, and the slope of this line $\frac{\Delta V}{\Delta P}$ is a reasonable estimate of lung compliance, expressed in liters per centimeter of water pressure. In the acutely ill patient in shock, measurements requiring patient cooperation cannot be made and another method of estimating compliance must be utilized.

Frequently, because of flail chest and other problems in which positive-pressure ventilatory support is necessary, a specific measure of lung compliance is also not possible. Under these conditions, one must settle for total thoracic compliance (pulmonary compliance plus thoracic cage compliance). A rough index of total thoracic compliance can be obtained by determining the peak airway pressures required to produce different tidal

---

granular pneumocytes (*GP 1, GP 2*) which are joined at *J* and show characteristic lamellar bodies (*L*) and microvilli (*MV*). The capillary (*C*) appears normal. There is marked widening of the interstitial space (*IN*) by edema fluid. A red cell (*E*) and fibrin (*F*) have been extravasated into the interstitium. A fibroblast (*FIB*) shows evidence of increased metabolic activity. (Reduced from ×16,800.) (Courtesy of Dr. Carl Teplitz.) (*Continued.*)

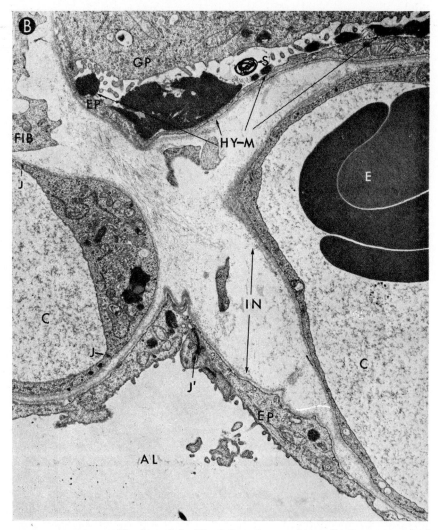

Fig. 3–2 (cont.). (B). (See legend for Fig. 3–2 *(A)* for case history.)—Severe interstitial edematous widening (*IN*) is present. Darkly stained fragments of inspissated serum protein and fibrin closely aligning the outer surface of alveolar epithelium (*EP*) constitute the ultrastructural counterpart of so-called hyaline membrane (*HY-M*). The intra-alveolar black whorled body (*S*) is phospholipid which is probably aggregated surfactant. The interendothelial capillary and epithelial junctions (*J* and *J'*) appear normal and are morphologically closed. Thus, the ultrastructural site of serum protein leakage into the alveolus cannot be ascertained. (Reduced from ×15,750.) (Courtesy of Dr. Carl Teplitz.) (*Continued.*)

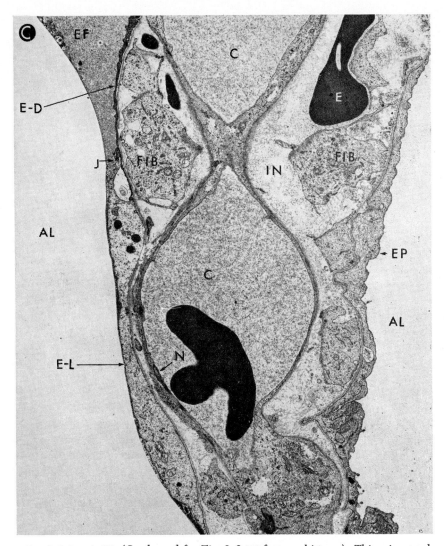

Fig. 3–2 (cont.). (C). (See legend for Fig. 3–2 (A) for case history.)—This micrograph illustrates pulmonary edema with capillary endothelial and epithelial injury. The darkly stained intra-alveolar protein-laden edema fluid (EF) has a denser concentration of serum protein than the lighter gray plasma in the capillary lumen (C). The light swollen epithelial cell (E-L) shows marked intracellular edema. The very dark thin epithelial cell (E-D) and the dark segment of capillary endothelium (N) are both demonstrating changes of early necrosis. The two injured epithelial cells still have an intact junction (J). The edematous interstitium (IN) contains an extravasated red blood cell (E). The interstitial fibroblasts (FIB) are showing ultrastructural evidence of increased activity. (Reduced from ×10,500). (Courtesy of Dr. Carl Teplitz.)

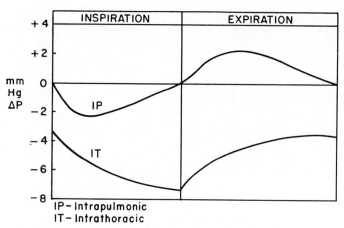

Fig. 3–3.—Intrathoracic and intrapulmonic pressure changes during one respiratory cycle.

volumes. This measurement is fraught with difficulties that limit its usefulness or interpretation. Many variables such as chest wall edema, abdominal distention, posture, and chest wall dressings will cause changes in total thoracic compliance. Although one must be cautious in relying too heavily on this measurement, nevertheless, in monitoring a patient supported on a ventilator, the development of a progressive increase in peak airway pressure at constant tidal volume suggests stiffening of the lung.

Compliance measurements have their greatest value when determined serially in a given individual under rigidly standardized conditions. A decrease in compliance means that more force is required to distend the lungs to a given volume. Many pathologic states, such as pulmonary edema and atelectasis, have been found to decrease compliance. A decrease in lung surfactant resulting in increased surface tension at the air-fluid interface of the lung also produces a decrease in compliance. Pathologic states that alter compliance frequently set up the conditions for the uneven ventilation-perfusion relationships so important in shock.

AIRWAY RESISTANCE AND BRONCHOMOTOR CONTROL

The pressure necessary to inflate the lungs is made up of two parts: (1) that necessary to overcome the elastic forces of the lung and thorax and (2) that necessary to overcome the resistance to flow of gas through the respiratory passages. Compliance is the index of the first of these and is measured under static conditions. The additional pressure necessary to produce gas flow may be further subdivided into two parts: (1)

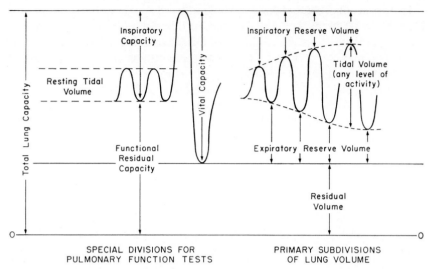

Fig. 3–4.—Subdivisions of lung volumes. (From Fed. Proc. 9:602, 1950.)

that necessary to produce laminar or streamline flow and (2) that necessary to produce turbulent flow. The pressure necessary to produce laminar air flow is entirely analogous to the pressure required to produce streamline blood flow through blood vessels and is described by Poiseuille's equation:

$$P = \dot{V}K_1 = \dot{V}\,\frac{8ln}{\pi r^4} = \text{Flow} \times \text{Resistance}$$

Therefore, resistance $= \dfrac{8ln}{\pi r^4}$ in which l is the length and r is the radius of the tube through which the gas is flowing and n is the coefficient of the viscosity of the gas. Since resistance is inversely proportional to the fourth power of the radius of the tube, it is apparent that the work of breathing will increase enormously with bronchial constriction, as in asthma. This fact also emphasizes the necessity for large-bore tubing in any apparatus through which the patient breathes.

When flow is turbulent, the pressure difference necessary to produce flow is proportional to the density of the gas and to the square of the flow. Thus for turbulent flow:

$$P = K_2\dot{V}^2$$

in which K_2 includes a term for density. For the situation in which both laminar and turbulent flow are present:

$$P = K_1\dot{V} + K_2\dot{V}^2$$

Evidence suggests that some turbulent flow is present in normal breathing and that a great deal more is present in conditions of airway obstruction. By substituting 80% helium and 20% oxygen for air, the work of breathing may be reduced under these conditions since the density of helium is less than that of nitrogen. Although the helium mixture has a higher viscosity than air and therefore increases slightly the work of producing streamline flow, when increased turbulence is present, the total work of breathing is reduced with the helium mixture. Considerable relief may be provided the patient with labored breathing brought about by obstruction by use of the helium mixture.

Physiologists have appreciated for some time that more than 90% of the airway resistance occurs distal to the carina. It is in this region of the lung that the radius of the airways is anatomically reduced, accounting for most of the resistance to air flow. It is also in this region of the lung that smooth muscle, surrounding the terminal airways and sensitive to numerous stimuli, can alter resistance by changes in airway dimensions. Bronchial smooth muscle, like other smooth muscle, responds to numerous neural and humoral stimuli. In general, sympathetic stimulation results in bronchial dilation whereas vagal (parasympathetic) stimulation results in bronchial constriction. Apparently bronchial smooth muscle contains very few alpha adrenergic receptors, since stimulation or blockade of these receptors with appropriate drugs has little influence on bronchomotor tone. In contrast, this tissue is exquisitely sensitive to stimulation by beta adrenergic receptor stimulants, which cause bronchial dilation. Beta adrenergic receptor blockade with propranolol will block bronchial dilation due to sympathetic stimulation and, in addition, will occasionally cause bronchial constriction in normal individuals, suggesting that beta stimulation helps to keep these tubules dilated in nonpathologic states.

Numerous other agents, such as histamine, serotonin, and parasympathomimetic agents, cause intense bronchial constriction. The fact that bronchial smooth muscle is constricted by most agents and dilated by beta adrenergic receptor stimulating drugs has led to the current and somewhat paradoxical hypothesis that bronchial asthma is due to diminished responsiveness of beta adrenergic receptors.

WORK AND ENERGY REQUIREMENTS OF BREATHING

Mechanical work is defined as the product of force and distance. It can be readily seen that the product of pressure $\frac{force}{cm^2}$ and volume (cm^3), has the units of mechanical work.

In our previous discussion, it was stressed that the lungs and the thoracic cage possess elastic properties. Work is performed by the inspiratory muscles as the volume of the thoracic cavity increases during inspiration and a given volume of gas is displaced due to the pressure gradient. Likewise, work is also performed during expiration as the potential energy generated during inspiration and stored in the elastic thoracic cage and

Fig. 3–5.—Energy cost, expressed as an increase in oxygen consumption, for a given increase in minute ventilation. (Courtesy of Arthur B. Lee, Jr., M.D.)

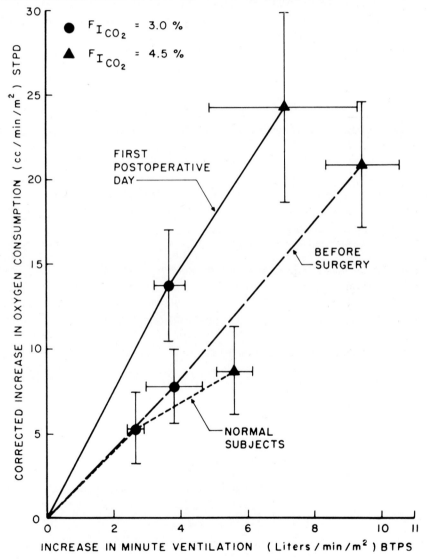

lungs is dissipated. Unlike the work of inspiration, work of expiration does not require active muscular contraction during normal resting breathing.

The energy requirements for the work of breathing have been approximated in terms of cubic centimeters of oxygen consumed per liter of ventilation (1 liter O_2 consumed $\simeq$ 4.86 kilocalories). At rest, respiratory musculature consumes about 0.5 to 1.0 ml oxygen per liter of ventilation. Lee has shown that with increased minute volumes the oxygen requirement per liter of ventilation is increased but considerably less than one would anticipate (Fig. 3-5). It is therefore highly unlikely that minute volumes of 5–15 liters place much additional burden upon the cardiovascular system, but severe hyperventilation may produce fatigue of the muscles of the respiratory system.

Surface Forces in the Lungs

In discussing compliance and work, we have considered the lungs as elastic structures somewhat analogous to a rubber balloon. Since the lungs are made up of millions of tiny air sacs lined with a liquid film, the surface tension forces in operation must also be considered and, in this sense, the alveolus is somewhat analogous to a soap bubble. The surface tension forces operating in a liquid-film bubble are expressed by the law of Laplace: $P = \dfrac{2T}{r}$. This means that more pressure is required to keep the small bubble inflated than the larger bubble and, when the two are connected, the small bubble will inflate the larger bubble (Fig. 3-6). This phenomenon suggests that there is an unusual problem of maintaining stability in the lungs, a highly complex interconnected system of liquid-film air sacs of varying sizes. What keeps the smaller alveoli from deflating

Fig. 3–6.—Surface tension forces in liquid film spheres illustrating the law of Laplace.

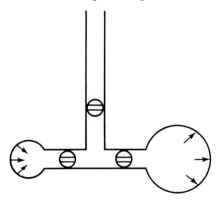

and inflating the larger alveoli much as the smaller bubble inflates the larger one?

The material in the liquid lining of the alveolus imparts an unusual property to the liquid film. Water has a surface tension of about 70 dynes per centimeter, and any surfactant added to water will reduce this surface tension to a lower value. The property required of the surfactant in the lungs, however, is not that of the usual detergent which simply decreases surface tension. The requirement is that the surface tension be decreased when the film is small (when the radius of the alveolus is decreased) and increased when the surface film is large (when the radius of the alveolus is increased). Clements demonstrated that the surfactant present in the film lining the alveoli of the lungs has these properties. Figure 3-7 is reproduced from the monograph, *Physiology of Respiration,* by Comroe, and demonstrates this unusual property of lung extract. In the absence of surfactant (see Fig. 3-1), it would be expected that many of the smaller alveoli of the lungs would collapse. A complex phospholipid, surfactant, is secreted by the type II alveolar cells (Fig. 3-2). Presumably, during inspiration, as the layer of phospholipid is thinned, it allows surface tension to increase; conversely, during expiration, as the layer thickens, it allows surface tension to decrease.

The physiologic importance of this substance cannot be overemphasized. Without surfactant the millions of small spherical alveoli would be inher-

Fig. 3–7.—Change in surface tension with changes in surface area. Note that water has a constant surface tension of about 70 dynes per centimeter despite changes in surface area. In contrast, surface tension decreases from 45 to below 5 dynes per centimeter with lung extract when the film area is reduced. (From Comroe, J.: *Physiology of Respiration* [Chicago: Year Book Medical Publishers, 1965, p. 108].)

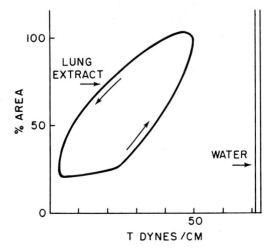

ently unstable because of their different sizes; small alveoli would empty into larger ones resulting in regional atelectasis and hyperinflated alveoli, the pressure required to overcome the surface tension during the initial phase of inspiration would be greatly increased, and the elastic recoil of the lungs during expiration would be considerably less. Absence or deficiency of surfactant has been linked to a number of clinical conditions that involve abnormal pulmonary function. Among these is hyaline membrane disease or respiratory distress syndrome of the newborn, oxygen toxicity, and respiratory difficulties following temporary occlusion of the pulmonary artery, as occurs in extracorporeal circulation with open heart surgery.

EXCHANGE AND TRANSPORT OF OXYGEN
AND CARBON DIOXIDE

An average man (body surface area $= 1.73$ M^2) at rest consumes about 250 ml of oxygen per minute. Depending on the type of food ingested and the state of the patient, for each cubic centimeter of oxygen consumed, approximately 0.8 ml of CO_2 is formed (respiratory quotient $= 0.8$). Since tissue oxygen reserves are virtually nonexistent, survival of cells is dependent upon efficient mechanisms for O_2 exchange and transport. Similarly, the buffering capacity of blood and tissue fluids is limited, and without adequate means of CO_2 disposal, profound and lethal acidosis would result. In the shock patient pulmonary damage is manifested by inadequate oxygenation; only terminally does CO_2 disposal become a significant problem.

Exchange of O_2 and CO_2 between alveolar air and blood occurs by simple diffusion in the lungs over a potential surface area of 50–100 M^2 and across a distance of 0.2–0.6 microns. The partial pressures of gases in air, alveolar air, and body fluids are given in Table 3-1.

Note that whereas the gradient for transport of O_2 between alveolar air and tissues is approximately 60 mm Hg, 80% as much CO_2 is transported in the opposite direction with a gradient of only 6 mm Hg. Fick's equation for diffusion states that the rate of diffusion is directly proportional to the

TABLE 3-1.—PARTIAL PRESSURE OF RESPIRATORY GASES (MM HG)

	O_2	CO_2	N_2	H_2O	TOTAL
Inspired air (dry)	159	0.3	600.7	0	760
Alveolar air	100	40	573	47	760
Arterial blood	95	40	573	47	755
Venous blood	40	46	573	47	706
Tissues	30–50	46	573	47	706

difference in concentration across the diffusion distance. CO_2 is twenty-two times as soluble as O_2 in tissue fluids and the concentration difference for each mm Hg difference is twenty-two times as great for CO_2 as it is for O_2. Because of this fact, impaired diffusion in the lungs often decreases O_2 transport but rarely interferes with CO_2 removal.

OXYGEN TRANSPORT

Oxygen is present in blood in two forms: (1) physically dissolved and (2) combined with hemoglobin. The solubility coefficient for O_2 in blood at 38°C is 0.00003 ml of O_2 per milliliter of blood per mm Hg partial pressure. Thus, arterial blood would normally contain 0.3 ml of physically dissolved O_2 in 100 ml of blood (vol%). One gm of hemoglobin can combine with 1.34 ml of O_2. Blood with 15 gm% hemoglobin would contain 20.1 vol% O_2 as HbO_2 if it were fully saturated. The relationship between partial pressure of O_2 and oxygen content of blood is shown in Figure 3-8, the well-known oxygen dissociation curves. Both the shape of these curves and the influence of acidity and temperature on the position of the curves are important clinically. Normally arterial blood is 97% saturated at Po_2 of 100 mm Hg. In blood containing 15 gm% Hb, this means an O_2 content (concentration) of 19.8 vol% of which 19.5 vol% is HbO_2 and 0.3 vol% is physically dissolved. If mixed venous blood is 70% saturated at a Po_2 of 40 mm Hg, its O_2 content is 14.2 vol% and 5.6 ml of O_2 is being delivered to the tissues by each 100 ml of blood. A cardiac output of 4.46 liters per minute would be required to deliver 250 ml of O_2 to the tissues per minute under these conditions.

Suppose that the patient has only 7.5 gm% Hb. What physiologic adjustments are available to allow continued delivery of 250 ml of O_2 per minute? This could be accomplished by either: (1) decreasing the venous and tissue Po_2 or (2) increasing the cardiac output or some combination of these two. With only 7.5 gm% Hb, arterial blood content would be 10 vol%, of which 0.3% is physically dissolved and 9.7% is HbO_2. If venous blood content decreased to 4.6 vol% (approximately 45% saturation), the required 5.6 vol% could be delivered with the same cardiac output. This would require a reduction in venous blood oxygen tension (and tissue tension) to between 25 and 33 mm Hg. On the other hand, if cardiac output increased to 9 liters per minute, the requisite 250 ml of O_2 per minute would be delivered with no decrease in tissue and venous blood tensions. Both of these mechanisms are likely to be operating in severe anemia.

This description illustrates the ease of estimating changes in cardiac output when arterial and mixed venous bloods are available. Since oxygen consumption equals the product of cardiac output and the difference in

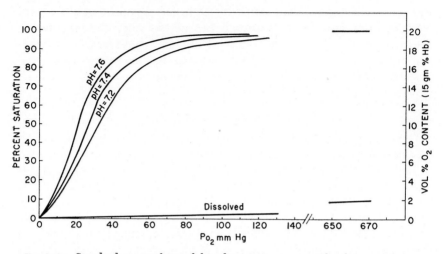

Fig. 3–8.—Standard oxygen-hemoglobin dissociation curves. The three upper curves are oxygen-hemoglobin dissociation curves at different pH. The straight line in the lower portion of the graph indicates the concentration of physically dissolved oxygen (ordinate on right side of graph).

oxygen content between arterial and venous blood, if O_2 consumption is constant, then cardiac output is inversely proportional to the difference between arterial and venous blood O_2 contents.

Figure 3-8 also illustrates that in blood of normal pH, O_2 saturation falls to only 90% at 60 mm Hg partial pressure and also that very little increase in HbO_2 content is accomplished by increasing Po_2 above 100 mm Hg. On the other hand, since dissolved oxygen is a linear function of Po_2, increasing Po_2 above 600 mm Hg by breathing 100% oxygen increases dissolved oxygen from 0.3 vol% to 2 vol% and, under these conditions, dissolved O_2 makes a significant contribution to O_2 delivery to tissues, but at the expense of producing lung damage due to oxygen toxicity.

CARBON DIOXIDE TRANSPORT

Carbon dioxide diffuses into the blood at the tissue capillaries under a diffusion gradient of about 6 mm Hg. Some of the CO_2 remains physically dissolved, some is hydrated ($CO_2 + H_2O \rightleftharpoons H_2CO_3$) and the acid formed reacts with buffer salts of weaker acids to form bicarbonate, and still another portion reacts with hemoglobin to form carbamino hemoglobin ($HbCO_2$). Hydration of CO_2 to carbonic acid proceeds slowly in plasma. The enzyme *carbonic anhydrase* is present in the red cells, however, and here hydration proceeds rapidly. The principal buffer taking up H^+

TABLE 3-2.—DIVISION OF TOTAL CO_2 INTO ITS VARIOUS FORMS BY ACTUAL
ANALYSIS OF ONE SAMPLE OF BLOOD (MM/L)

	ARTERIAL BLOOD	VENOUS BLOOD	% OF TOTAL PRESENT (VENOUS)	AMOUNT GIVEN UP TO ALVEOLAR AIR	% OF TOTAL CARRIED IN EACH FORM
$H_2CO_3 + CO_2$	1.05	1.19	5.1	0.14	8.3
$HbCO_2$	0.97	1.42	6.1	0.45	26.7
HCO_3^-	19.51	20.60	88.8	1.09	65.0
Total	21.53	23.21	100	1.68	100

Adapted from Davenport, H. W.: *The ABC of Acid-Base Chemistry* (Chicago: University of Chicago Press, 1958).

and forming bicarbonate is hemoglobin, and most of the bicarbonate formed originates in the red cells. A portion of the HCO_3^- formed in the red cells migrates out of the red cells into the plasma by exchanging for plasma chloride—the chloride shift.

Table 3-2 gives the division of total CO_2 into its various forms by actual analysis of one sample of human blood. Concentration here, and in the discussion to follow, will be in terms of millimoles per liter, unless otherwise indicated. To convert volumes percent to millimoles per liter, divide the former by 2.226 (the molar volume of carbon dioxide is 22.26 liters). Total CO_2 concentration of blood is the total amount of CO_2 that can be extracted under vacuum and by addition of acid, per unit volume of blood, or the total of the four forms mentioned in Table 3-2: physically dissolved CO_2, H_2CO_3, HCO_3^-, and $HbCO_2$. As indicated in Table 3-2, about 90% of the CO_2 in the blood is in the form of bicarbonate, and this is the principal form in which CO_2 is transported.

Carbon dioxide dissociation curves or, as they are more commonly called, carbon dioxide absorption curves, may be constructed in a fashion similar to oxygen dissociation curves. Such curves are represented in Figure 3-9. In order to make the units comparable to those of the oxygen dissociation curves presented previously, the ordinate is given in vol% on the left. The more commonly used units, millimoles per liter (mM/L), are given on the right. The position of the curve is influenced by the degree of oxygenation of the hemoglobin. Maximum CO_2 content at a given CO_2 tension, other factors remaining constant, will be present in completely reduced blood, and minimum content will be present in oxygenated blood. Just as addition of CO_2 to blood by decreasing pH aids in the transport of oxygen, the addition of oxygen aids in the release of CO_2 in the lungs. More CO_2 will be absorbed by the blood at a given tension when the hemoglobin is reduced by loss of oxygen than would have been the case if reduction had not taken place. Oxygen has this influence on CO_2 trans-

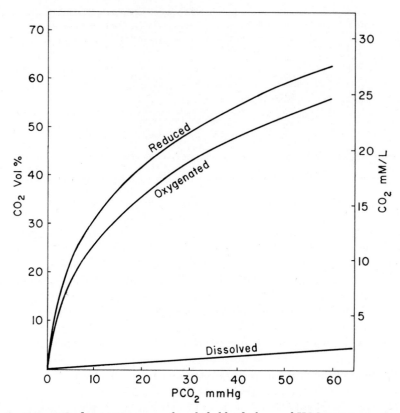

Fig. 3–9.—CO_2 dissociation curves for whole blood of normal HCO_3^- concentration.

port because reduced hemoglobin is a weaker acid than oxyhemoglobin and takes up H^+ to form bicarbonate more readily from H_2CO_3 than does oxyhemoglobin. Reduction of hemoglobin also increases its affinity for CO_2 as carbamino hemoglobin. A summary of the chemical reactions taking place in the exchange of gases in the lungs is presented in Figure 3-10. A similar diagram could be constructed to show the reactions that take place in tissue capillaries.

REGULATION OF BREATHING

It is common for patients in trauma or in septic shock to exhibit a pronounced ventilatory drive even after the hypoxemia has been corrected and CO_2 tensions are already depressed. This seemingly inappropriate respiratory drive is particularly common following head injury, septic

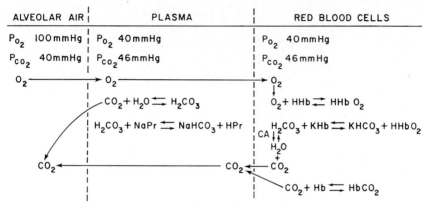

Fig. 3–10.—Chemical reactions taking place in pulmonary capillary blood during exchange of O_2 and CO_2 with alveolar air.

shock, and hemorrhage. The respiratory alkalosis which follows may be extremely difficult to control. Increasing the inspired CO_2 simply produces an added ventilatory drive, although the arterial P_{CO_2} remains significantly low. It appears as though the respiratory center has been reset at a new and lower P_{CO_2} level. Upon withdrawal of ventilatory assistance, these patients will often hyperventilate during the following 12–24 hour period. The mechanisms for these symptoms are not entirely clear at present, but considerable insight may be gained by reviewing some of the known factors that regulate respiration.

CENTRAL NERVOUS SYSTEM REGULATION

A certain degree of voluntary control of breathing is exercised almost continuously during consciousness and is exhibited in speaking, singing, breath holding, etc. The regulation of rhythmic breathing, however, is predominantly under involuntary control and will occur after ablation of nervous tissue cephalad to the pons.

Experimentally, at least three regions in the brain-stem portion of the central nervous system can affect changes in the rate and depth of breathing. These regions are the *respiratory center*, located in the medulla oblongata; and the *apneustic* and *pneumotaxic centers*, located in the lower and upper portion of the pons respectively (Fig. 3-11).

It is generally considered that the respiratory center, made up of two components, the *inspiratory region* and the *expiratory region*, serves as the primary integration center for respiration. The respiratory center receives numerous afferent impulses from central and peripheral respiratory

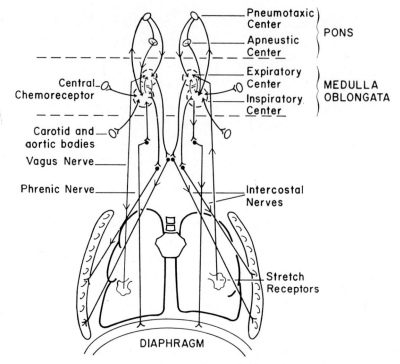

Fig. 3–11.—The neural control of breathing.

receptors that provide feedback on a moment-to-moment basis so that an appropriate stimulus will be initiated and propagated from this center to the respiratory musculature. Reciprocal innervation exists between the inspiratory and expiratory regions since the discharge of motor impulses from one leads to inhibition of the other.

The apneustic and pneumotaxic centers serve to modulate the depth and rate of breathing. The apneustic center, discharging continuously and independently of surrounding structures, keeps the inspiratory region of the respiratory center in a facilitated state, thus insuring that inspiration will take place once the inhibitory influence of expiration is over. In contrast, the pneumotaxic center serves to enhance rhythmic breathing by stimulating the expiratory region of the respiratory center shortly after inspiration, thus helping to insure that the organism will not remain in a state of continuous inspiration (apneusis).

Permanent or temporary dysfunction of any of these centers due to head trauma, hypotension, drugs, anesthesia, or other causes may result in various forms of disturbed breathing, including apnea.

RESPIRATORY RECEPTORS

Respiratory receptors can be broadly grouped into those sensitive to chemical stimuli and those sensitive to mechanical stimuli. These receptors are strategically located, and upon stimulation they send afferent impulses to the respiratory (integrative) center.

CHEMICAL RECEPTORS

Receptors that are extremely sensitive to CO_2 tensions or, more specifically, to hydrogen ion concentration, are located on the lateral surface of the fourth ventricle. Since these receptors are bathed with cerebrospinal fluid (CSF) instead of blood, an increase in the CO_2 tension of arterial blood causes a delayed but powerful response in terms of rate and depth of breathing. Until recently, it was felt that these receptors were predominantly CO_2 sensitive. Further investigation has suggested that they respond to changes in hydrogen ion concentration caused by the rapid diffusion of CO_2 into the CSF. Since the CSF, in contrast to blood, lacks hemoglobin to buffer CO_2, an increase in CO_2 tension in the CSF decreases the pH more than it would in blood. Conversely, a reduction in the CO_2 tension in CSF increases the pH in CSF more than would be true for fluid containing hemoglobin.

Evidence suggests that when the pH in CSF is altered by an increase or decrease in CO_2 tension, HCO_3^- is transported into or out of the CSF in a direction to restore pH toward normal. This adjustment (compensation) requires several hours or days for completion, and it provides an explanation for the continued drive to hyperventilation after removal of the initial stimulus in the patient in whom hyperventilation has been present for several hours. For example, if an initial stimulus of low arterial oxygen tension results in overbreathing to produce a decreased arterial blood CO_2 tension, pH in blood and CSF will increase. With time, HCO_3^- will be actively transported out of the CSF and pH will decrease. When the hypoxic stimulus is removed, ventilation will decrease and P_{CO_2} will rise. Increase of P_{CO_2} in CSF in the presence of the reduced HCO_3^- concentration, however, results in a decrease of pH in CSF which stimulates the central chemoreceptors to continue the increased breathing. The hyperventilation will continue until CSF (HCO_3^-) has been restored to normal. This increased sensitivity to CO_2 and the maintained hyperventilation have been demonstrated in subjects after 24 hours of passive hyperventilation in a body respirator.

In addition to the central receptors, there are peripheral chemoreceptors in the aortic and carotid bodies which are very near the aortic arch and at the junction of internal and external carotid arteries in the region of the carotid sinus. In proportion to their weight these bodies have a very large blood flow. Until the function of the carotid and aortic bodies was elucidated, the manner in which a decrease in oxygen tension produces an increase in respiratory ventilation was unexplained. These peripheral chemoreceptors are stimulated by low oxygen tension, increased CO_2 tension, and increased hydrogen ion concentration. The most important ordinarily is the response of these centers to decreased oxygen tension. When a human breathes mixtures containing decreasing concentrations of oxygen, very little respiratory response is observed until the inspired oxygen concentration is reduced to about 16%. As the oxygen concentration of the inspired mixture is decreased still further, a maximum minute volume of two to three times resting may be obtained. This appears, therefore, to be a relatively insensitive mechanism, but it is the only means by which low oxygen tension can increase respiration.

In the absence of the peripheral chemoreceptors, a reduction in oxygen tension produces a decrease in ventilation since anoxia depresses the central centers, just as it depresses most other tissues in the body. Relatively larger increases in CO_2 tension and/or hydrogen ion concentration are necessary to stimulate the carotid and aortic bodies. When they are stimulated by any means, afferent impulses are discharged over a branch of the ninth nerve (in the case of the carotid bodies) and over a branch of the tenth nerve (in the case of the aortic bodies) to the medulla, where they stimulate the inspiratory portion of the respiratory center. The importance of these peripheral receptors should not be underestimated because they lack sensitivity to small changes in oxygen tension. Frequently, when central receptors are depressed due to drugs, hypoxia, or anesthesia, these peripherally located O_2 receptors are predominantly responsible for maintenance of rhythmic breathing and survival. In addition, it has been shown that decreased O_2 tensions, incapable of primary respiratory stimulation, serve nevertheless to potentiate the respiratory stimulating effects of CO_2.

MECHANICAL RECEPTORS

It has become clear in the past decade that muscle spindles (gamma system) scattered throughout the respiratory musculature in a parallel arrangement serve an important role in regulating the extent of contraction of inspiratory muscles (Fig. 3-12). A sudden reduction in tidal volume induced by decreasing total compliance results in an immediate compensatory response designed to restore tidal volume. Changes in blood gases do not occur as rapidly as this and therefore are not likely to be responsible for this response, nor is this response affected in man or animal by vagot-

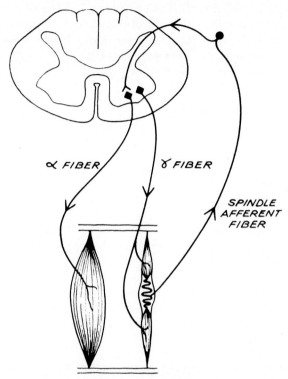

α FIBER   γ FIBER

SPINDLE
AFFERENT
FIBER

Fig. 3–12.—Nerve fibers innervating main muscle fibers (extrafusal fibers) and muscle spindles (intrafusal or fusiform fibers). (From Comroe, J.: *Physiology of Respiration* [Chicago: Year Book Medical Publishers, 1965, p. 86].)

omy. Other studies indicate that patients undergoing transection of sensory roots in the cervical and thoracic region of the spinal cord for relief of pain due to cancer develop temporary paralysis of inspiratory muscles deprived of local sensory input.

Observations such as these suggest an important role for the muscle spindles and their nerves in regulating the depth of breathing through a local feedback system causing facilitation of the anterior horn cells (Fig. 3-12). Removal of this local excitatory system renders other available afferent impulses (perhaps from the respiratory center itself) upon these anterior horn cells inadequate to excite them.

Several reflexes alter respiration. The best known and probably the most significant in quiet breathing is the Hering-Breuer reflex. Stretch receptors in the lung parenchyma increase their rate of firing during inspiration (inflation of the lung). Impulses generated from these receptors travel over the vagus nerve, stimulate the expiratory region of the respiratory center, and cause cessation of the inspiratory effort. Expiration then takes place passively. Although not essential for rhythmic breathing, ablation of this reflex by vagotomy will result in abnormally slow and deep breathing.

OTHER RECEPTORS

Numerous other receptors influence the rate and depth of breathing. The anterior hypothalamus is capable of increasing breathing in response to elevated body temperature. Receptors for pain, cold, proprioception, and pressure all may influence respiration by sending afferent impulses to the respiratory center.

PULMONARY CIRCULATION

Normally, right ventricle and left ventricle outputs are equal (i.e., pulmonary blood flow = systemic blood flow), and since mean pulmonary artery pressure (MPAP) is about one-eighth that of mean aortic pressure, pulmonary vascular resistance is one-eighth that of systemic vascular resistance. The pulmonary circulation may be thought of as a low resistance, low pressure, high flow system.

PHYSICAL FACTORS CONTROLLING PULMONARY BLOOD FLOW AND DISTRIBUTION

It has been appreciated for some time that the lungs possess large reserves of tissues that are underperfused and underventilated at rest. With the use of radioactive O_2 and CO_2, and by external counting during breath holding, the uptake of either gas is proportional to the rate of blood flow. In the normal upright subject, the rate of disappearance of radioactive CO_2 varies from about 20% per second at the base of the lungs to virtually nothing at the apex. Presumably, the differences in the perfusion pressure available at the capillary level account for the predominance of blood flow in the dependent portions of the lung in the upright position. It can be readily visualized that little or no blood flow can occur through the apical regions of the lung while the subject is standing at rest because the pressure required to elevate blood to the apical areas often exceeds mean pulmonary artery pressure. These differences in perfusion between the apical and basal regions of the lung can be eliminated by having the subject assume either the supine or the prone position.

Because of the large reserves of underperfused lung tissue, pulmonary blood flow may increase twofold or threefold in conditions such as exercise whereas vascular resistance declines proportionately and pulmonary artery pressure increases only a few mm Hg. Apparently, increases in blood flow through this organ are predominantly accommodated by recruiting and perfusing large reserves of previously underperfused vessels and, to a lesser extent, by increasing the dimensions of resistance elements. Removal of large amounts of lung tissue (e.g., pneumonectomy) therefore does not result in pulmonary hypertension under normal resting conditions.

Other factors, such as extravascular pressure on the caliber of pulmonary and intrathoracic vessels, effect changes in cardiac output and therefore in pulmonary blood flow. This is especially true when assisted positive-pressure ventilation (PPV) is required. It has been well documented that cardiac output is frequently reduced with either controlled or assisted PPV. The predominant mechanisms for this reduction in cardiac output with PPV is thought to be impairment of venous return to the right side of the heart. Another important aspect of PPV probably is its effect on the local distribution of pulmonary capillary blood flow.

Considerable work has been done on the effects of mechanical compression (atelectasis, pneumothorax) on the distribution of pulmonary blood flow. Atelectasis produced experimentally is accompanied by reduced blood flow to the collapsed tissue. After bronchial obstruction, the rate of gas reabsorption depends on blood flow, surface for diffusion, and composition of gases present. As the gas content of the lung decreases, blood flow is reduced secondary to mechanical compression of pulmonary vessels, especially capillaries in the collapsed alveoli. After total collapse of the lung tissue, often requiring many hours, measurements reveal that blood flow may be reduced by 80–90% of control values. Pneumothorax and chronic underventilation of lung segments also result in reduced blood flow, which seems to correspond well with the extent of pneumothorax or the degree of collapse with underventilation. Of greater importance in the shock patient is the development of large numbers of perfused but unventilated or poorly ventilated alveoli resulting in venous admixture.

HUMORAL FACTORS CONTROLLING PULMONARY BLOOD FLOW AND DISTRIBUTION

Much attention has been focused on the effects of chemical factors in altering resistance in the pulmonary vasculature, the most notable being the alveolar P_{CO_2}, P_{O_2}, and pH in the area of the resistance vessels. Pulmonary vascular resistance increases when alveolar CO_2 tension is high or when alveolar O_2 tension is low. In addition, pulmonary vascular resistance increases with infusion of acid and appears to depend upon the degree of acidosis at the resistance vessels rather than upon specific anions of the administered acid. These observations have led some investigators to theorize that at least part of the effects of acute hypoxia and acute hypercapnia on pulmonary resistance vessels is mediated by changes in pH in the environment of the pulmonary resistance elements. Hypoxia theoretically could result in a buildup of lactic acid, which lowers pH and results in vasoconstriction, whereas hypercapnia decreases pH due to the formation of carbonic acid with resultant vasoconstriction.

Conceptually one could visualize a highly efficient system whereby alveolar CO_2 and O_2 tensions locally autoregulate pulmonary vascular resistance, thereby guaranteeing perfusion in proportion to ventilation by shunting blood from poorly ventilated alveoli to adequately ventilated alveoli. This would insure even alveolar ventilation and perfusion, which is so vital for efficient respiration. Whatever the mechanisms for even and synchronous alveolar blood flow and ventilation, they are clearly upset in shock and many other disease processes and lead to respiratory dysfunction.

HUMORAL FACTORS

Aviado has reviewed the various agents that alter pulmonary artery pressure and has noted a paucity of agents that reduce pressure and an abundance of agents that increase pressure. There is little argument that agents such as norepinephrine and epinephrine are capable of increasing pulmonary artery pressure and that acetylcholine and isoproterenol reduce pulmonary artery pressure. Where these agents mediate their effects (pulmonary veins, arterioles, or distal to the pulmonary veins) is a matter of contention. For example, norepinephrine clearly increases pulmonary artery pressure in man due to an increase in left atrial pressure and not because of an increase in vascular tone of pulmonary arterioles; whereas hypoxia increases pressure by inducing vasoconstriction in vessels proximal to the pulmonary veins (Fig. 3-13). If one calculates resistance according to the formula:

$$\text{Resistance} = \frac{\overline{PA} - \overline{LA}}{\text{Flow}}$$

where $\overline{PA}$ equals mean pulmonary artery pressure and $\overline{LA}$ equals mean left atrial pressure, then norepinephrine causes no change in pulmonary vascular resistance whereas hypoxia increases pulmonary vascular resistance. Many evaluations of the effects of these agents on calculated resistance are confusing because of differences in preparations, in species of animals studied, and in failure to consider the effects of vasoactive substances on left atrial pressure.

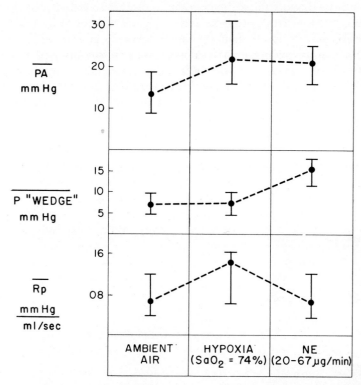

Fig. 3–13.—The effects of acute hypoxia and norepinephrine on mean pulmonary arterial pressure (PA), mean pulmonary arterial wedge pressure (P "WEDGE"), and mean pulmonary vascular resistance (Rp) in 13 normal humans. Note that despite the increase in pulmonary artery pressure with infusion of norepinephrine, pulmonary vascular resistance decreased. (From Goldring, R. M., *et al.*: The catecholamines in the pulmonary arterial pressor response to acute hypoxia, J. Clin. Invest. 41:1211, 1962.)

Some broad generalizations about the effects of vasoactive agents can be made if one limits his observations to the intact dog and man. Norepinephrine and epinephrine increase pulmonary artery pressure in the intact dog and man predominantly by passive back pressure from the left heart. It is also reported that these agents cause pulmonary venous constriction, but this effect is hard to evaluate in intact man or animal. Acetylcholine and isoproterenol reduce pulmonary vascular resistance in man and dog by reducing vascular tone in vessels proximal to the pulmonary veins. In the dog, massive doses of histamine will cause pulmonary hypotension and a precipitous drop in systemic blood pressure. In man, serotonin in small and tolerable doses apparently has no discernible effect on pulmonary artery pressure.

Some investigators think that serotonin may cause pulmonary venoconstriction, but the data arise from isolated perfusions of lungs and cannot
be extrapolated to intact man or animal. Bradykinin appears to constrict
the pulmonary veins in the intact dog proximal to the venoatrial junction,
thereby causing passive distention of vessels upstream to the pulmonary
veins. Recently, the effects of the fibrinopeptides (products from the action of thrombin on fibrinogen) on the intact dog, lamb, and rabbit have
been studied. Injections of minute amounts of these agents into the lesser
circulation of these animals causes profound effects on this vascular bed.
Pulmonary hypertension occurs with decreased effective pulmonary blood
flow and elevation in resistance. These effects occur immediately after injection and persist for as long as an hour. Clement's group thinks that
these agents are produced continuously, in vivo, and that they may accumulate in excess in pathologic states such as shock, respiratory distress
syndrome, oxygen toxicity, or following cardiopulmonary bypass, and account for elevated pulmonary resistance and resultant respiratory dysfunction. If this concept is valid, it may explain the common lung lesion found
in these various entities.

Neural Factors Controlling Pulmonary Blood Flow and Distribution

Although the pulmonary vasculature is richly innervated and some pulmonary reflex adjustments can be demonstrated, neurogenic regulation of
pulmonary blood flow under normal circumstances seems to be minimal.
Recent investigations, however, suggest that certain pathologic conditions
may cause lung damage and dysfunction through reflex control of the
pulmonary vasculature. For example, the totally denervated (excised and
reimplanted) lung may be more resistant to congestive atelectasis following hemorrhagic shock in the dog. Cervical cordotomy appears to prevent
pulmonary edema and right to left shunting across the lung with arterial
hypoxemia during increased intracranial pressure in this same animal. It
should be stressed that these studies are only suggestive that neural factors
play a role in mediating these pathologic responses and do not localize the
disturbance to the pulmonary vasculature.

Transcapillary Pressure Relationships

The mean pulmonary capillary hydrostatic pressure (MPCHP) in the
lung is dependent upon the pressure gradient across the pulmonary capillaries and the tone of the precapillary and postcapillary sphincters. By
means of indirect techniques, MPCHP has been found to be approximately

6–10 mm Hg, whereas the mean systemic capillary hydrostatic pressure is approximately 20–25 mm Hg. Provided the plasma protein concentrations are within normal limits, colloid osmotic pressure exerts an inward force of 25–30 mm Hg, which greatly exceeds the hydrostatic force of 6–10 mm Hg outward and, therefore, little net filtration takes place across the lung capillaries. Because of this and also because of a rich network of lymphatics, the normal lung remains in a "dry" state, favoring optimal respiratory function.

VENTILATION-PERFUSION RELATIONSHIPS

One of the major requirements for effective and efficient respiration is the regional synchronization of ventilation with blood flow. Regional synchronization requires that the amount of ventilation to each of 300,000,000 alveoli be matched to the amount of blood perfusing the capillaries of each of these alveoli. Under normal conditions, this matching of blood and gas occurs with enough uniformity to insure arterialization of pulmonary capillary blood. In numerous pathologic conditions, including shock, gross mismatching of blood and gas occurs, leading always to arterial hypoxemia and to variable carbon dioxide tensions in arterial blood.

DISTRIBUTION OF VENTILATION

The distribution of ventilation has been widely studied by means of external counters and various radioactive gases. Using radioactive xenon 133, West quantitated the distribution of ventilation and perfusion in man in relation to the various lung regions (Fig. 3-14). In erect man, the major fraction of minute volume is distributed to the dependent regions of the lung where blood flow is also predominantly distributed.

The mechanisms whereby ventilation is preferentially distributed to the perfused regions of the lung are still poorly understood. The previously mentioned factors that alter airway resistance through bronchomotor tone and the factors that alter lung compliance are certainly important, especially in pathologic situations. Under physiologic conditions, regional residual volume (RVr) and regional functional residual capacity (FRCr), which are a function of pleural pressure, seem to play a major role in the distribution of ventilation (Fig. 3-15). RVr and FRCr constitute respectively about 35 and 66% of apical region total lung capacity (TLC), whereas in the basal regions RVr and FRCr, respectively, account for approximately 6 and 23% of TLC. Regional vital capacity (VC) appears to be greatest in regions that are normally less distended (lower FRC).

Thoracic cage expansion and contraction are undoubtedly important in

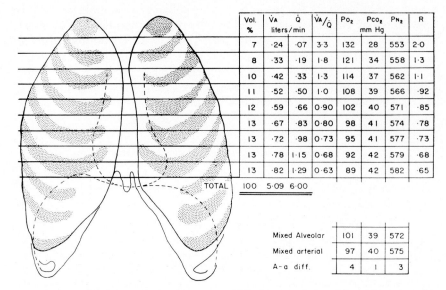

Vol. %	$\dot{V}_A$ liters/min	$\dot{Q}$	$\dot{V}_A/\dot{Q}$	Po_2	Pco_2 mm Hg	PN_2	R
7	·24	·07	3·3	132	28	553	2·0
8	·33	·19	1·8	121	34	558	1·3
10	·42	·33	1·3	114	37	562	1·1
11	·52	·50	1·0	108	39	566	·92
12	·59	·66	0·90	102	40	571	·85
13	·67	·83	0·80	98	41	574	·78
13	·72	·98	0·73	95	41	577	·73
13	·78	1·15	0·68	92	42	579	·68
13	·82	1·29	0·63	89	42	582	·65
TOTAL	100	5·09	6·00				

	Po_2	Pco_2	PN_2
Mixed Alveolar	101	39	572
Mixed arterial	97	40	575
A-a diff.	4	1	3

Fig. 3–14.—Quantitative values for regional alveolar ventilation ($\dot{V}_A$), perfusion ($\dot{Q}$) and gas tensions (Po_2, Pco_2, PN_2), and respiratory exchange ratio (R) in erect man. (From West, J. B.: Regional differences in gas exchange in the lung of erect man, J. Appl. Physiol. 17:893, 1962.)

determining which areas of the lung are ventilated most effectively. The lowermost portion of the thoracic cavity, including the region of the diaphragm, undergoes the greatest volume change during inspiration and expiration and accounts for the predominance of ventilation in this region.

It seems likely that in shock the compliance of the lung varies from one area to another; the engorged and less-compliant dependent portions accepting less ventilatory volume than the more compliant and less-engorged anterior portions, thus leading to an imbalance between ventilation and perfusion.

VENTILATION-PERFUSION RATIOS

The "normal" or "optimal" ventilation-to-perfusion ratio ($\dot{V}_A/\dot{Q}$) at rest is about 0.8 (alveolar ventilation of 4 liters per minute, cardiac output of 5 liters per minute). Provided alveolar ventilation is regionally matched with alveolar blood flow, the oxygen content of arterial blood will be maximal for a given alveolar Po_2 (Fig. 3-16). Under these conditions, the alveolar gas-arterial blood (A-a) gradient for O_2 will be small, and for CO_2 it will be approximately zero. These conditions are reasonably well met normally. Although blood flow occurs predominantly through the depen-

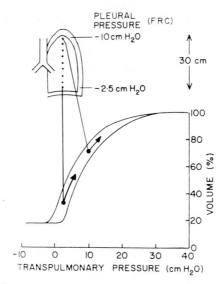

Fig. 3–15.—Intrapleural pressure is greater in the dependent portions of the lung due to the forces of gravity. At normal resting lung volume (FRC), alveoli are at different points on the pressure volume curve and for a given change in transpulmonary pressure more air will go into the lower than upper alveoli. (From Bates, D. V.: Import of radioactive gas studies of the lung on surgery and postoperative care, Bull. Am. Coll. Surgeons 54:355, 1969.)

dent portions of the lungs, ventilation also predominates in this region.

Under certain conditions, ventilation may be imperfectly matched with perfusion. Gerst has demonstrated convincingly the effects of decreased pulmonary blood flow secondary to hemorrhage on ventilation-perfusion relationships. Holding tidal volume (VT) constant with a respirator, the control ventilation-perfusion ratio was 0.73. With a progressive decrease in blood volume and secondary reduction in pulmonary blood flow, the ventilation-perfusion ratio increased two to threefold (Fig. 3-17). Concomitantly, the physiologic dead space increased from a control level of 0.3 to 0.5 VT due to the overventilation of a large number of alveoli with reduced perfusion.

Under conditions when the ventilation-perfusion ratio is greater than 0.8 due to low flow states and ventilation is regionally matched with perfusion, pulmonary capillary blood becomes appropriately saturated for the existing alveolar O_2 tension, but the Pa_{CO_2} will be markedly decreased (Fig. 3-16). Essentially the same changes in blood gases and physiologic dead space occur with hyperventilation and normal pulmonary blood flow (Fig. 3-16). The difference between the two states is that primary

FAMILIES OF ALVEOLI IN DAMAGED LUNG

A. NORMAL PERFUSION AND VENTILATION

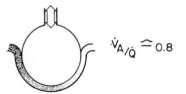

$$\dot{V}_{A/\dot{Q}} \cong 0.8$$

Alveolar Capillary

B. IMPAIRED VENTILATION – VENOUS ADMIXTURE

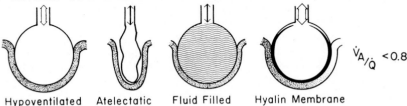

$$\dot{V}_{A/\dot{Q}} < 0.8$$

Hypoventilated   Atelectatic   Fluid Filled   Hyalin Membrane

C. IMPAIRED PERFUSION

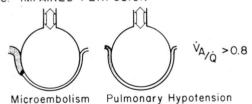

$$\dot{V}_{A/\dot{Q}} > 0.8$$

Microembolism   Pulmonary Hypotension

D. HYPERVENTILATION

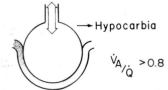

→ Hypocarbia

$$\dot{V}_{A/\dot{Q}} > 0.8$$

Fig. 3–16.—Relation of alveolar ventilation to pulmonary capillary perfusion in normal and pathologic states.

respiratory alkalosis will occur with simple hyperventilation in contrast to primary metabolic acidosis when blood flow is markedly reduced.

In simple hypoventilation, regional ventilation is matched with blood flow, but the ventilation-perfusion ratio is considerably less than 0.8 (see Fig. 3-16). Most commonly, this occurs secondary to drugs or anesthesia in CNS-depressed patients. Under these conditions, arterial hypoxemia

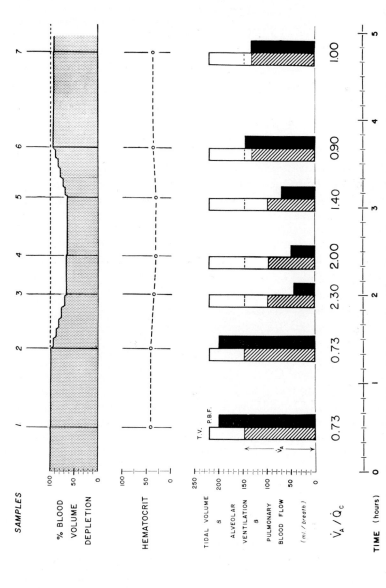

Fig. 3–17.—Changes in pulmonary blood flow (black columns) and alveolar ventilation (cross-hatched portion of V_T) during control period (1, 2), following hemorrhage (3, 4, 5) and after blood restoration (6, 7). Tidal volume (V_T) is divided into alveolar ventilation ($\dot{V}_A$) and dead space (white portion of V_T). The dead space is subdivided by the broken line into "anatomic" dead space above and "alveolar" dead space below. (From Gerst, P. H., *et al.*: Effects of hemorrhage on pulmonary circulation and respiratory gas exchange, J. Clin. Invest. 38:524, 1959.)

and arterial hypercapnia occur, regardless of the absolute values for alveolar ventilation or pulmonary blood flow. These blood-gas changes are due to underventilation of segments of the lung being perfused. Under these conditions, the alveolar P_{CO_2} is elevated and the P_{O_2} decreased, leading to arterial hypoxemia and hypercarbia.

Uneven Ventilation and Perfusion

The extreme aberration in altered ventilation-perfusion relationships would occur if the main-stem bronchus of one lung and the pulmonary artery to the opposite lung were occluded. The over-all ventilation-perfusion ratio would still be 0.8, but this condition is obviously not compatible with survival since no gas exchange could occur. Varying degrees of uneven ventilation in relation to blood flow is probably the most common cause of respiratory dysfunction in disease states. In these situations arterial hypoxemia always occurs, but the arterial CO_2 tension may be increased or decreased.

Consider a hypothetical situation in which a subject breathing room air has a cardiac output of 5 liters per minute, with 3 liters of blood flow distributed to the right lung and 2 liters to the left lung (Table 3-3). Suppose that because of retained secretions, atelectasis, and decreased compliance in the left lung, the effective alveolar ventilation of 4 liters occurs exclusively in the right lung. The result will be a ventilation-perfusion ratio of 4/3 in the right lung and 0/2 in the left. Pulmonary venous blood entering the left atrium from the left lung will have gas tensions of mixed venous blood, whereas venous drainage from the right lung will be fully oxygenated and have a reduced CO_2 tension due to overventilation of that lung. When these bloods are mixed in the left atrium, the P_{CO_2} and P_{O_2} will be approximately 36 and 60 mm Hg respectively.

Here is a paradoxical situation in which both Pa_{O_2} and Pa_{CO_2} are decreased in a patient breathing air. The explanation for this situation is found in the oxygen and carbon dioxide dissociation curves. The CO_2 curve (Fig. 3-9) is essentially linear over the range of 20 to 60 mm Hg,

---

TABLE 3-3.—Illustration of Effects of Uneven Ventilation
and Blood Flow on Left Atrial Blood Gases

Blood Sample	$\dot{V}_A/\dot{Q}$	P_{O_2}	%Hb Sat.	O_2 Content Vol%	P_{CO_2} mm Hg	Total CO_2 Content mM/L
Right pulmonary vein	4/3	120	100%	20.5	30	19.1
Left pulmonary vein	0/2	40	70%	14.2	46	23.5
Left atrial blood	—	60	88%	17.9	36	20.9

meaning that blood perfusing overventilated alveoli will lose CO_2 in proportion to the Pa_{CO_2} of those alveoli. Since the blood perfusing nonventilated alveoli will have the CO_2 content of mixed venous blood (Pco_2 46 mm Hg), the blood from the overventilated areas may be able to more than compensate for the admixture (Table 3-3). The Pa_{CO_2} and CO_2 content of the mixed arterial blood will depend on the degree of hyperventilation and the proportion of cardiac output perfusing the hyperventilated areas.

The situation for oxygen is very different. Increasing Pa_{O_2} from 100 to 120 mm Hg by hyperventilation increases blood O_2 content by a negligible amount. The O_2 dissociation curve (Fig. 3-9) is very flat in this area, and a 20 mm Hg increase in Pa_{O_2} increases O_2 content only 0.06 vol%. Thus, blood perfusing hyperventilated alveoli gains very little by virtue of the hyperventilation. Conversely, blood perfusing underventilated or nonventilated alveoli will have a reduced O_2 tension and content. The final mixture then will always be hypoxemic whereas the CO_2 tension may be normal or low under these conditions. This situation of low arterial O_2 tension accompanied by low CO_2 tension is seen frequently in the shock patient.

Venous Admixture

Venous admixture refers to the mixing of venous blood with arterialized blood. Under normal circumstances, the amount of venous blood entering the arterial circuit is approximately 2% of the total cardiac output. A portion of this venous blood arises from the bronchial circulation, which drains into the pulmonary veins, and that part of the coronary circulation which drains via the left ventricular thebesian veins. Unevenness of alveolar ventilation in relation to blood flow and anatomic right to left shunts occurring normally in the lung account for the remaining venous admixture. The amount of mixing of venous blood with arterial blood is significantly increased in certain disease states and shock, primarily through mismatching of alveolar ventilation with blood flow.

Mechanisms of Pulmonary Edema

Failure of the Left Ventricle

Probably the most common cause of pulmonary edema in shock is failure of the left ventricle. Primary failure of the left side of the heart most frequently follows extensive myocardial infarction, whereas secondary failure is also common and complicates many forms of severe shock regardless of origin. Left ventricular end-diastolic pressure (LVEDP) increases and results in a high mean left atrial pressure (MLAP). Passive distention of the vessels, upstream to the left atrium, occurs with elevation of the mean pulmonary capillary pressure. When mean capillary pressure exceeds plasma oncotic pressure, net filtration takes place across pulmonary capillaries, and when the rate of filtration exceeds the capacity for lymphatic drainage, fluid accumulates in the interstitial space and alveoli.

Acute, intense, sympathetic stimulation of the peripheral resistance vessels may produce a high central aortic pressure, and reflex bradycardia leading to increased left ventricular end-diastolic pressure and a high mean left atrial pressure and may cause pulmonary edema. Decreased contractility (negative inotropic effects) due to vagal stimulation of the heart probably accounts for the elevation in the end-diastolic pressure and the mean atrial pressure. Essentially, heart failure occurs under these conditions and provides a plausible explanation for pulmonary edema due to excessive vasopressor administration or increased sympathetic activity following elevation of intracranial pressure. The beta adrenergic blocking agent, propranolol, operating by a different mechanism, has also been shown to reduce contractility in the stressed or marginally compensated heart and can lead to pulmonary edema by passive distention of vessels upstream from the heart.

Cottrell *et al.* have recently evaluated the acute microscopic alterations in alveoli with the electron microscope after pure hemodynamic pulmonary edema in dogs. Increased interstitial fluid was primarily localized to the collagen-containing portions of the alveolar septum, whereas the endothelium of capillaries, alveolar epithelium, and respective basement membranes were structurally intact. Therefore large areas of the air-blood barrier were unaffected in these crucial studies. The hypoxemia and venous admixture found during pulmonary edema are most likely accounted for by continued perfusion of alveoli which are distended with protein-rich edema fluid. The oncotic forces due to the extravascular plasma protein maintains fluid within the alveoli in contradistinction to non-colloid-containing alveolar fluid which can be rapidly drawn back into the vascular space.

PULMONARY VEIN CONSTRICTION

For many years it was felt that the pulmonary veins merely functioned as passively distensible conduits offering little or no resistance between pulmonary capillaries and the left atrium. Recently it has become evident that these veins are not passive conduits and may actually account for as much as 30% of the resistance between the pulmonary artery and the left atrium under normal conditions. Histologically it has been known for some time that in man the pulmonary veins are richly innervated and contain smooth muscle fibers arranged longitudinally and circularly in groups. Extrapulmonary veins appear to have more smooth muscle than intra-pulmonary vessels.

Various studies have shown that small pulmonary veins respond by constriction to many stimuli, such as stellate ganglion or cervical vagosympathetic trunk stimulation. They have been shown to be actively constricted by bradykinin infusion in the dog. Substances such as catecholamines, serotonin, and histamine constrict isolated strips of these vessels when bathed with these agents. Because of these findings, it has been suggested that these vessels may aggravate or initiate pulmonary edema in certain disease states.

Aviado has proposed that pulmonary edema resulting from respiratory burns and edema after alloxan administration are due to pulmonary vein constriction. Whether this response is mediated by humoral agents is unknown at present. Radiologic observations on patients with mitral valve disease and high mean left atrial pressure have shown pulmonary veins in the basal lobes to be constricted whereas those in the apical region are widely patent. Braunwald and his associates feel that pulmonary venous constriction plays a major role in altering the distribution of pulmonary blood flow in patients with mitral valve disease.

The precise role of the pulmonary veins in initiating or aggravating pulmonary edema or in altering the distribution of pulmonary blood flow in shock can only be guessed at at present, due to insufficient information. Studies to define the role of these vessels in the intact human in shock is exceedingly difficult. Perhaps by correlating pulmonary wedge pressures taken simultaneously with mean left ventricular diastolic pressures, a rough index of the pressure gradient between pulmonary capillaries and the left atrium could be obtained. The mean left ventricular diastolic pressure is approximately equivalent to mean left atrial pressure in the absence of mitral valve disease, whereas pulmonary artery wedge pressure evaluates pressure distal to the small pulmonary arteries.

OVERHYDRATION

Another frequent cause of lung edema is inadvertent overload of the vascular space with blood, colloid, or crystalloid solutions. This occurs frequently in shock patients, particularly when adequate monitoring (serial determination of body weight or central venous pressure) is not carried out, or when myocardial reserve is marginal or acute renal failure is present. The lung is more susceptible to pulmonary edema after large quantities of non-colloid solutions, such as Ringer's lactate, because of dilution of the plasma proteins (decrease in colloid osmotic pressure) with the resulting extravascular distribution of these fluids. Guyton and Lindsey vividly showed the importance of plasma protein concentration in protecting the lung from increased hydrostatic pressure. They found that dogs with normal plasma proteins did not accumulate lung fluid until left atrial pressures exceeded 25 mm Hg. When the plasma protein concentration was reduced by approximately 50%, however, fluid accumulation occurred at left atrial pressures of 10 mm Hg.

Non-colloid-containing fluids such as Ringer's solution rapidly distribute into the interstitial space. Within minutes after administration, less than one-third of the administered volume remains in the vascular tree. The lung may accumulate more than its share of this type of fluid because of its loose anatomic characteristics. These two factors may, in part, explain the "wet lung syndrome" observed so often in Vietnam and in civilian practice after resuscitation of shock victims with massive quantities of Ringer's lactate solution.

INCREASED CAPILLARY PERMEABILITY

Altered capillary permeability may create pulmonary edema as a result of the leakage of colloids into the interstitium of the lung. The forces necessary to keep the lung dry are upset by damage to the capillary endothelium, and net filtration occurs because of excess extravascular colloids. This is frequently seen in burn victims in whom both smoke inhalation and thermal injury occur to the pulmonary tissue. Recent evidence obtained by Kistler suggests that the site of the dominant toxic effects of high oxygen tensions on the lung may be the capillary endothelium. Electronmicrographs of lung tissue taken from rats exposed to 98.5% oxygen at 1 atmosphere of pressure for 6–72 hours revealed a progressive thickening of the air-blood barrier from the normal of 1.5–3.0 microns after exposure to oxygen for 3 days. Thickening of the air-blood barrier was primarily due to accumulation of edema fluid, cells, and fibrin in the interstitial space. Approximately 50% of the capillaries were destroyed, many endothelial cells were fragmented, and 65% of alveoli were obliterated by a heterogenous exudate. In contrast, little damage or structural change was noted in the epithelial cells lining the alveolae.

Many humoral agents (histamine, bradykinin) are known to alter capillary permeability. These substances have been identified in shock states, particularly endotoxin shock, and could account for pulmonary edema of noncardiac origin. Other substances, such as the neutral proteases of human leukocytes, have been shown to damage capillaries in vivo and actually digest vascular basement membranes in vitro at neutral pH. These neutral proteases are released during phagocytosis, especially when sepsis supervenes in the lung.

The role of overt or subclinical infection in altering capillary permeability is well known. Pneumonitis frequently occurs in the obtunded shock patient and may account for pulmonary edema when present. The mechanisms whereby inflammation alters local capillary permeability have not been fully elucidated, but agents such as bradykinin, serotonin and histamine, all of which alter capillary permeability, are released in areas of sepsis. After fat embolism, it appears that the lung damage is brought about by fatty acids that are intensely damaging to the capillary endothelium.

MECHANICAL VENTILATION

Prolonged mechanical ventilation has recently been suggested as a cause of water retention and pulmonary edema. This concept is difficult to document because of the complex underlying disease leading to the need for prolonged ventilation. A retrospective study of 100 patients on prolonged mechanical ventilation showed that 19 patients developed water retention and radiologic signs of pulmonary edema without evidence of cardiac failure or excess fluid administration. Hemodilution and hyponatremia were present in these patients. These changes were rapidly reversed with negative water balance and diuretics. Several causes for this syndrome must be considered, including relative water overload, subclinical heart failure, or a rise in antidiuretic hormone production due to stimulation of volume receptors in the left atrium by mechanical ventilation. The latter mechanism appears very attractive, and the following evidence tends indirectly to strengthen such a hypothesis.

The area of the left atrium which adjoins the pulmonary veins is believed to be the site of low pressure volume receptors. Stimulation of these receptors gives rise to discharge of vagal afferent fibers which alter ADH release in the posterior pituitary gland. Positive-pressure respiration and hemorrhage have been found to reduce the rate of firing of these receptors and result in increased circulating ADH levels, whereas negative-pressure breathing and volume expansion increase the rate of firing and reduce the ADH level.

Mechanisms for Atelectasis

MECHANICAL PLUGGING OF BRONCHIOLES

Probably the most common cause of atelectasis in shock patients is retention of secretions causing plugging of small bronchioles. Collapse may occur in minutes or may take hours, depending on the amount of blood flow to the alveoli distal to the obstructed airway, composition of the gases present, and area for diffusion. The next result is a "shunt unit" (Fig. 3-16) which, depending on blood flow, leads to varying degrees of venous admixing of left atrial blood.

In the past decade considerable attention has been focused on the important role that proper humidification plays in keeping bronchial secretions liquefied. Under ordinary circumstances, inspired air is rapidly warmed and saturated with water in the upper airways. This prevents dehydration of small distal airway secretions. Without proper humidification, secretions become concentrated, tenaceous, and crusted and may lead to occlusion of small bronchioles. In addition, the drying effects of inadequately humidified air causes irritation of airway epithelium, leading frequently to excessive thick secretions.

Recently, attention has been focused on the depressing effects that 100% oxygen concentrations have on ciliated respiratory epithelium. Prevention of secretions from collecting in the dependent regions of the lung is largely a function of small beating cilia lining the airways. Raised oxygen concentrations directly decrease the motion and, therefore, the ability of these cilia to transport secretions out of the small airways. Secretions may be retained in small air passages and lead to airway plugging. Aspirations, after vomiting or simply as a result of failure to clear nasotracheal secretions in an obtunded patient, add to the likelihood of atelectasis in the shock patient.

Large droplets of respiratory secretions are normally cleared from the airways mechanically. Coughing or "clearing one's throat" causes the forceful expulsion of loose airway secretions, thereby facilitating the cilia in cleaning and maintaining patent airways. This can be accomplished adequately only with an intact glottis and considerable muscular effort. In patients with tracheostomy, painful surgical incisions, muscular weakness, or depression of the central nervous system, secretions are often retained, resulting in plugging of bronchioles.

Parasympathetic and sympathetic stimulation of numerous glandular structures as well as of the secretory cells of the airway leads to changes in rate and consistency of secretions. The well-known parasympathetic blocking agent, atropine, decreases secretions, whereas recent studies suggest that the pure β-adrenergic receptor stimulating drug, isoproterenol, may cause excessive secretions. Studies by Baue suggest that prolonged administration of this agent will lead to accumulation of large volumes of tenaceous secretions in the form of casts, causing blockade of airways.

DEPRESSED SURFACTANT ACTIVITY

Well over a dozen laboratories have now established that pulmonary alveolar surfactant activity is significantly diminished following a few hours of hemorrhagic shock in laboratory animals. Other investigators have shown that ligation of the pulmonary artery for 4 or more hours subsequently reduces surfactant activity. Clements has shown that if this substance is exposed to air, it loses its activity after 3 or 4 hours, suggesting that it must be continuously replenished in the alveoli. Others have shown that edema fluid, blood, plasma or, more specifically, fibrinogen, destroy surfactant activity. It would appear that adequate pulmonary blood flow is necessary for synthesis of surfactant and that a "dry" lung is essential if accelerated degradation is to be prevented.

Henry and associates, in attempting to unravel the role of surfactant, studied the effects of hemorrhagic shock on oxygen uptake by lung tissue, surfactant activity, and the incorporation of radioactive ^{32}P by the lung inorganic phosphate and phospholipid phosphate fractions. Using fasted dogs with ligated pancreatic ducts, they attained prolonged survival after severe shock. Severe atelectasis was noted 18–72 hours following shock, which correlated well with significantly depressed air deflation curves on pressure-volume plots performed on lobes of lung. Oxygen uptake by whole lung tissue and by separated mitochondria was depressed by 50% as early as 4 hours after shock. Incorporation of ^{32}P into lung-phospholipid phosphate was severely curtailed in shock lungs, whereas incorporation of ^{32}P into lung-inorganic phosphate was increased. These investigators concluded that since depressed tissue respiration and defective phospholipid metabolism preceded the development of diminished surfactant activity and severe atelectasis, perhaps decreased pulmonary blood flow and ischemia of lung tissue caused impaired surfactant production and the subsequent pathologic sequence. Other possibilities are that increased levels of inorganic phosphate in lung tissue, observed by these investigators, or circulating toxins could account for these metabolic deficits. Inorganic phosphate has been known to decrease respiration in numerous tissues.

The observation that edema fluid destroys surfactant activity points out mechanisms other than decreased surfactant production, which may account for a deficiency of this material in the lung. Recent studies in the dog have suggested that total vascular occlusion or complete denervation of the lung protects the treated lung from developing edema or generalized atelectasis during hemorrhagic shock. The basis for this protection is still being sought. It has been postulated, however, that these maneuvers may protect the lung against pulmonary edema and thereby prevent the rapid degradation of surfactant. Isolation of the lung from vasotoxic materials during shock may also be involved in this mechanism. Accelerated degradation of surfactant may prove to be the more significant mechanism by which surfactant activity is depleted and leads to atelectasis in shock.

LACK OF DEEP BREATHING OR SIGHING

It is clear that persistent shallow breathing and absence of sighing and coughing can severely impair normal respiratory function. It was traditionally felt that under conditions of normal quiet breathing, tidal volume and frequency were fairly constant, but continuous monitoring with a strain-gauge pneumograph demonstrates the irregularity of normal breathing. Tidal volumes vary from 200 to 2,000 cc, along with marked variations in rate during quiet breathing. It appears that variability is a prime requisite for maintenance of good pulmonary function. Sighing, "clearing one's throat," laughing, coughing, and changes in posture all serve to vary tidal volume and to intermittently expand underventilated lung tissue and prevent atelectasis.

After trauma or operation, pain with splinting is frequent and, as a result, movement is inhibited and respiration tends to be shallow and regular. Sighing and deep breathing are rare, and very little alteration in volume or frequency of respiration occurs. Observations have been made on intact humans by Ayres and Giannelli by strapping the chest to prevent deep breathing. Within one hour of chest strapping, arterial oxygen

Fig. 3–18.—Change in arterial hemoglobin saturation produced by chest strapping. Presumably the arterial hypoxemia is due to perfusion of collapsed alveoli. This state is readily reversed by deep breathing. (From Ayers, S. M., and Gianelli, S., Jr.: *Care of the Critically Ill* [New York: Appleton-Century-Crofts, 1967, p. 37].)

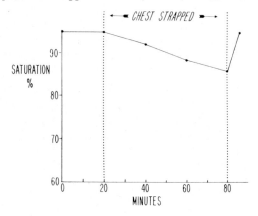

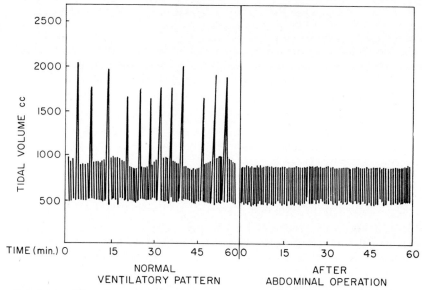

Fig. 3–19.—The effects of abdominal surgery on sighing and tidal volume in man. (Courtesy of Arthur B. Lee, Jr., M.D.)

saturations fell from a normal value of 95–98% saturation to an abnormal value of 85% (Fig. 3-18). This has also been observed in humans and dogs during anesthesia on constant ventilation. Although this type of respiratory dysfunction, presumably due to collapse of alveoli (atelectasis), may be rapidly reversed with deep breathing in a normal individual, it has not been established that atelectasis due to maintained constant tidal volume in the shock patient is readily reversible. (Modern respirators and good nursing care provide for frequent sighing of the patient.)

The basis for postoperative atelectasis and pulmonary dysfunction after abdominal surgery has recently been evaluated by Lee. Again, the one factor which was strikingly absent in these patients was the lack of sighing or deep breathing (Fig. 3-19). Whether these patients lose the ability or stimulus to sigh naturally, or whether pain limits the patient's willingness to breathe deeply after abdominal surgery, remains to be determined. The latter would appear to be the more important factor, since it has been shown empirically that vigorous physical therapy (preoperative training in coughing and deep breathing) significantly lowers the incidence of respiratory complications. The importance of postoperative atelectasis can scarcely be overemphasized since it represents the first stage in the development of postoperative pneumonitis.

Increased Pulmonary Vascular Resistance following Shock

In the preceding discussion, it was emphasized that pulmonary vascular resistance was only about one-eighth that of systemic vascular resistance. After hemorrhage in the anesthetized dog, the percentage decrease in pulmonary artery pressure is much less than that of systemic arterial pressure, and the elevation in pulmonary vascular resistance is much more pronounced than that of the peripheral vascular resistance (TPR). Often after sustained hemorrhagic hypotension, pulmonary vascular resistance reaches values five times control level. With retransfusion, peripheral vascular resistance frequently becomes normal, but pulmonary vascular resistance may remain at two or three times control levels.

Explanations of this phenomenon vary, depending on the interest of the investigator. Some investigators feel that reduced vessel size from mechanical compression (atelectasis) can account for the elevated resistance whereas others feel that capillary plugging from thrombi, fat, leukocytes, or platelet emboli may be important. That acidosis, hypoxia, and humoral and neural factors can reduce the caliber of resistance vessels in this circuit should be considered when evaluating this response. Finally, Clement's group has observed that fibrinopeptides released during intravascular coagulation cause sustained pulmonary hypertension and may have considerable influence on the pathogenesis of the lung changes in shock.

Case Histories

Case 1.—A 49-year-old healthy female was involved in an automobile-train collision. The patient, who was the sole occupant and driver of the automobile, was found lying about 30 feet from the point of impact between the car and the train. Initial emergency care given at the local hospital consisted in intravenous administration of 500 ml of dextran and splinting of fractures.

She was transferred to the University of Kansas Hospital approximately 3 hours following injury and, upon admission, was in severe circulatory and respiratory distress. Blood pressure was 80/60 mm Hg, pulse 136 beats per minute, respiratory rate 30 per minute and labored. A flail chest was grossly evident on the left side, secondary to multiple rib fractures (Fig. 3-20). Multiple cutaneous lacerations were also present along with fractures involving both forearms, left humerus, and left femur.

Initial therapy consisted in placing an endotracheal tube, positive-pressure breathing, and administration of Ringer's lactate solution and blood. The patient promptly improved. Under general anesthesia (2 hours), debridement and primary closure of the lacerations were carried out, and the fractures were treated by closed reduction and traction. A tracheostomy was performed.

The patient was then transferred to the intensive care unit and was progressing satisfactorily with arterial oxygen tensions approximating 100 mm Hg on room

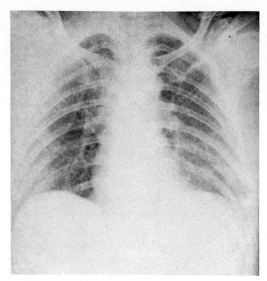

Fig. 3–20.—Admission x-ray, 8/15/68 (Case 1).

Fig. 3–21.—Summary of blood gases and acid-base studies (Case 1).

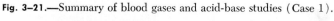

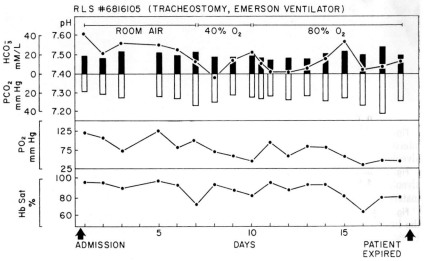

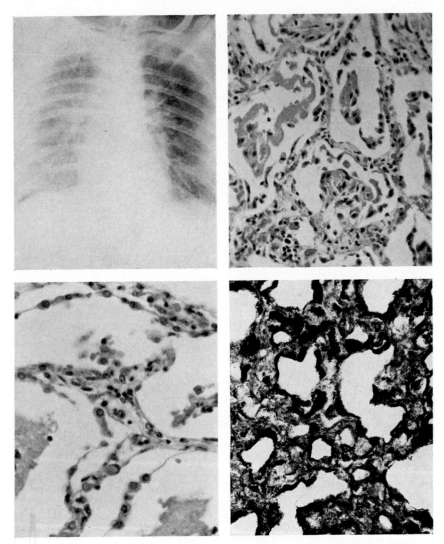

Fig. 3–22 (above left).—Thirteenth day after admission (Case 1).

Fig. 3–23 (above right).—Lung section 17 days after injury. Note thickening of alveolar interstitium by proliferating fibroblasts. Alveolar macrophages are prominent in the alveolar hyaline membranes (Case 1).

Fig. 3–24 (below left).—Respiratory distress syndrome. Seventeen days after injury, the alveolar interstitium is thickened by edema and proliferating fibroblasts. Proteinaceous material fills the alveoli (Case 1).

Fig. 3–25 (below right).—Fat embolism. Sudanophilic material in this thick section of the lung is shown black and is seen within blood vessels and lining the alveolar walls (Case 1).

air and a clear chest (Fig. 3-21) until the second day after admission when a pleural effusion developed on the left side. A thoracentesis was performed, with removal of 200–300 ml of blood-tinged fluid. Three days after admission, the patient became febrile. Intensive respiratory care and antibiotics were given. On the seventh day following admission, the tidal volume was increased and 40% oxygen had to be substituted for room air because of arterial hypoxemia (Fig. 3-21). By the tenth day following admission, the inspired oxygen concentration was increased to 80%, again because of progressive arterial hypoxemia. Despite elevation of the inspired oxygen concentrations, increased volume and rate of ventilation, steroids and the administration of phenoxybenzamine, the patient's respiratory status continued to deteriorate, progressive bilateral pulmonary infiltrates were present (Fig. 3-22) and she expired on the eighteenth day following admission.

Autopsy revealed, in addition to numerous fractures, hemorrhagic and consolidated lungs along with numerous hyaline membranes (Fig. 3-23) thickening of the alveolar wall (Fig. 3-24), and fat emboli (Fig. 3-25). Cause of death was progressive respiratory insufficiency and sepsis.

This case represents a common sequence: shock, followed by recovery; then mild evidences of reduced gas exchange responding initially to increased $F_{I_{O_2}}$ and tidal volume. In the final phase, the alveolar-oxygen tension difference was so great that saturation of hemoglobin could not be obtained with 100% oxygen.

CASE 2.—A 32-year-old female sustained multiple long-bone and rib fractures and a flail chest in an automobile accident. The patient was taken to the local hospital where pain medication was given and splinting of fractures was performed.

Fig. 3–26.—Summary of blood gases and acid-base studies (Case 2).

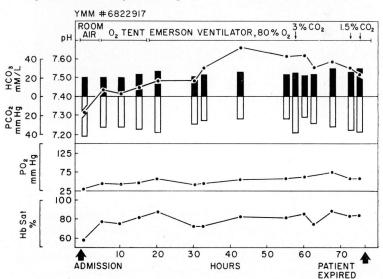

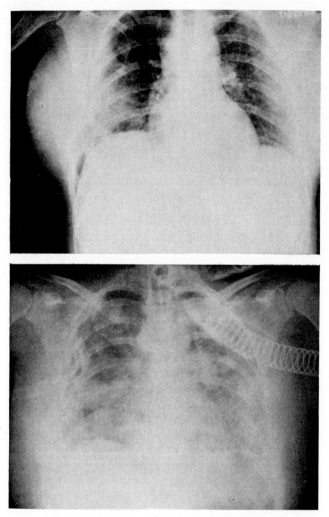

Fig. 3–27 (above).—Admission x-ray (Case 2).
Fig. 3–28 (below).—Case 2, 48 hours after admission.

Eighteen hours after injury the patient was transferred to the University of Kansas Hospital. Physical examination revealed the patient to be in severe distress with a blood pressure of 70/50 mm Hg, pulse 160 beats per minute, respiration 28 breaths per minute. There was some flailing of the anterior chest, most severe on the right side. In addition, a right pneumothorax was present.

Initially, the patient was given dextran solution, Ringer's lactate, and whole blood; and a chest tube was placed into the right pleural space. She responded to the fluid replacement, showing improvement in blood pressure and urine vol-

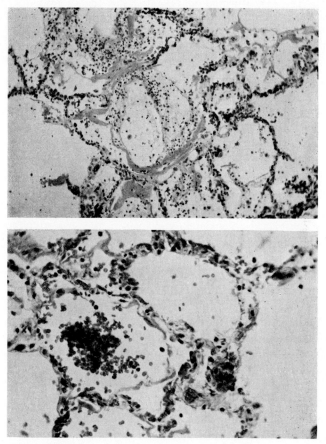

Fig. 3–29 (above).—Hyaline membrane formation (Case 2).
Fig. 3–30 (below).—Edema of the capillary wall, hyaline membrane formation, and hemorrhage (Case 2).

umes greater than 50 ml per hour. Her fractures were reduced and plaster casts were applied. She was transferred to the intensive care unit.

During the early course of her hospitalization, the patient was placed in an oxygen tent. Blood gases revealed severe arterial hypoxemia despite what was thought to be satisfactory ventilation clinically (Fig. 3-26). A tracheostomy was performed, and the patient was placed on an Emerson ventilator with 40% inspired oxygen. Despite ventilatory support, arterial hypoxemia persisted. Chest x-ray revealed diffuse bilateral pulmonary infiltrate in contrast to a relatively normal chest x-ray on admission (Figs. 3-27, 3-28). The inspired oxygen concentration was increased to 80%, and the volume and rate of ventilation manipulated with little improvement in the patient's respiratory status. Because of severe respiratory alkalosis secondary to hyperventilation, CO_2 was added to the inspired air. The patient would not tolerate either the 3% inspired CO_2 or a reduction in the rate and volume of ventilation (see Fig. 3-26). An attempt was then made to reduce the rate and volume of respiration by manually ventilating the patient with an Ambu bag. This appeared to be well tolerated by the patient, but shortly after it was initiated, the patient developed cardiac arrest. She could not be resuscitated.

Autopsy revealed, in addition to the injuries already described, marked bilateral edema and hemorrhage of the lungs. Microscopic evaluation revealed hyaline membranes throughout the lung (Fig. 3-29) and intra-alveolar hemorrhage (Fig. 3-30).

Pathophysiology of the Heart in Shock

It is difficult to overestimate the importance of the heart in human shock, whether it be primarily involved or secondarily damaged as a result of hypotension, hypoxemia, or sepsis. A low or reduced cardiac output is commonly associated with shock, and even in the hyperdynamic state of septic shock, impaired cardiac performance can often be demonstrated. Primary involvement of the heart occurs in cardiogenic shock in which low cardiac output and depressed cardiac contractility are frequently the result of myocardial infarction. Here the venous filling and venous return to the heart are adequate, but the contractility of the left ventricle is so poor that adequate peripheral perfusion cannot be maintained. Recently, attention has been directed to secondary myocardial dysfunction in shock associated with hemorrhage, sepsis, and burns. Lefler has demonstrated a low-molecular-weight, heat-stable, dialysable polypeptide which acts as a myocardial depressant factor in experimental animals subjected to hemorrhagic shock. Siegel has noted the frequent occurrence of myocardial failure in patients with septic shock. In experimental preparations, some investigators have shown that *Escherichia coli* endotoxemia exerts a detrimental effect on left ventricular performance. Often in the advanced case with lung damage, it is difficult to decide whether the low output is due to heightened resistance in damaged lungs and failure of the right side of the heart or to reduced left ventricular function. Soon both factors operate conjointly as the lowered Pao_2 damages the myocardium and the failing left ventricle further damages the lungs (terminal positive feedback).

Cardiogenic shock usually follows myocardial infarction when the systolic blood pressure falls below 80 mm Hg. Failure of peripheral perfusion with marked oliguria, pallor or cyanosis, diaphoresis, cold skin, and dulling of the sensorium attest to the generalized state of lowered perfusion. Left ventricular end-diastolic pressures are usually markedly raised and may reach 40–50 mm Hg (normal 4–12 mm Hg). Left atrial pressures are also high in most cases of cardiogenic shock (normal 4–12 mm Hg). Pulmonary artery (normal 10–20 mm Hg) and central venous pressures (normal 4–8 mm Hg) are also usually raised.

HEMODYNAMIC MEASUREMENTS IN CARDIOGENIC SHOCK

Measurements in cardiogenic shock have revealed a decreased cardiac output and slightly to markedly elevated total peripheral resistance. It is of interest, however, to note that the cardiac output of patients with myocardial infarction who are in shock may differ significantly from the cardiac output of patients with infarction who are not in shock. Patients with infarction who have a cardiac index below 1.3 liters per square meter are almost always hypotensive and exhibit manifestations of reduced tissue perfusion. Patients with cardiac indices between 1.3 and 2.6, however, may show no evidences of cellular hypoxia. On the other hand, patients who are chronically ill from cardiac disease may have extremely low cardiac indices and yet lack the peripheral circulatory findings present in cardiogenic shock. For example, many patients with severe mitral or aortic valvular disease studied at cardiac catheterization have extremely low cardiac indices (Table 3-4). Yet these patients are ambulatory and not oliguric. In general, they do not have the impaired tissue perfusion usually present in shock.

Patients with myocarditis or in chronic severe congestive heart failure due to arteriosclerotic heart disease also have extremely low cardiac indices without shock. Thus, low cardiac index alone may not be the total explanation for cardiogenic shock. The gradual fall in cardiac output in the chronic cardiac patient is in some way rendered tolerable by adaptive reactions that are not clear. On the other hand, an acute fall in cardiac output, such as follows myocardial infarction, is very poorly tolerated. Marginal but adequate perfusion of vital organs is maintained in

TABLE 3-4.–LOW CARDIAC INDEX IN
MITRAL VALVE DISEASE

DIAGNOSIS	CARDIAC INDEX L/min/m²
Mitral stenosis	2.1
Mitral stenosis	2.1
Mitral stenosis	1.6
Mitral stenosis	1.5
Mitral insufficiency	1.6
Mitral stenosis	1.7
Mitral stenosis	1.7
Mitral stenosis	2.4
Mitral stenosis	1.6
Mitral insufficiency	2.4

the chronic cardiac with low output, but not when shock follows myocardial infarction, although the levels of cardiac output in the two groups may be comparable. In general, patients who are in cardiogenic shock have an extremely small stroke volume and a marked tachycardia. Thus a reduced stroke volume may define more critically the hemodynamic abnormality in cardiogenic shock than does low cardiac output.

Papillary muscle dysfunction, such as occurs with acute myocardial infarction, can interfere with the four cardiac phases, due to marked incompetence of the mitral valve. In addition, ventricular aneurysm is not an infrequent development with acute myocardial infarction, and asynchrony of ventricular contraction or impaired contractility of an infarcted segment may interfere markedly with cardiac performance.

MYOCARDIAL FUNCTION

Many indicators of myocardial function are available to the cardiac physiologist. Some of these are based on the Starling principle and relate left ventricular work to an indicator of left ventricular stretch such as end-diastolic pressure. The Starling principle implies that the strength of contraction increases in proportion to the initial length and tension of the fibers. If the diastolic volume in the left ventricle is augmented by increased venous return to the heart, the stroke volume will also be augmented. As a result, in a steady state the output of the left and the right ventricles are equal; the total blood volume remains distributed in the proper way between systemic and pulmonary circulations. In cardiogenic shock the heart usually shows an abnormal left ventricular function curve; and very high end-diastolic pressures are required to produce small increases in left ventricular stroke volume and stroke work (Fig. 3-31). Cohn has shown that this abnormal left ventricular function frequently exists in hemorrhagic and septic shock as well.

Another indication of myocardial function is ventricular dp/dt or the rise in pressure with time. This measurement is available in a cardiac catheterization laboratory or physiology laboratory, where the rate of left ventricular pressure rise may be accurately determined by an intracardiac micromanometer. Normal values are approximately 1,000 mm Hg per second. Weissler and others have developed noninvasive techniques for measuring myocardial function. One of these relates left ventricular function to the pre-ejection period as measured on the phonocardiogram. A prolonged delay between electrical and mechanical events, i.e., between the QRS complex and the carotid pulse upstroke, is associated with a failing myocardium.

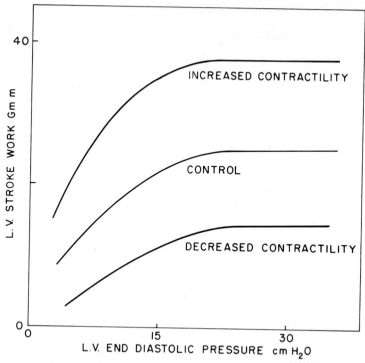

Fig. 3–31.—The relationship between filling pressure and stroke work in the determination of myocardial function.

A common clinical test of myocardial function is based on measuring the response of central venous pressure and stroke volume to small fluid loads. In general, if the central venous pressure rises markedly with a small increase in stroke volume, ventricular function is impaired. It has recently been suggested that central venous pressure is not a reliable indicator of left ventricular filling pressure. Since central venous pressure or right atrial pressure is dependent on elevated pulmonary pressure and failure of the right ventricle, there may be some time delay between elevations in left atrial and right atrial pressures. Information regarding this point is very scanty in the human during cardiogenic shock; however, in the cardiac catheterization laboratory, patients with rheumatic valvular disease are seen with left atrial pressures approaching pulmonary edema levels, and yet they are able to maintain normal right atrial pressures. Examples of lack of relationship between left atrial and right atrial pressure can be seen in Table 3-5. Other clinical indications of myocardial fail-

TABLE 3-5.—Simultaneous Measurement of Left and Right
Atrial Pressures in Mitral Valve Disease

DIAGNOSIS	RA PRESSURE mm Hg	LA PRESSURE mm Hg
Mitral insufficiency	14	18
Mitral stenosis	3	20
Mitral stenosis	5	21
Mitral stenosis	8	34
Mitral stenosis	5	20
Aortic stenosis	6	24
Mitral stenosis	8	26
Mitral stenosis	3	18
Mitral stenosis	4	21
Aortic stenosis	7	28
Mitral stenosis	$\begin{cases}3\\4°\end{cases}$	$\begin{cases}18\\24°\end{cases}$

° After fluid expansion.

ure are pulmonary edema and pulmonary venous congestion as demonstrated by chest x-ray. Detection of moist rales or gallop rhythm by auscultation may be additional important clinical signs of left heart failure.

Altered Blood Volume Distribution

The normal blood volume is distributed between the pulmonary circulation and systemic circulation in an unequal fashion. According to Burton, a blood volume of 5.2 L is normally distributed as follows:

Pulmonary arteries, 400 ml
Pulmonary capillaries, 60 ml
Pulmonary venules, 140 ml
Pulmonary veins, 700 ml
Heart, 250 ml
Aorta, 100 ml
Systemic arteries, 450 ml
Systemic capillaries, 350 ml
Systemic venules, 200 ml
Systemic veins, 2050 ml
Liver and spleen reservoirs, 550 ml

It is apparent that the pulmonary veins and venules, together with the systemic veins and venules, account for the major portion of the blood volume. The venous system acts as a huge reservoir for blood and, under certain pathologic circumstances, even larger volumes of blood may be sequestered in the venous circulation.

In cardiogenic shock, the total blood volume may be increased. Signs of pulmonary venous congestion are seen on chest x-ray as evidence of increased blood volume in the pulmonary circuit. There may be a redistribution of cardiac output so that blood flow to the brain and heart is maintained while the flow to limbs, kidney, and mesentery is markedly diminished.

Altered Structure of the Heart

Shock which occurs following an acute myocardial infarction may correlate with the extent of gross muscle necrosis. However, cardiogenic shock may also occur with only small areas of necrosis. Sampson found small areas of myocardial damage in a "trigger area" near the apex of the left ventricle in fatal cases of myocardial infarction and shock.

Recent advances in defining the ultrastructure of the heart allow better understanding of the pathophysiology of cardiogenic shock. The myocardial muscle cells are arranged in orderly columns, which can be clearly delineated with light microscopy. Electron microscopy has clearly demonstrated the presence of myofibrils which are the basic contractile elements present in the myocardial cells. The myofibril, in turn, is divided into smaller functional units called sarcomeres. Under the electron microscope, a sarcomere is delineated by Z lines, has a dark A band in the center, and two relatively lighter I bands on either side. An intricate system of transverse and longitudinal tubules also exists in close apposition to the Z lines (Fig. 3-32). The sliding-filament concept of cardiac contraction suggests that myosin filaments interdigitate with actin filaments to form the A, I, and Z bands (Fig. 3-33).

In cardiogenic shock, as in other forms of cardiac failure, change in sarcomere length is primarily related to increases of I band length. Spot-

Fig. 3–32.—Relationship of sarcomere length and filament pattern.

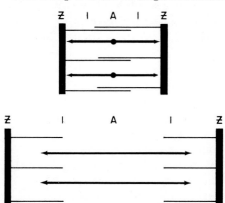

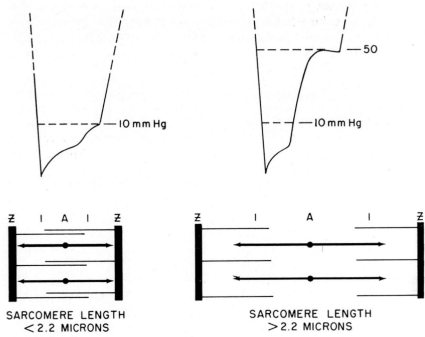

SARCOMERE LENGTH
< 2.2 MICRONS

SARCOMERE LENGTH
> 2.2 MICRONS

Fig. 3–33.—The relationship between left ventricular end diastolic pressure and sarcomere length.

nitz has shown that left ventricular function depends directly on the length of the sarcomere. With normal left ventricular function, the length of the sarcomere is less than 2.2 microns; in the failing myocardium, the length is increased. With elevated left ventricular filling pressures of 50 mm Hg, the length of the sarcomere is greater than 2.3 microns. Thus, overstretching of the myofibrils with disruption of the intricate system of transverse and longitudinal tubules and displacement of energy-synthesizing mitochondria may provide an explanation for the failing myocardium on an anatomic basis. In addition, dehiscences of intercalated disks may also occur. The result of these dehiscences is that contact of cells is lost, large interspaces develop, and the mechanical contraction of the sarcomeres may become ineffective. Hypoxia causes reversible swelling of mitochondria, due to intracellular ionic changes, with a rapid appearance of mitochondrial granules. The most important disruption of mitochondrial function takes place in the mitochondrial membrane in which the phospholipid fraction of the mitochondrial membrane is altered during ischemia. The mechanical-chemical properties of this membrane are adversely influenced, and a significant fall in the cardiolipin percentage of the mitochondria occurs.

ENERGY UTILIZATION AND METABOLISM IN SHOCK

In many cases of acute myocardial infarction with cardiogenic shock the heart does not appear to be dilated, and overstretching of myofibrils may not occur. In these circumstances, a biochemical lesion pertaining to the transfer of chemical to mechanical energy is postulated. One such lesion has been postulated to be an ATPase deficiency since the release of ATP is vital in energy utilization. In addition, a markedly reduced concentration of norepinephrine has been repeatedly demonstrated in cardiac tissue of a failing myocardium, suggesting impairment of catecholamine synthesis. Decreased neuronal uptake and binding of circulating norepinephrine has also been demonstrated in acute left heart failure. The conversion of chemical to mechanical energy may thus fail, due to one of these chemical deficiencies.

The energy sources for the myocardium are primarily dependent upon aerobic metabolic processes. Bing found that the oxygen consumption of arrested heart muscle is 4.8 ml per minute per 100 gm of heart muscle. The oxygen consumption of the beating heart has a fairly constant relationship to heart rate and blood pressure so that:

Oxygen consumption = k · heart rate × blood pressure × stroke volume
The linear relationship of oxygen consumption and cardiac work may be altered by the administration of catecholamines.

Many substrates are available to the heart for nutrition. These include glucose, pyruvate, lactate, fatty acids, acetates, ketones, and amino acids (Fig. 3-34). The prime substrates are fatty acids and pyruvic acids, which are oxidized in the myocardial mitochondria. The energy thus liberated is eventually stored as ATP and creatine phosphate. With myocardial energy sources highly dependent on oxidative processes, any process such as shock (in which myocardial hypoxia occurs) will severely interfere with energy kinetics. Experimentally produced myocardial infarction and shock results in a marked depression of myocardial extraction and utilization of myocardial glucose. These data are derived from simultaneous arterial and coronary sinus sampling.

In the normal human heart, approximately one-third of the energy for work is derived from the oxidation of carbohydrates. Since myocardial utilization of these substrates is dependent on their arterial concentration, glucose and lactate are used in approximately equal amounts and pyruvate utilization is significantly lower. Bing has estimated that the normal human heart utilizes approximately 11 gm of glucose and 10 gm of lactate per day. The blood insulin level is an important additional factor in regulating the myocardial consumption of glucose. Acidosis and alkalosis also influence myocardial carbohydrate metabolism. In the presence of

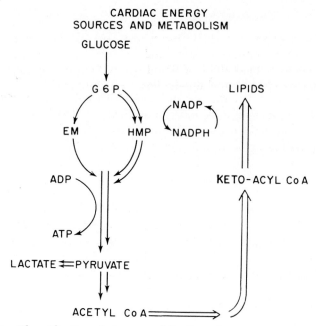

Fig. 3–34.—The utilization of glucose and lipids in the generation of adenosine triphosphate (ATP) in the heart.

acidosis there is an increase in the blood concentration of glucose, but a diminished myocardial uptake of the substrate. In the presence of alkalosis there is a marked increase in blood lactate and pyruvate, and the myocardial uptake of these substrates is markedly increased.

Normal cardiac metabolism is much more dependent on fatty acids than on glucose. In the presence of low blood glucose, the heart may utilize lipid metabolism almost exclusively. The metabolism of other noncarbohydrate substrates such as phospholipids, cholesterol, and ketone bodies may also increase. In the presence of anoxia, the concentration of ATP falls whereas ADP and AMP are increased. There is also a marked increase in the concentration of inorganic phosphate. This breakdown of nucleotides releases free adenosine, which in turn may have a direct coronary-dilating effect and augment coronary blood flow. In the presence of myocardial anoxia, glycogen disappears very rapidly due to glycolytic enzymes. Lactic acid is generated in increased amounts since hypoxia results in a marked increase in NADH, and the following equation is shifted to the right:

$$\text{Pyruvate} + \text{NADH} \underset{}{\overset{\text{LDH}}{\rightleftharpoons}} \text{lactate} = \text{NAD}$$

THE CORONARY CIRCULATION IN SHOCK

The volume of blood flow in the coronary circulation is approximately 5% of the cardiac output. Both right and left coronary arteries have a comparable volume of blood flow of 80 ml per 100 gm per minute. With the use of miniaturized electromagnetic flow transducers, it has been demonstrated that flow in the left coronary artery falls precipitously with ventricular muscle contraction due to extravascular compression. Consequently 70 to 90% of coronary flow occurs in diastole, indicating the importance of the diastolic pressure in regulating coronary blood flow. A slowing of the heart theoretically would be expected to increase coronary flow because of an increased duration of diastole. An increase in the heart rate may reduce coronary flow.

Autoregulatory mechanisms are important in adjusting coronary flow to metabolic demand. Coronary vessels respond by vasodilation to myocardial hypoxia, and presumably this is the mechanism for autoregulation of coronary flow. It is also known that some nervous influences are important. For example, vagal stimulation may result in an increase in coronary blood flow due to slowing of the heart rate. The question of vasoconstriction versus vasodilation with sympathetic stimulation is still unresolved. There are alpha and beta receptors in the coronary circulation, and both vasoconstriction and vasodilation have been described following sympathetic stimulation in an arrested heart. Stimulation of cardiac sympathetic nerves via the stellate ganglion produces a rather marked dilatation of the coronary vessels primarily on a metabolic basis. Epinephrine has a direct effect on coronary smooth muscle, resulting in vasodilation. Much more important, however, are the indirect effects of epinephrine (increased aortic pressure and increased myocardial oxygen consumption) that further increase coronary blood flow (Fig. 3-35). Presumably, thyroxin also augments coronary blood flow due to an increase in metabolic rate and oxygen consumption of the heart muscle. Pitressin has a definite direct vasoconstrictor effect on the coronary circulation and diminished coronary flow.

In shock, the coronary vascular bed becomes markedly dilated when the aortic pressure falls. This vasodilation presumably is produced by the action of metabolites on precapillary arterioles. Vasodilator metabolites such as adenosine, histamine, potassium, bradykinin, carbon dioxide, and hydrogen ions have been postulated as responsible for this response. Braunwald has emphasized that autoregulation, which is present in normal coronary beds, is abolished by coronary shock because of the extreme metabolic vasodilatation. Ross has shown that under these circumstances, the coronary blood flow is almost entirely pressure dependent. Accordingly, impairment of coronary perfusion during severe hypotension may

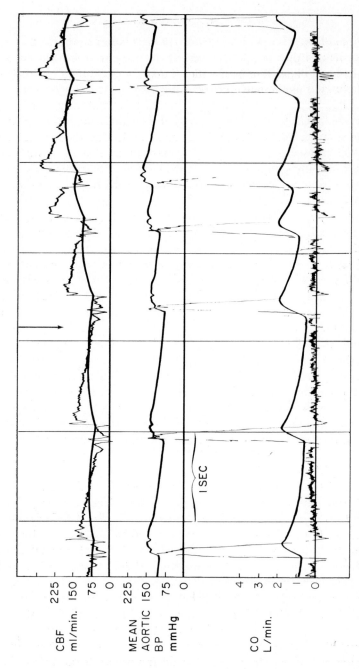

Fig. 3-35.—The effects of epinephrine on coronary blood flow in a conscious dog. 25 μg of epinephrine were administered (*arrow*) into the superior vena cava 8 seconds prior to any increase in the flow. Note that increases in coronary blood flow are associated with changes in mean aortic blood pressure and heart rate. (Courtesy of K. L. Goetz and A. S. Hermreck.)

perpetuate and further depress myocardial performance. An increase in aortic pressure is essential for adequate myocardial perfusion in cardiogenic shock, but unfortunately provides an unfavorable increase in the afterload of an already failing left ventricle. This passive perfusion is therefore markedly dependent on a critical perfusion pressure. The critical closing pressure in the coronary system is thought by Braunwald to range between 15 and 60 mm Hg. When the mean pressure begins to approach the critical closing pressure, the coronary vessels may collapse and perfusion cease.

Effect of Hypoxia on Cardiac Function

The profound effects of hypoxia and acidosis on myocardial performance are important in understanding the pathophysiology of the heart in shock. Acidosis itself may cause a significant depletion of myocardial norepinephrine stores and the deterioration of ventricular performance on this basis. Hoppel, working with the isolated perfused rat heart, found that below a critical extracellular pH of 7.1, there was a marked fall in cardiac rate and peak pressures due to decreased mechanical efficiency of the heart.

The importance of correcting the acidosis that is commonly associated with shock due to any cause is clear. In the same way, hypoxia, by limiting the aerobic metabolism of the myocardium, also interferes with cardiac performance and must be corrected. Lundsgard states that the primary cause of heart damage in shock is a deficient oxygen supply to the myocardium. One prime indicator of myocardial hypoxia is the level of the coronary sinus Po_2 and oxygen saturation. Normal coronary sinus oxygen content is approximately 5–7 vol%. The critical level of the coronary sinus Po_2 is 20 mm Hg and corresponds to a hemoglobin saturation of less than 20%. Po_2 below this level indicates that anaerobic metabolism is occurring and the heart is suffering from severe hypoxia.

Another indicator of hypoxic metabolism in the myocardium is the coronary sinus lactate. Normal coronary sinus lactate levels are approximately 1.0 mM per liter. With hypoxic metabolism, there is a marked increase in coronary sinus lactate. Bing, and others, utilize the fall in redoxpotential difference between the coronary vein and arterial blood to assess the degree of myocardial hypoxia. In severe myocardial hypoxia the redox potential, or the delta E_H, is always negative. The myocardial cells, damaged by anoxia, release enzymes detectable in the coronary sinus and peripheral blood. The enzymes include mallic dehydrogenase, various forms of transaminase, citric acid dehydrogenase, and creatine phosphokinase. Anoxia and failure of glucose extraction alter the permeability of the cell membrane, allowing leakage of myocardial enzymes. This may be the most subtle index of hypoxia and injury, but it does not always correlate with myocardial performance, in that focal damage may release extracellular enzymes such as serum glutamic oxalacetic transaminase (SGOT) without serious impairment of myocardial function as a whole.

PULMONARY FUNCTION IN CARDIOGENIC SHOCK

Abnormal pulmonary function is frequently observed in cardiogenic shock. This abnormal function results in a depressed Pao_2. MacKenzie and others have noted a Pao_2 in the range of 40–50 mm Hg in patients with cardiogenic shock which were not increased to normal tensions by administration of 100% oxygen. This arterial hypoxemia is due to shunting or venous admixture, and is probably due to atelectasis and to interstitial and alveolar edema. A positive feedback develops from myocardial failure and results in pulmonary edema and hypoxia which, in turn, further depresses myocardial metabolism and myocardial contractility.

ANIMAL MODELS

Experimental animal models for cardiogenic shock can be produced by surgical ligation of the coronary vessels or by embolization by plastic microspheres in coronary arteries of dogs. Binder has produced experimental coronary shock in the dog by the injection of plastic microspheres into the coronary arteries during temporary cardiac arrest. In these animals, as in patients with clinical cardiogenic shock, there was a prompt and dramatic fall in cardiac output and usually an accompanying rise in total peripheral resistance. In experimental myocardial infarction produced by Jennings in dogs, changes in the nucleoplasm and cytoplasm of cells occurred within 5 minutes after the surgical occlusion of a coronary vessel. Within 20 to 40 minutes after the onset of ischemia, myocardial cells ceased contracting and could not be restored by oxygenated blood. In 4 to 7 hours, the cell boundaries of ischemic myocardial cells were destroyed as the sarcolemma and endoplasmic reticulum disappeared. Accompanying these anatomic changes were specific metabolic changes. In the first 2 hours after experimental infarction, intracellular acidity increased, cellular glycogen disappeared, high-energy organic phosphates were lost, and potassium escaped from the cell. It is interesting that in humans the signs of severe failure of the left side of the heart may not develop immediately with the onset of myocardial infarction pain and a time delay of 2–6 hours may exist between the onset of the infarction and the development of shock. The metabolic and structural changes that have been observed in the experimental animal offer a logical explanation for this time delay.

Bing has produced coronary shock in animals and has demonstrated rather significant falls in blood pressure and cardiac output with a generalized increase in total peripheral resistance. In Bing's experiments, there was no change in the coronary vascular resistance following the onset of cardiogenic shock.

THERAPEUTIC CONSIDERATIONS

The problems in cardiogenic shock relate mainly to impaired contractility, but severe tachycardia or bradycardia may contribute to myocardial failure. Certain generalizations may be made about therapy. The object of cardiac support is to control the heart rate at a level which provides optimal filling, to improve myocardial contractility, and to provide the coronary vessels with blood having a high O_2 content at optimal aortic pressures.

Surgical, mechanical, and drug approaches have been used to augment ventricular contractility in cardiogenic shock. Years ago, Gordon Murray and Heimbecker suggested that emergency infarctectomy could be effective in saving lives of patients who develop coronary shock. They were able to demonstrate that in experimentally produced myocardial infarction in calves there was a striking improvement in both left ventricular function and survival following surgical removal of the infarcted area of myocardium. The electrical, biochemical, and mechanical advantages of infarctectomy increased the survival in calves from 0 to 47%.

Mechanical means of circulation support have also received considerable interest. One of these means is counterpulsation. By this technique, blood is let into a reservoir during arterial systole and is pumped back into the circulation during diastole. This method does not require a thoracotomy and does diminish the work load of the left ventricle. Total cardiopulmonary bypass has also been recommended. With the current imperfection in this technique, total bypass has only limited application. It can be maintained for only short periods, and it requires extensive operative intervention.

Hyperbaric oxygenation has also recently gained widespread attention. Theoretically, this technique has the advantage of reversing ischemia in areas of myocardium with marginal blood supply that have not yet become infarcted. Although the results in experimental animals and in limited patient experiences are encouraging, actual measurements show a fall in cardiac output and a rise in peripheral vascular resistance with hyperbaric oxygen. In addition, patients can remain in the hyperbaric chamber for only short periods without serious pulmonary and cerebral complications.

Another mechanical means of augmenting the cardiac output of the failing myocardium is the use of temporary transvenous pacing. Since the stroke volume of the failing myocardium is severely limited, a bradycardia will result in an even further reduction in total cardiac output. Pacing the heart within physiologic rates up to 100 per minute may provide a moderate augmentation of cardiac output by these means. Cohn has advocated use of the central venous pressure catheter as the means for allowing cautious volume expansion in certain patients in cardiogenic shock. By an application of the Starling principle, increased venous return to the heart should augment stroke volume and total cardiac output. Unfortunately, many patients in cardiogenic shock have already reached a plateau on the Starling curve, and further increases in filling pressure do not augment stroke volume. Recently, Nixon has reported a significant improvement in myocardial function in cardiogenic shock using 5% dextrose solution. He has been successful in improving cardiac output and survival even when the central venous pressure has become markedly elevated (25 cm of water).

A wide variety of vasoactive drugs have been advocated in the treatment of cardiogenic shock. Commonly used alpha adrenergic drugs include methoxamine and phenylephrine. Although these drugs are effective in increasing blood pressure by augmenting arterial resistance, the work load of the left ventricle is markedly increased and tissue perfusion may be reduced. It is generally felt that pure alpha adrenergic drugs do not prove beneficial in the treatment of shock due to myocardial infarction since they do not improve myocardial contractility and do increase the afterload. Angiotensin resembles the alpha adrenergic stimulating drugs in its actions.

Beta adrenergic stimulating drugs include isoproterenol and mephentermine. These drugs augment cardiac output and heart rate, but their effects on blood pressure are somewhat variable. Isoproterenol is usually administered by continuous intravenous perfusion at a dose rate of 3–10 μg per minute. Its most serious drawback has been the precipitation of ventricular arrhythmias. Commonly used drugs such as metaraminal and norepinephrine have combined alpha and beta adrenergic stimulating actions. In small doses these drugs may be predominantly beta adrenergic stimulants, but in large doses they become predominantly alpha stimulating and cause a marked increase in blood pressure due to peripheral vasoconstriction. Braunwald has suggested that these drugs are the ideal vasoactive drugs for use in cardiogenic shock since they augment cardiac output and raise systemic blood pressure and could, thereby, augment coronary blood flow. It has been recommended that they be used to maintain arterial blood pressure at a level 20–30 mm below the preshock level.

Alpha adrenergic blocking drugs such as phenoxybenzamine and phentolamine have had only limited clinical trials in patients with cardiogenic shock. When these drugs have been used, they have the ability to augment cardiac output despite a decrease in blood pressure. Increases in skin temperature and in urine flow have been attributed to improved tissue perfusion. Volume expansion is often required when these drugs are used, or serious volume deficits may result. Beta adrenergic blocking drugs, such as propranolol, are useful in alleviating cardiac arrhythmias, but they may have an adverse effect in cardiogenic shock. The fall in cardiac output with even further increases in total peripheral resistance is undesirable and should be avoided in most circumstances, except when rate control is a dominant concern. Since left heart failure is invariably present in patients with cardiogenic shock, the ideal drug is one which improves the efficiency and contractile strength of the myocardium. This drug is most closely approximated by digitalis. Patients in cardiogenic shock should be given digitalis, using a rapid-acting intravenous preparation. This is frequently beneficial in augmenting cardiac output and in improving blood pressure and peripheral perfusion.

The clinician must make evaluations of myocardial function based on physical signs and available physiologic data. Gallop rhythm, poor quality heart tones, and moist rales generally indicate poor left ventricular function. The most readily available physiologic data to evaluate myocardial function are based on the Starling principle and allow stroke volume to be plotted against filling pressure. Details of treatment are given in Chapter 7.

Liver

Since the liver is the major site for conversion of lactate to pyruvate, the accumulation of lactate in shock patients suggests a severe degree of impairment of liver blood flow. This is supported by the work of Schimassek, who found lactate accumulation in isolated perfused rat livers at a flow of 0.6 ml per minute per gram through the portal vein. Drappanas, using the calf liver, reported lactate accumulation with flows less than 0.79 ml per minute per gram. Ballinger found cessation of lactate metabolism at arterial pressures of 40 mm Hg. It seems clear that low flow and portal venous desaturation concomitantly impair the ability of the liver to handle the excess lactate load developing in shock. Studies of liver ultrastructure by Hift and Strawitz (1961) revealed that the mitochondria were enlarged and swollen and that this change involved the intramitochondrial matrix with a "loosening" of the internal structure.

Central Nervous System Failure in Shock

Many classifications of shock include the term *neurogenic shock,* or vasovagal collapse. This is usually associated with emotion, pain, or the bleeding of blood donors. Clinical features are restlessness, pallor, a feeling of warmth, loss of consciousness, a fall in pulse rate and blood pressure, and warm, moist skin. This sequence is often considered to be due to a loss of peripheral arteriolar resistance resulting from reflex dilatation in areas of skeletal muscle. The pooling of blood in peripheral vascular beds with loss of vascular tone results in inadequate venous return, a fall in cardiac output, and subsequent reduction in arterial blood pressure. Since marked improvement usually occurs with a minimum of treatment, there is little quantitative data to substantiate this sequence of hemodynamic events.

The earliest clinical sign of cerebral hypoxia in the shock patient is restlessness. The cause for this may not be readily apparent in that arterial Po_2 may be within normal range and even the blood pressure may be within low normal levels. As the arterial blood pressure falls, restlessness gives way to apathy, stupor and, finally, coma.

The study of patients with trauma to the central nervous system has provided useful information for evaluating clinical shock problems. The patient with closed head injury does not usually demonstrate hypotension, tachycardia, decreased urinary output, and other signs of hypovolemic shock. The appearance of clinical shock in the patient with head injury emphasizes the need for detailed search for blood loss or trauma in the chest, abdomen, or extremities. An often unrecognized but important complication in stuporous patients is vomiting with aspiration injury to the lung, leading to severe hypoxemia. The presence of a closed head injury with diffuse cerebral damage is not a contraindication to performing emergency surgical procedures elsewhere in the body. Special attention should be paid to the amount of blood loss, since a significant number of these patients may show a normal blood pressure but are already hypovolemic and vasoconstricted from associated injury. One investigator has estimated that the most common cause of death during the course of intracranial surgery for trauma is sudden blood loss from cranial vessels in a patient who is already hypovolemic, followed by shock, diffuse hypoxia, and cardiac arrest.

The frequency of hyperventilation in shock has already been referred to, and the resulting respiratory alkalosis may have potential significance in the shock patient since cerebral blood flow decreases in a linear fashion with a decrease in arterial CO_2 tension. When the arterial Pco_2 is reduced to 20 mm Hg, the cerebral blood flow is approximately half or 20–30 ml per minute per 100 gm of brain tissue. The significance of these changes for the function of nervous tissue is poorly understood, but several observations are of interest. When the P_{CO_2} is reduced to half normal by hyperventilation, abnormal changes are observed in the electroencephalographic tracings of conscious subjects. Respiratory alkalosis of this degree in anesthetized man is followed by the appearance of anaerobic glucose utilization in the brain. The marked decrease in cerebral blood flow under these conditions may be an important factor in the shift toward anaerobic cerebral metabolism. In addition, respiratory alkalosis results in a movement of the oxygen dissociation curve to the left, thus impairing the release of oxygen from hemoglobin.

The Adrenal Gland and Adrenergic Agents

The central position of the adrenal gland in the reaction to injury warrants an outline of its normal function as well as its role in shock.

GLUCOCORTICOIDS

Glucocorticoid production by the adrenal gland is directly under the influence of the adrenocorticotrophic hormone (ACTH) from the anterior pituitary gland. Lack of ACTH due to pituitary dysfunction or inhibition of release of ACTH by administration of 11-hydroxylated glucocorticoids rapidly results in atrophy of the zona fasciculata cells of the adrenal. In contrast, increased endogenous ACTH release secondary to stress or administration of exogenous ACTH causes adrenal hypertrophy and increased glucocorticoid production.

Glucocorticoid preparations have profound and well-known metabolic effects. In physiologic concentrations these substances stabilize carbohydrate metabolism by their gluconeogenic effects. In addition, they dampen the effects of insulin on tissues. In pharmacologic doses they alter fat and protein metabolism. It is common to see iatrogenic Cushing's disease with prolonged administration of these agents. The mechanisms whereby the glucocorticoids mediate some of their metabolic effects is still unclear. Recent evidence suggests that they may act, like many other hormones, by way of cyclic adenosinemonophosphate (AMP), which has been shown to influence enzyme activity in numerous tissues (Fig. 3-36).

Less-well understood are the circulatory and metabolic effects of glucocorticoids under stress and shock states. Actual acute pathologic changes in the adrenal gland in shock are rare except for the adrenal necrosis in meningococcemia sepsis (Waterhouse-Friedrichsen syndrome). Bolstered by the knowledge that the adrenalectomized animal tolerated minor injury poorly, a parallel was sought in human shock, and for years various

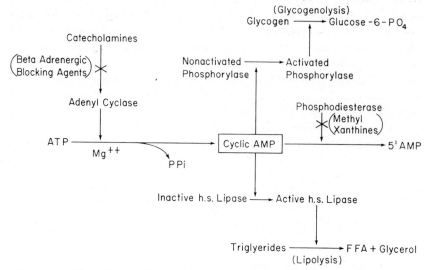

Fig. 3–36.—The influence of catecholamines on the formation of cyclic AMP and some of the important influences of this substance on glycogenolysis and lipolysis.

natural and synthetic adrenal steroids have been used in treatment. Nevertheless, measurements of adrenal cortical function in shock have consistently failed to show impaired function. Quantitative evidence for the participation of the adrenal glands in shock has been presented by numerous investigators. Studies in animals and humans with hemorrhagic shock have demonstrated increased glucocorticoid production with hemorrhagic hypotension; this response could be reversed by replacement of blood volume. Studies by other investigators on endotoxin shock in animals and on septic states in humans have shown that output by the adrenal cortex remained elevated until immediately before death. Several studies suggest that as long as the blood supply is adequate to the adrenal gland under these stressful conditions, the response to corticotropin is comparable to that seen in healthy subjects.

Despite the demonstration of adequate adrenal function in shock, there is considerable evidence in experimental hemorrhagic and endotoxin shock models that pretreatment with glucocorticoids increases survival rates. It should be pointed out, however, that pretreatment with a number of unrelated substances such as epinephrine, endotoxin, and dibenzyline offer similar protection, but the basis for this remains only speculative.

In physiologic amounts, glucocorticoids keep vascular smooth muscle in a reactive or responsive state to catecholamines. Also, it is well known now that glucocorticoids are necessary to induce the enzyme, phenylethanalamine-N-methyl transferase, which is necessary to convert norepinephrine to epinephrine in the adrenal medulla. Steroids given in larger doses have been reported to function as vasodilators, but there is considerable inherent variability in this type of response. Other studies suggest that corticoids increase myocardial contractility in physiologic doses and depress the mechanical ability of the heart in high concentrations.

Recent work by Shumer has revealed that glucocorticoids given in pharmacologic doses to monkeys in hemorrhagic shock decreased the amount of lactate production. Monkeys treated with steroids consistently had higher arterial pH, Pco_2, HCO_3^-, and survival rates. Whether this action is due to improved circulation or direct metabolic effects is unclear.

The powerful anti-inflammatory properties of steroids may also explain some of their postulated beneficial effects in low-flow states. It is well established clinically and experimentally that glucocorticoids help to maintain the integrity of the blood brain barrier and reduce cerebral swelling in cerebral trauma and also decrease capillary permeability in many inflammatory conditions. Janoff et al. have demonstrated that steroids stabilize the lysosomal membranes in cells during shock periods. Lysosomes contain numerous lytic enzymes which, if released, have a deleterious effect on cellular enzyme function. While any real value of these agents in the management of clinical shock remains to be established, hazards such as liability of spread of infection and potentiation of stress ulceration of the stomach are well recognized.

MINERALOCORTICOIDS

The outer layer of the adrenal cortex (zona glomerulosa) is the site of production of the powerful salt-retaining hormone, aldosterone. This steroid directly affects the ability of the renal tubular cells to reabsorb sodium and secrete potassium. It mediates these effects on the tubular cells most likely by enhancing production of ribonucleic acid (RNA) which, in turn, increases the amount of substrate available for active reabsorption of sodium.

The mechanisms for the regulation of aldosterone production, in contrast to glucocorticoid production, have proved to be quite complex. Aldosterone secretion increases with acute hemorrhage, low salt, or high potassium intake, and in many other situations. Although ACTH does play a role in maintaining the integrity of the glomerulosa cells to produce maximal amounts of aldosterone, experimental work has made it clear that other factors are far more important. Early work suggested that after hypophysectomy in experimental animals, the zona glomerulosa cells of the adrenal gland were maintained and even increased in size upon salt restriction. Animals undergoing hypophysectomy did not die from salt loss as did animals with adrenalectomy. The eventual conclusion that aldosterone regulation was associated with the renin-angiotensin system stemmed from work accomplished in several laboratories. It is now clear that the zona glomerulosa cells of the adrenal gland secrete aldosterone predominantly in response to the powerful octapeptide (angiotensin II). Angiotensin I, a decapeptide, is formed from the alpha$_2$-globulin fraction of plasma by the proteolytic enzyme renin. Inactive angiotensin I is converted into active angiotensin II by a converting enzyme located predominantly in the lung. The factors responsible for renin release by the juxtaglomerular cells of the kidney are illustrated in Figure 3-37.

Aldosterone levels are raised in shock during the postoperative period and in many other conditions and cause retention of sodium and water. Altered aldosterone secretion by the adrenal gland, whether increased or decreased, has not been shown to jeopardize the patient in shock.

CATECHOLAMINES

The medullary portion of the adrenal gland is a part of the autonomic nervous system. Made up of chromaffin cells with catecholamine-containing droplets, the adrenal medulla responds to preganglionic stimuli by predominantly releasing epinephrine, and to a lesser degree, norepinephrine. These amines, as well as numerous synthetic adrenergic agents that are used in the support of the shock patient, have extremely important metabolic and circulatory effects.

Fig. 3–37.—Possible mechanisms for the release of renin. (From Vander, A. J.: Control of renin release, Physiol. Rev. 47:359, 1967.)

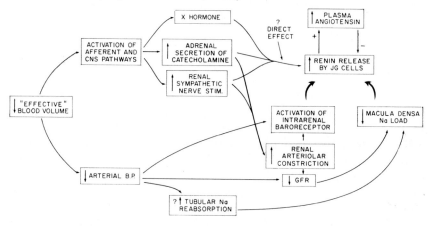

CLASSIFICATION OF ADRENERGIC AGENTS

Ahlquist in 1948 devised a classification for adrenergic agents based upon hypothetical receptors stimulated in target organs. Observing that closely related sympathomimetic amines had differing potencies on various functions, e.g., vasoconstriction, stimulation of the heart, and pupillary constriction, Ahlquist developed the concept of specific alpha and beta receptors to account for the different patterns of pressor amine activity. Adrenergic agents such as norepinephrine, epinephrine, isoproterenol, and methoxamine are classified as either alpha or beta adrenergic stimulating agents. Many adrenergic drugs such as norepinephrine and epinephrine have both alpha and beta stimulating properties; whereas drugs like isoproterenol and methoxamine are pure beta and alpha adrenergic receptor stimulating agents respectively. This classification has considerable practical value when the types of receptors that populate different effector organs and the response elicited upon stimulation of these receptors are known. The action of most of these drugs then becomes predictable. Table 3-6 is a listing of the various effector organs, the receptors that populate these organs, and the response with stimulation.

Additional evidence supporting Ahlquist's alpha and beta receptor theory has evolved with the development of highly specific adrenergic receptor blocking agents that produce a differential blockade on either alpha or beta receptors. The beta adrenergic receptor blocking agent propranolol and the alpha adrenergic receptor blocking drug phenoxybenzamine are commonly used to reduce the effects of increased sympathetic activity on various components of the cardiovascular system.

CARDIOVASCULAR EFFECTS

According to the classification devised by Ahlquist, adrenergic drugs may be termed alpha or beta receptor stimulants or alpha or beta receptor blocking agents, depending on the receptor stimulated or blocked. Methoxamine represents a prototype of the alpha adrenergic receptor stimulating drugs. As shown in Table 3-6, the peripheral vascular tree (veins and arteries) is conceived to be richly populated with, and the heart devoid of, alpha adrenergic receptors. Consequently, this drug causes intense peripheral vasoconstriction with a marked rise in arterial blood pressure and reflex slowing of the heart. Venous tone and central venous pressure are increased. Despite the increase in central venous pressure, cardiac output decreases, most likely due to the reflex vagal bradycardia and increased vascular resistance against which the heart must work. Blood flow

TABLE 3-6.—RESPONSES OF EFFECTOR ORGANS TO ADRENERGIC STIMULI

EFFECTOR ORGAN	RECEPTOR TYPE	RESPONSE
Heart		
Sinoatrial node	Beta	Increase in heart rate
Atrioventricular node and conduction system	Beta	Increase in conduction velocity and shortening of functional refractory period
Atria	Beta	Increase in contractility and conduction velocity
Ventricles	Beta	Increase in contractility, conduction velocity, automaticity and rate of idiopathic pacemaker
Arteries		
Coronary	Alpha & Beta	Constriction; dilation
Skin and mucosa	Alpha	Constriction
Skeletal muscle	Alpha & Beta	Constriction; dilation
Cerebral	Alpha	Constriction (minimal)
Pulmonary	Alpha & Beta	Constriction; dilation
Abdominal viscera	Alpha & Beta	Constriction; dilation
Veins		
Systemic veins	Alpha & Beta	Constriction
Lungs		
Bronchial muscle	Beta	Relaxation
Gastrointestinal Tract		
Motility		
Stomach	Beta	Increase
Intestine	Alpha & Beta	Decrease
Sphincters		
Stomach	Alpha	Contraction
Intestine	Alpha	Contraction
Urinary Bladder		
Detrusor	Beta	Relaxation
Trigone & sphincter	Alpha	Contraction
Eye		
Radial muscle; iris	Alpha	Contraction (mydriasis)
Ciliary muscle	Beta	Relaxation (negative accommodation)
Skin		
Pilomotor muscles	Alpha	Contraction
Sweat glands	Alpha	Sweating of palms of hands & plantar surfaces of feet

(From Koelle, G. B.: Drugs Acting at Synaptic and Neuroeffector Junctional Sites, in Goodman, L. S., and Gillman, A. [eds.]: *The Pharmacological Basis of Therapeutics* [3d ed.]. [New York: The Macmillan Company, 1965], Chap. 21.)

to most organs is decreased due to the intense vasoconstriction and decreased cardiac output.

Isoproterenol at the opposite pole of the adrenergic receptor stimulating drugs is a prototype of the pure beta adrenergic receptor stimulating drugs. All components of the cardiovascular system are subserved by the beta adrenergic receptors (Table 3-6). The response seen with a beta adrenergic stimulating agent is almost directly opposite to that seen with an alpha stimulating agent. Peripheral vasodilation occurs with a slight increase in systolic blood pressure but a decrease in diastolic pressure. Venous tone is enhanced and blood is shifted centrally. Central venous pressure decreases, however, due to the positive inotropic and chronotropic effects of isoproterenol on the heart. Blood flow is augmented to most organs as a result of the increased cardiac output and decreased peripheral vascular resistance. Unfortunately, only a few adrenergic drugs can be classified neatly as pure alpha or beta adrenergic receptor stimulating agents. Most of these agents, such as norepinephrine and epinephrine, have varying degrees of alpha and beta activity and will be considered individually in the therapy section.

METABOLIC EFFECTS

Recent studies have begun to elucidate the important metabolic effects of the catecholamines. These metabolic effects cannot be classified as clearly as the hemodynamic effects on the basis of alpha or beta receptors. Elevation of blood glucose and lactate, and a decrease in the glycogen content of the liver and skeletal muscle, are well-known effects of catecholamines, but the control of vital metabolic processes exercised by catecholamines has only recently been subjected to a unitarian hypothesis. The common process underlying the various actions of catecholamines is apparently an acceleration of the synthesis of cyclic (3′, 5′) AMP, the formation of which is catalyzed by adenyl cyclase, an enzyme affected by catecholamines (see Fig. 3-36). In muscle, cyclic AMP converts nonactivated phosphorylase to activated phosphorylase, which in turn brings about the breakdown of glycogen to yield glucose 6-phosphate. Since muscle lacks glucose 6-phosphatase, glucose 6-phosphate is metabolized to lactic acid, causing an increase in blood lactate levels. In the liver, however, glucose 6-phosphatase is present and converts glucose 6-phosphate to glucose, thereby raising blood glucose.

Catecholamines also raise the blood concentration of free fatty acids by activation of a specific hormone-sensitive lipase in adipose tissue which converts triglycerides to glycerol and free fatty acids. This may be accomplished by the activation of the same cyclic AMP system which is involved in glycogenolysis. It has been demonstrated that epinephrine increases the activity of adenyl cyclase as well as levels of cyclic AMP in adipose tissue and that cyclic AMP has the same lipolytic effects as catecholamines. Catecholamines have many other less clear metabolic effects that are most likely mediated via cyclic AMP. It should be pointed out that most adrenergic receptor stimulating agents increase caloric expenditure from 15 to 20 percent.

Evidence is also accumulating which suggests that cyclic AMP may be involved in the inotropic response of the heart. In addition, many other hormones besides catecholamines are thought to mediate their effects on target organs by controlling the rate of vital enzyme reactions through cyclic AMP. On experimental grounds, the hypothetical beta receptor is thought to be the enzyme adenyl cyclase.

Kidney

The fall in urine output in most shock states is often taken as an index of tissue perfusion. Initial changes in urine output in shock more accurately reflect the degree of peripheral sympathetic activity and other factors responsible for the maintenance of extracellular fluid volume. If the shock state continues unabated, alterations in renal function will most likely represent severe chemical and structural damage to the renal parenchyma. Most of the changes in renal function observed in shock can now be explained at least partly in physiologic terms.

Functional Anatomy

The functional units of the kidney are the nephrons along with their surrounding vasculature (Fig. 3-38). Approximately 1.5 million nephrons of various lengths exist in each kidney. The proximal portion of the nephron is made up of a capillary tuft (glomerulus) separated from the nephron lumen only by the capillary endothelial cells, the glomerular membrane, and the surrounding epithelial cells (Fig. 3-39). This membrane functions as if pores are present, ranging in size from 80 to 100 Å in diameter and occupying about 5% of the total functional membrane area. These glomerular membranes act as a filter and are readily permeable to substances with molecular weights below 5,000. Substances with molecular weights up to that of hemoglobin (68,000) or serum albumin (40,000) permeate less readily. Essentially an ultrafiltrate of plasma, free only of plasma proteins, is formed upon passing through these membranes and begins its voyage down the nephron where, ultimately, after various processes such as active reabsorption and secretion of solutes, and passive reabsorption of solvent and solutes, it becomes urine. Various regions of the nephron, characterized anatomically, have unique functions in that specialized processes occur in these areas and humoral agents exert pro-

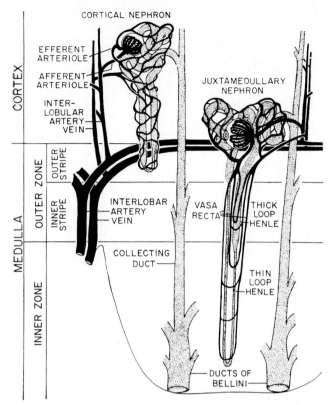

Fig. 3–38.—The blood supply and loops of Henle in the cortical and juxtamedullary regions of the kidney. (From Pitts, R. F.: *Physiology of the Kidney and Body Fluids* [2nd ed.; Chicago: Year Book Medical Publishers, 1968, p. 19]. Reproduced by permission.)

found specific effects on the capacity of the tubular cells to carry out specialized functions (Figs. 3-40 and 3-41).

FILTRATION RATE

The kidneys under normal conditions receive about 20–25% of the total cardiac output. This amounts to about 1,000–1,500 ml of renal blood flow during a 1 minute period. Only about 18–20% of the renal plasma flow (120 ml per minute) is filtered by the glomeruli. During a 24 hour period, approximately 50 gallons of plasma is filtered or the entire circulating plasma is processed fourteen times. Only about 1% of the total filtrate is eventually excreted as urine in the normal individual.

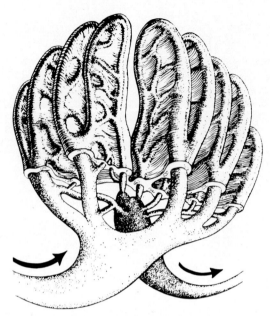

Fig. 3–39.—Anatomy of the glomerulus demonstrating the afferent and efferent arterioles, capillary lobules with the enveloping glomerular basement membrane. (From Pitts, R. F.: *Physiology of the Kidney and Body Fluids* [2nd ed.; Chicago: Year Book Medical Publishers, 1968, p. 16]. Reproduced by permission.)

The primary factor determining glomerular filtration rate (GFR) is filtration pressure. A minimal filtration pressure of about 45–50 mm Hg is required to overcome the colloid osmotic pressure of plasma (35 mm Hg) and the tubular hydrostatic pressure (10–15 mm Hg) to form an ultrafiltrate of plasma. The afferent arterioles of the glomeruli play a major role in determining filtration pressure. With high perfusion pressures, such as in hypertension and catecholamine administration, afferent arteriolar constriction reduces the effective filtration pressure and, conversely, with lower perfusion pressures, afferent arteriolar dilation may enhance filtration pressure. Similarly, efferent arteriolar dilation and constriction can also decrease and enhance filtration pressure.

URINE OUTPUT

Urine output is regulated by the processes responsible for the maintenance of extracellular fluid volume. In general, since the sodium ion is responsible for maintaining extracellular volume, it assumes a primary role

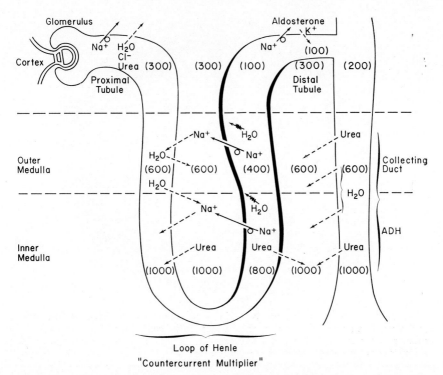

Fig. 3–40.—Summary of passive and active exchange of water and solute in the nephron and the sites of action of ADH and aldosterone. Note that the ascending loop of Henle is relatively impermeable to H_2O, allowing the formation of a hyperosmolar zone in the medullar region of the kidney. Concentrations of tubular urine and peritubular fluid in milliosmoles per liter, solid lines indicate active reabsorption and dashed lines, passive exchange of water and solute.

in the ability of the kidneys to maintain fluid volume control and, therefore, urine output. In shock and other unfavorable states such as severe water deprivation, urine output is reduced to a minimum in an attempt to maintain extracellular fluid volume even at the expense of other important renal functions.

Perfusion pressure and, therefore, glomerular filtration rate, along with the influence of the humoral agents, antidiuretic hormone, aldosterone, and changes in the ability of the tubular cells to reabsorb solutes such as sodium or glucose are the main determinants of urine production in the normal individual. A low glomerular filtration rate, along with high levels of ADH and aldosterone, results in very little urine formation. In contrast, a high filtration rate, the lack of ADH (diabetes insipidus), a reduction in the reabsorption of sodium or glucose, or the presence of mannitol will

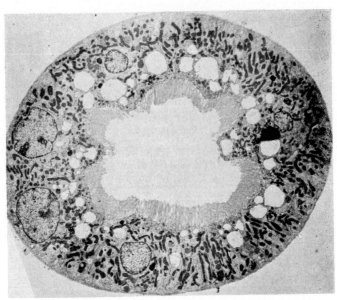

Fig. 3–41.—Low magnification (× 1300) electron micrograph of the proximal tubule in the rat. The numerous dense spherical bodies in the cell represent mitochondria. The tubular lumen is lined with brush border which greatly increases the absorptive area. (Courtesy of Dr. Jared Grantham.)

result in diuresis. Therefore urine output is not necessarily a reliable index of renal blood flow.

Renal Blood Flow

At rest, kidney vascular resistance is not substantially influenced by the sympathetic nervous system; therefore, denervations of this organ cause very little alteration in blood flow or function. This organ, like other organs, has considerable inherent ability to autoregulate blood flow, most likely by an intrinsic myogenic mechanism.

By contrast, when sympathetic activity is great, such as in exercise and stress, renal blood flow is decreased considerably. In early hemorrhagic shock, renal blood flow falls in proportion to perfusion pressure and vascular resistance remains at control levels or even lower. With prolonged shock, however, renal blood flow is reduced and vascular resistance increased far more on a percentage basis than is blood flow to other organs. In normal persons, upon administration of sublethal amounts of bacterial pyrogen, dramatic renal hyperemia occurs after a latent period of 40–80 minutes; this response may occur in septic patients with high cardiac output, low vascular resistance, and normovolemic shock. However, oliguria may be present in septic patients due to low-perfusion pressures or even renal damage. Also, if peripheral sympathetic activity is great, this renal hyperemia response may be overridden by the powerful vasoconstricting effects of norepinephrine. It would therefore appear that in shock and stressful conditions the sympathetic nervous system exerts a dominant role in the reduction of renal blood flow, a response that can be blocked with the powerful alpha adrenergic receptor blocking agent phenoxybenzamine.

Many agents commonly used in the treatment of shock profoundly alter renal blood flow. Norepinephrine, methoxamine, and epinephrine cause severe vasoconstriction of the kidney, whereas bradykinin, isoproterenol, histamine, and acetylcholine cause vasodilation. Of interest is the recent finding that dopamine, after alpha adrenergic receptor blockage of the kidney with phenoxybenzamine, will cause vasodilation. This response cannot be blocked with the beta adrenergic receptor blocking drug propranolol. Consequently, the recent hypothesis suggests that dopamine receptors present in the kidney can be manipulated or blocked with haloperidol and chlorpromazine.

Antidiuretic hormone has long been held suspect in altering the distribution of renal blood flow. Some feel that lack of ADH, in addition to decreasing water reabsorption in the collecting duct, can alter the distribution of renal blood and affect the ability of the kidneys to handle sodium and water.

Various ions, for example sodium, in the range of 160 mEq per liter induce striking vasodilation of renal vasculature. The mechanism for this is not entirely understood at present. It should also be noted that serum potassium concentrations ranging from 5 to 10 mEq per liter elicit the same response, whereas potassium concentrations below 3 mEq per liter cause vasoconstriction.

In essence, renal blood flow, like blood flow to other organs, can be altered by a multitude of agents. In shock states, when hypovolemia frequently exist in the presence of increased sympathetic activity and high concentrations of catecholamines, renal blood flow is severely curtailed and is most likely an important factor contributing to the anuric state so frequently observed.

DISTRIBUTION OF RENAL BLOOD FLOW

The distribution of renal blood flow is of considerable importance in determining water and salt excretion by the kidney. Normally, about nine-tenths of the total renal blood flow is distributed to the cortical portions of the kidney and the remainder to the medullary area. With a moderate increase in sympathetic activity, renal blood flow is shifted away from the outer cortex, where short nephrons predominate to the inner cortex populated mainly by long nephrons (Fig. 3-38). Sodium and water conservation results. If one administers the alpha adrenergic receptor blocking agent phenoxybenzamine under these conditions, blood flow is redistributed to the outer cortical region of the kidney. Increased salt and water excretion occurs. This redistribution of renal blood flow with altered sympathetic activity may play an important role in fluid volume control.

Studies on the distribution of renal blood flow under conditions of shock and hypovolemia, when intense sympathetic activity is present, are controversial. Early workers, using qualitative methods, felt that selective cortical ischemia occurred with a shifting of blood flow to the medulla in shock states. Pathologists have also frequently observed the paleness of the renal cortex and the plethoric appearance of the medulla in shock states. These observations have led to the hypothesis that shunting of renal blood flow away from the glomeruli in the cortex to the medullary region occurs in shock. Numerous workers using more quantitative methodology have not been able to substantiate the presence of such shunts or altered distribution of renal blood flow in shock.

Oxygen Requirements of the Kidney

Unlike many other organs, the kidney performs no immediately critical metabolic or mechanical function. It functions to maintain fluid, osmolar, and acid-base balance and to rid the body of waste products. It is not surprising therefore that these organs receive far more blood than is required to meet the local metabolic requirements. Of considerable interest is the observation that as renal blood flow decreases and glomerular filtration falls, so does renal oxygen consumption, since less-active reabsorption of sodium occurs. Renal vein blood remains between 80 and 90% saturated with oxygen at blood flows ranging from 50 to 75% below normal to 50% above normal. This does not mean that all areas of the kidney are equally supplied with oxygen. In contrast there is good evidence that the tissue oxygen tension of the medullary region is about 40% less than cortical oxygen tensions. Some investigators feel that the ability of the loop of Henle to reabsorb sodium is dependent upon the availability of oxygen.

Water Excretion

About 1 to 1.5 liters of urine is formed daily in a normal individual. This urine usually contains about 5 to 15 gm of urea, 20 to 40 mEq per liter each, of sodium, potassium, and chloride. Hydrogen ions and the anions bicarbonate, phosphate, and sulfate are excreted in varying concentrations, depending on the diet and acid-base status of the patient. Water excretion by the kidney is dependent upon fluid intake, the influence of ADH on the collecting duct cells, glomerular filtration rate, and the amount of unreabsorbed solutes such as sodium. At least 400 ml per day of water excretion is necessary in normally functioning kidneys to rid the body of urea and other waste materials.

SODIUM EXCRETION

Sodium excretion is dependent upon glomerular filtration rate, effects of aldosterone on the distal nephron, and the ability of tubular cells to actively reabsorb this ion in the proximal tubule, ascending loop of Henle, and distal nephron (see Fig. 3-38). Renal physiologists in the past 10 years have been working intently on the control of sodium reabsorption by the proximal tubule (see Fig. 3-39). A unique phenomenon, known as glomerular-tubular balance (G-T balance), occurs in this region of the kidney. In the nonhydropenic individual, about 65% of the filtered sodium is actively reabsorbed in the proximal tubule despite wide variations in the glomerular filtration rate. This phenomenon is of considerable importance, since the major portion of sodium reabsorption occurs in this region. Of interest to the physician caring for the critically ill patient is that G-T balance is upset with administration of saline and other sodium-containing solutions. Proximal tubular reabsorption of the filtered sodium is reduced considerably with saline administration, leading to saline diuresis. The nonreabsorbed sodium in the tubular lumen sets up the conditions for diuresis. Many of the modern diuretics exert their effects in the proximal tubule by depressing active sodium reabsorption.

Considerable investigation has been carried out to elucidate the basis for G-T balance (ability to reabsorb sodium in the proximal tubule). Several investigators have postulated the presence of a "natriuretic hormone" which is released after extracellular volume expansion with saline-containing fluids which selectively blocks the ability of the proximal tubules to reabsorb sodium. More recently, Earley and associates have presented convincing evidence that impaired proximal tubular sodium reabsorption, after expansion of the extracellular space with sodium-containing fluids, is primarily due to alterations in Starling's forces (tissue colloid osmotic pressure and capillary hydrostatic pressures in the peritubular capillaries, and renal parenchyma in the proximal tubular region).

Other mechanisms, besides the effects of the renin-angiotensin-aldosterone system, are equally important in the ability of the kidneys to maintain sodium balance. Recently, Goetz and Hermreck have shown that considerable changes in renal sodium and water excretion occur with selective tamponade of the atrium. Low-pressure stretch receptors are present in the atrium, and changes in the activity of these receptors result in dramatic changes in salt and water excretion by the kidney (Fig. 3-42). This mechanism may explain why renal sodium and water excretion is altered in conditions in which blood volume is decreased due to mild hemorrhage or increased with administration of iso-osmotic, iso-oncotic fluids.

Fig. 3–42.—The effects of altering atrial transmural pressure by selective atrial tamponade on urine flow and sodium excretion in a stable hydrated conscious dog. Note that changes in atrial transmural pressure are not accompanied by any measurable changes in other circulatory variables. (From Goetz, K. L., *et al.*: Contribution of atrial receptors to diuresis following plasma expansion in conscious dogs, Fed. Proc. 28:584, 1969.)

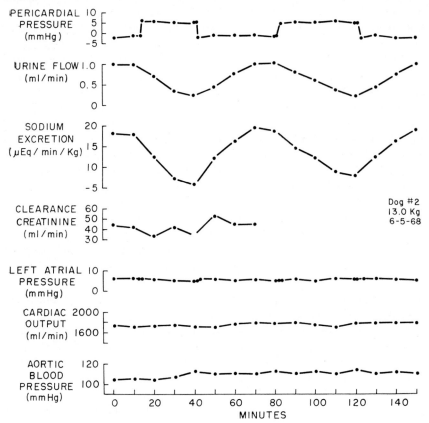

POTASSIUM EXCRETION

An almost obligatory amount of potassium of approximately 40 mEq per day is lost in the urine in a fasting individual and must be continually replaced to prevent hypokalemic alkalosis, adynamic ileus, muscular weakness, and cardiac arrhythmias when the heart is under the influence of digitalis. The major portion of filtered potassium is thought to be reabsorbed. Most of the potassium excreted in the urine is secreted by the distal tubule. Aldosterone potentiates this secretion, and one frequently sees hypokalemic alkalosis in primary aldosteronism (Conn's syndrome). The diuretic, spironolactone, blocks the potassium-secreting effects of aldosterone.

An association between hydrogen and potassium ion excretion in the distal tubule has been noted for some time. Berliner proposed that hydrogen and potassium ions compete for a single secretory pump in distal tubular cells. This concept is no longer tenable since recent observations suggest that the transtubular potential difference of the distal tubule, and the tubular cell concentration of potassium, are the main factors in determining potassium secretion. A large potential difference in the distal tubule (-70 to -90 millivolts) created by the active reabsorption of sodium out of the distal tubule and poorly reabsorbed anions (HCO_3^-, PO_4^-, SO_4^-) left behind leads to enhanced potassium secretion. Secretion of hydrogen ions by the distal tubule may curtail potassium secretion by reducing the potential difference of the distal tubule, hence the relationship between potassium and hydrogen ion secretion. The other explanation to account for the association between hydrogen and potassium ion excretion in distal tubular cells stems from the work of Fenn et al., Brown et al., and others. This work indicates that, with alkalosis, potassium is taken up by cells and hydrogen ions are released. Theoretically this would result in a lowering of intracellular hydrogen ion concentration and an increase in intracellular potassium concentration. High intracellular concentrations of potassium would favor its secretion from tubular cells into urine, due to the chemical gradient. Acidosis would have just the opposite effect. Although neither of the mechanisms has been proved to exist in the clinical situation, there is considerable experimental evidence to suggest that they may be important.

Hypokalemic alkalosis with hypochloremia cannot be corrected readily with non-chloride-containing potassium salts ($KHCO_3$, KNO_3, etc.) since these anions are poorly reabsorbed, leading to a continued high tubular potential difference and a high potassium secretion. Correction of this disorder requires the administration of chloride, preferably KCl, which is highly diffusible in the distal tubule. The movement of chloride out of the tubule tends to reduce the potential difference and maintain it at a low level. This depresses potassium secretion and aids in the correction of the disorder.

Numerous diuretic agents directly or indirectly affect potassium excretion by the kidney. Spironolactone, as previously mentioned, blocks the potassium-secreting effects of aldosterone and decreases potassium excretion. Triamterene, a rather weak diuretic, depresses potassium secretion and, therefore, is free of the side effect of increased urinary potassium loss. Carbonic anhydrase inhibitors lead to excessive potassium loss by decreasing hydrogen secretion into the urine, elevating the potential difference of the distal tubule, and augmenting potassium secretion. Other diuretics, such as the thiazides and ethacrynic acid, which inhibit sodium reabsorption in the proximal portions of the nephron, enhance potassium loss.

Acid-Base Balance

Immediate changes in acid-base disturbances are compensated for by changes in respiration and the action of the blood and tissue buffers. The kidney's ability to compensate for respiratory acid-base changes becomes evident several hours after the disturbance.

The rate of H^+ secretion by the kidney is the primary process by which this organ can alter the acid-base status of the patient. Bicarbonate excretion or reabsorption is entirely dependent upon the rate of hydrogen ion secretion by the kidney. Figure 3-43 shows the relationship between hydrogen ion secretion and HCO_3^- reabsorption. When H^+ is secreted into the tubular lumen of the nephron where filtered HCO_3^- is present, the following reaction takes place:

$$H^+ + HCO_3^- \overset{\text{C.A.}}{\rightleftharpoons} H_2O + CO_2$$

Carbonic acid is formed, but is readily converted to water, and CO_2 from the action of carbonic anhydrase (CA), which is thought to be attached to the tubular cell membranes. Carbon dioxide rapidly diffuses into the tubular cell where it is rehydrated under the influence of cellular carbonic anhydrase to H_2CO_3. Ionization of this acid occurs, and the HCO_3^- is returned to the plasma. The net result of this whole process is one HCO_3^- removed from the urine and returned to the plasma.

Hydrogen ion secretion and, therefore, HCO_3^- reabsorption, is extremely sensitive to arterial CO_2 tensions. Elevation in arterial P_{CO_2}, causing mild acidosis, results in an excess H^+ secretion by the kidney, reabsorption of most of the filtered HCO_3^-, and titration of the buffers $\dfrac{HPO_4-}{H_2PO_4}$ and $\dfrac{NH_3^+}{NH_4}$, forming an acid urine. Low arterial CO_2 tensions, resulting in mild

TUBULAR CELL

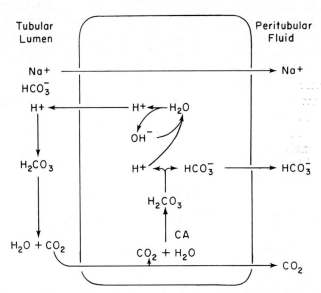

Fig. 3–43.—Bicarbonate reabsorption in the proximal tubular cell of the nephron.

alkalosis, depress H^+ secretion. Filtered HCO_3^- is not totally reabsorbed, due to the lack of H^+; therefore the urine remains alkaline. When the arterial P_{CO_2} is low in response to severe metabolic acidosis from shock, H^+ secretion is reduced because of the low arterial P_{CO_2}, but plasma HCO_3^- is also severely reduced. Under these conditions H^+ secretion, although diminished, is always in excess of the filtered HCO_3^-. Total reabsorption and conservation of HCO_3^- results with the remaining excess H^+ being buffered with $\dfrac{HPO_4^-}{H_2PO_4}$ and $\dfrac{NH_3}{NH_4^+}$ in the urine.

Clinical Characteristics of Acute Renal Insufficiency

Acute renal insufficiency usually follows a catastrophe such as severe trauma, shock, transfusion reactions, and occasionally occurs in the elderly after a mild hypotensive period or administration of nephrotoxic drugs. The renal response to injury varies considerably and, therefore, the diagnosis is not always obvious. Characteristically, there is anuria (less than 20 ml urine per 24 hours) or oliguria (less than 350–400 ml urine per 24 hours) but a considerable diuresis (high output renal failure) may even be seen concomitantly with a rising blood urea nitrogen. Renal conservation of sodium is usually impaired and, therefore, sodium concentrations in urine may approach that of serum. Urine sodium concentration may be very low, however, even with tubular necrosis and acute renal insufficiency due to continuing function in some nephrons. Osmolality of the urine is also very near that of plasma in the majority of cases, but it is not a reliable guide to the existence of acute tubular necrosis or to the extent of renal damage. A rising BUN in the face of adequate hydration and arterial blood pressure indicates acute renal parenchymal damage.

The gross and microscopic changes in the kidneys of an oliguric shock patient in renal failure often do not adequately explain the severe functional disorder. Electron microscopy, micropuncture studies, and histochemical analysis may be more informative in the future. In any event, acute renal insufficiency is usually a reversible lesion with time. With the development of peritoneal and hemodialysis, prevention of the lethal complications of renal shutdown can be accomplished and recovery expected in a large number of these cases.

MECHANISMS FOR ACUTE RENAL INSUFFICIENCY

The basis for acute renal insufficiency aside from such factors as ureteral obstruction, renal artery or vein thrombosis, or the direct cellular toxins such as mercuric chloride, which causes tubular necrosis, is still poorly understood. Numerous mechanisms have been postulated, such as ischemia, nephron blockade with debris, renal vasospasm, and intravascular coagulation, to account for the tubular necrosis and renal insufficiency following shock. These factors will be considered below.

ACUTE TUBULAR NECROSIS

Acute tubular necrosis has been observed both clinically and experimentally following ingestion of toxins such as mercuric chloride or potassium chromate. Previously, acute proximal tubular necrosis often resulted in oliguria, uremia, and death. If the basement membranes remain intact, however, and a few viable cells are present, the kidney has an amazing ability to regenerate tubular epithelium, and recovery results when appropriate support such as dialysis is given.

Acute tubular necrosis is most frequently seen clinically following hypotensive episodes and has been termed *ischemic necrosis,* although ischemia is usually not the sole causative factor in many cases. The experimental models of acute tubular necrosis are generally rather gross. Total occlusion of the renal vascular supply is necessary for 1.5–3 hours, or large amounts of serotonin and norepinephrine must be infused locally. It seems unlikely that these models represent a satisfactory account of the lesion found in man. Clinically, several factors acting together seem to be important. These include underlying chronic vascular disease, plugging of the nephrons with cellular casts, intense sympathetic activity, and intravascular coagulation. The kidney has an abundant blood supply, and although flow may drop to 25% of normal, renal vein oxygen content is often surprisingly high. Shunting or redistribution of blood flow in the kidney with focal ischemia, hypoxia, and tubular damage during shock could account for the tubular necrosis, in spite of what appears to be grossly adequate oxygenation. Whether or not these patients regain renal function depends upon the integrity of the basement membranes and the presence of viable tubular cells to regenerate and repopulate the nephrons.

Renal Vasospasm

Initially, in shock, blood flow is reduced proportionately with pressure, and after 30–60 minutes it falls even more while calculated resistance increases severalfold. When systemic arterial pressure and blood volume return to normal, renal blood flow may persist at a reduced level for varying periods. Indirect measurement of kidney blood flow in humans with acute renal insufficiency suggests that flow is reduced to about 35% of normal. Seldom is there any evidence of microscopic thrombi or other obstructive vascular lesions to account for this high renal vascular resistance. One is left with the impression that intense afferent arteriole vasoconstriction is present and, therefore, accounts for the elevated renal vascular resistance, lack of urine formation and renal insufficiency. As stated earlier in this discussion, intense afferent arteriolar vasoconstriction reduces the filtration pressure below a critical level, resulting in a failure of filtration and urine formation. Early local infusion of a vasodilator may be of benefit under these specific conditions.

High Interstitial Hydrostatic Pressure

Severe edema of the kidney with increased interstitial hydrostatic pressure must also be considered as a mechanism for the high renal vascular resistance, oliguria, and renal failure. High interstitial hydrostatic pressure may mechanically collapse vessels and nephrons. The effective filtration pressure would be considerably greater under these conditions since tubular hydrostatic pressure might be 50–60 mm Hg instead of 10–15 mm Hg, and effective filtration pressure would have to be 80–90 mm Hg instead of 40–50 mm Hg. In addition, renal vascular resistance would increase considerably under these conditions. It is obvious in instances of acute renal insufficiency characterized by a high output of a protein-free plasma-like urine that neither elevated interstitial hydrostatic pressure nor vasospasm of the afferent glomerular arterioles is responsible for this pathophysiologic condition. Malfunctioning injured tubular cells must account for this clinical picture of high-urine-output renal failure.

Total Reabsorption of Filtrate

A peculiar aspect of renal hemodynamics is that the hematocrit and colloid osmotic pressure of blood is greatly increased in the efferent arteriole and early postglomerular peritubular capillaries. With an individual kidney blood flow of 600 ml per minute, hematocrit of 45% and glomerular filtration rate of 60 ml per minute the hematocrit will increase from 45% to 61% while colloid osmotic pressure also increases about 22% in the efferent arteriole. This is merely due to the loss of 60 ml of protein-free plasma from the blood into the lumen of the nephron. Because of the increased colloid osmotic pressure in the peritubular capillaries, some investigators feel that almost all the glomerular filtrate is immediately reabsorbed in the proximal nephron when the tubular cells are injured due to ischemia or other factors. They feel that the injured tubular cells and fragmented basement membrane function as a less effective barrier to prevent reabsorption of glomerular filtrate. Therefore reabsorption takes place rapidly, reconstituting the peritubular capillary blood to its original hematocrit and colloid osmotic pressure, and no urine is formed. There is little, if any, quantitative data to substantiate this theory, and in view of what is known about how the normal proximal tubule behaves, it is doubtful that this could occur. Inhibition of active reabsorption of sodium in the proximal tubule by metabolic inhibitors leads to massive diuresis rather than to reabsorption of the filtrate. This massive diuresis is seen in some cases of acute renal injury when the tubular cell activity is altered. If the nephron is occluded by cellular debris and casts, total reabsorption of the filtrate may take place.

Mechanical Block of the Nephron

Fourteen cases of acute renal failure have been reported following the use of low-molecular-weight dextran (dextran-40) in humans. It has been suggested that with low-flow states the urine viscosity increases and tubular stasis with blockade results.

Myoglobin may exert its disastrous effects on the kidney in much the same manner. Myoglobin (molecular weight 17,000) is readily filtered by the glomerular membranes. Large amounts of this substance in the form of myoglobin cast may cause mechanical blockade of the tubular lumen and resultant renal insufficiency. It should be noted that these substances produce these effects only when urine output is minimal. Administration of dextran-40 or myoglobin in the face of adequate urine output is harmless.

Circulating free hemoglobin is probably not damaging to the normal kidney, but in low-flow states the combination produces severe disturbances in renal function and tubular necrosis. Less than 3% of hemoglobin is normally filtered, and with normal urine flow hemoglobin does not accumulate significantly in the urine. Recent work in man suggests that hemoglobin is relatively harmless in transfusion reactions whereas the antigen-antibody complex from the incompatible red blood cell stroma and naturally occurring endogenous antibodies leads to acute renal damage. Red blood cell stroma from compatible donors is harmless. Hemoglobin has been reported experimentally to result in tubular damage, but only when severe reductions in renal blood flow had been brought about.

INTRAVASCULAR COAGULATION

Hardaway and others have suggested that acute renal insufficiency may be on the basis of diffuse microscopic intravascular coagulation within the kidneys. As indicated previously, a hypercoagulable state is often seen in shock and other conditions. Although microthrombi are occasionally found to be causative, other investigators have failed to identify them in the majority of cases. Autopsy specimens of victims of acute renal insufficiency occasionally reveal microthrombi, but these lesions are also present in specimens of patients with intact renal function up to the time of death.

A recent report suggests that epsilon amino caproic acid can induce acute renal insufficiency by massive intravascular coagulation of the glomerular capillaries. For this reason, this agent is administered in conjunction with heparin when excessive fibrinolysis is present.

METABOLIC FACTORS

Clinicians have noted a high incidence of renal failure in patients with hepatic dysfunction from hepatitis, obstructive jaundice, and other conditions. The importance of this problem is brought out by the findings that 50% of patients who die after surgical procedures for obstructive jaundice die with renal failure. In jaundice, a hypotensive or shock period has usually been associated with the renal failure.

Recent clinical and experimental work has clarified this problem considerably. Bile is a powerful vasodilator, and vasodilation of the kidney results in excess sodium and, therefore, water loss. Intravenous administration of as little as 8 cc of bile (comparable to a 0.6 mg per 100 ml increase in concentration) will cause a temporary three to fourfold increase in excretion of filtered sodium and increased water excretion. The high incidence of renal complications in jaundiced patients can be prevented with adequate preoperative hydration and with the use of mannitol. More recent evidence verifies that the kidneys in patients with the hepatorenal syndrome are functionally intact. The use of several of these organs as transplant kidneys was followed by excellent renal function in the recipient.

Deficits of various ions in the body, particularly potassium, have been shown to impair renal function. The chronic use of many currently available diuretic agents is usually responsible for these conditions. The structural and chemical aberrations in the kidney caused by low potassium levels are unknown, but correction of these deficits usually results in improved renal function.

Many antibiotics used in the control of septic conditions have toxic effects on the renal tubules and can cause acute renal insufficiency. The aminoglycoside group of agents (kanomycin, gentamicin, streptomycin, etc.) are the most commonly used antibiotics that have renal toxic effects. Again, the precise chemical or morphologic alterations in the kidneys by these drugs is poorly understood. Proper assessment of renal function should always accompany the use of these antibiotics, and if renal function is impaired the dosage should be adjusted.

CASE HISTORY

A 19-year-old male sustained a severe crush injury of his entire right leg in a tractor accident. He was pinned under the machine an estimated 5 hours before help arrived. The tractor was removed, and he was taken to his local hospital where he was immediately transferred to the University Hospital.

Physical examination revealed the patient to be in severe cardiovascular distress. Blood pressure 65/40, pulse 150 beats per minute, and respiratory rate 25 breaths per minute. The crushed leg was cold, cyanotic, and swollen from the inguinal region distally. A catheter was placed into the bladder, and 300 ml of urine was recovered. Fluids were administered over the next 30–60 minutes, with considerable improvement in the patient's hemodynamic status. Clinically, the circulation to the leg appeared to be intact. Despite fluids, mannitol, and reconstitution of the blood pressure to 110/75, no urine formed. The serum potassium was 5.5 mEq per liter upon admission and rose to 8.6 mEq per liter with fluid administration and improvement in the peripheral circulation. A decision was made to remove the crushed limb; a tourniquet was applied and the patient was transferred to the operating room.

A mid-thigh amputation was carried out. The elevated serum potassium was temporarily reduced with intravenous administration of insulin, glucose, and K-Exolate enemas. The cardiac effects of hyperkalemia were reduced by administration of calcium gluconate.

During the 72 hours following injury, the patient excreted a total of 200 ml of dark chocolate-colored urine which contained myoglobin. During the following 22 days, the patient was totally anuric (Fig. 3-44). Almost continuous peritoneal dialysis was carried out initially to control the serum potassium and, subsequently, because of renal insufficiency. The patient's course was complicated by peritonitis secondary to dialysis, further necrosis of the remaining right limb requiring debridement, massive gastrointestinal bleeding requiring surgery, severe thrombocytopenia, and sepsis. On the twenty-third day following injury, urine volumes averaging from 50 to 100 ml per 24 hours were obtained (see Fig. 3-44). On the thirtieth day following injury renal biopsy revealed some glomeruli with occasional foci of hypercellularity and dilated nephron tubules lined with flattened cuboidal cells (Fig. 3-45). Despite the favorable biopsy report, the patient remained oliguric, required dialysis, and finally expired on the forty-first day from peritonitis with severe sepsis.

Fig. 3–44.—Summary of renal function and serum potassium levels in Case 1. X denotes periods of upper gastrointestinal hemorrhage; 1 denotes revision of amputation stump; 2 denotes time of hip disarticulation; and 3 denotes time of vagotomy and pyloroplasty to control hemorrhage.

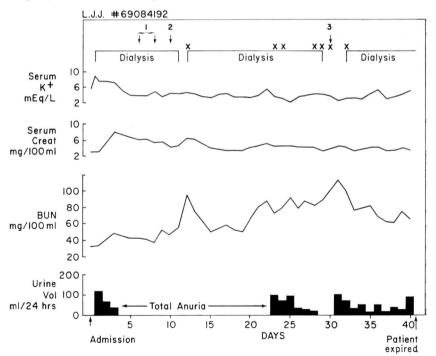

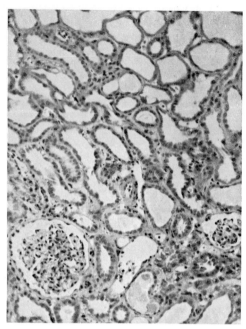

Fig. 3–45.—Renal biopsy, taken on the thirtieth day following injury, showed a hypercellular glomerulus and dilated nephron tubules lined with flattened cuboidal tubular cells (Case 1).

Gastrointestinal Tract in Shock

Extensive destruction of the mucosal layer of the gastrointestinal tract characterizes all forms of shock in the dog but is exceptionally rare in the human, making comparisons based on canine shock tenuous when applied to the clinical problem. On the other hand, terminal gastrointestinal hemorrhage from superficial ulceration of the stomach and duodenum is not rare, especially in septic shock.

Dog studies from Gurd's group demonstrated that when hemorrhagic hypotension progressed beyond a certain point, reinfusion of oxygenated blood could restore normal blood flow and almost-normal oxygen consumption in the liver and limbs, but not in the intestine. In vivo studies of the rate of turnover of ^{32}P in nucleotides and inorganic phosphate present in the acid soluble fraction of the intestinal wall revealed severe impairment in both the biosynthesis of ATP and in the rate of oxidative phosphorylation within the mucosal cells. The reduced metabolism of these mucosal cells impaired the energy-dependent defense mechanisms that protect the epithelial cells of the mucosa from dissolution by intraluminal proteases and from damage by other intraluminal toxins. If the intestinal lumen of a dog with hemorrhagic shock was previously washed with saline, pathologic changes and metabolic depression were prevented. Trasylol, a protease inhibitor, when applied intraluminally, was also capable of preventing the hemorrhagic enteritis usually seen in this experimental preparation. One explanation offered by Gurd for the difference between intestinal pathology in shock in man and dogs is the greatly reduced quantity of trypsin in the human intestine when compared to that of the dog.

Reticuloendothelial System in Shock

Clinical experience points to the heightened susceptibility of shock patients to pneumonia, wound infection, and septicemia. Depression of the detoxifying, phagocytic, and antibody (complement and bactericidal) functions of the reticuloendothelial system have been documented in both man and experimental animals following hemorrhage, sepsis, burns, and the experimental administration of endotoxin. Along these lines, Rittenbury has demonstrated reduced uptake of standard fat emulsion given intravenously after burns and has correlated the degree of depression of reticuloendothelial clearing ability with the ultimate mortality rate. Similarly, Moncrieff has shown preservation of the anamnestic response to tetanus toxoid in burn patients. On the other hand, the ability to form antibody to new antigen is reduced, and leukocytes exposed to endotoxin fail to exercise normal phagocytic function. The basis for this damage to the reticuloendothelial system following shock, according to Fine, is reduction in blood flow through the liver and spleen. The liver, which is the largest aggregate of reticuloendothelial cells, suffers extensive damage during protracted periods of hypotension, manifested by a diminished phagocytic capacity of the Kupffer cells which function subnormally for 4–5 days in surviving animals. Blockade of the reticuloendothelial system with colloidal material such as India ink or thorotrast further suppresses phagocytic activity and renders these animals far more sensitive to the effects of trauma and hemorrhage. The inability to contain infection in the shock patient limits survival by allowing spread of microorganisms which, under normal circumstances, would be isolated and controlled.

In the experimental animal a state of tolerance to shock is seen after repeated sublethal insults of various types leading to an adaptive change characterized by a heightened resistance to injury. Resistance can be diminished by reticuloendothelial blockade with particulate material. Jacob Fine, in particular, has stressed the importance of the reticuloendothelial system in endotoxin shock, showing that after the induction of shock the spleen is unable to clear endotoxin and that the effect of endotoxin or hemorrhage can be greatly mitigated by substitution of a normal spleen or by previous ablation of the sympathetic supply to the spleen. Repeated sublethal exposure producing tolerance to endotoxin often renders the animal tolerant to trauma or hemorrhage, illustrating the nonspecific nature of this response. The reverse also applies; repeated sublethal drum trauma establishes a resistance to lethal amounts of endotoxin. Repeated exposure to endotoxin has a number of nonspecific effects; the lymph nodes enlarge, the follicles become hyperplastic, and there is a more efficient uptake of material from the blood stream. As Zweifach points out, these findings may prompt the idea that the improved status of these animals may be due to more efficient removal of vasotoxic material from the blood stream but isolated preparations, using portions of the vascular tree of tolerant animals, when tested in vitro are also resistant to vasotoxic material. Fine explains the lack of specificity of the tolerant animal by suggesting that shock-inducing injury shares the common property of releasing endotoxin from the gut. He suggests that tolerance is in fact specific for endotoxin.

REFERENCES

LUNG

General references

Ayres, S. M., and Giannelli, S., Jr.: *Care of the Critically Ill* (New York: Appleton-Century-Crofts, Inc., 1967).

Bendixen, H. H., Egbert, L. D., Hedley-Whyte, J., Laver, M. B., Pontoppidan, H.: *Respiratory Care* (St. Louis: C. V. Mosby Company, 1965).

Comroe, J. H., Jr.: *Physiology of Respiration* (Chicago: Year Book Medical Publishers, 1965).

Comroe, J. H., Forster, R. E., II, Dubois, A. B., Briscoe, W. A., and Carlsen, E.: *The Lung: Clinical Physiology and Pulmonary Function Tests* (2nd ed.; Chicago: Year Book Medical Publishers, 1962).

Eiseman, B., and Ashbaugh, D. G. (eds.): Pulmonary effects of nonthoracic trauma, J. Trauma 8:623, 1968.

Erlanger, J., and Gasser, H. S.: Studies in secondary traumatic shock: II. Shock due to mechanical limitation of blood flow; III. Circulatory failure due to adrenalin, Am. J. Physiol. 49:151, 345, 1919.

Fenn, W. O., and Rahn, H. (eds.) Respiration, Vols. I and II, *Handbook of Physiology*, Section 3 (Washington, D.C.: American Physiological Society, 1965).

Fishman, A. P.: Dynamics of the Pulmonary Circulation, in Hamilton, W. F. (ed.): *Handbook of Physiology: Sec. 2. Circulation*, Vol. II (Washington, D.C.: American Physiological Society, 1963), p. 1667.

Moore, F. D., Lyons, J. H., Pierce, E. C., Jr., Morgan, A. P., Jr., Drinker, P. A., MacArthur, J. D., and Dammin, G. J.: *Post-Traumatic Pulmonary Insufficiency* (Philadelphia: W. B. Saunders Company, 1969).

Special references

Abel, F. L., Waldhausen, J. A., Daly, W. J., and Pearce, W. L.: Pulmonary blood volume in hemorrhagic shock in the dog and primate, Am. J. Physiol. 213:1027, 1967.

Abrams, M. E., and Taylor, F. B., Jr.: Isolation and quantitative estimation of pulmonary surface active lipoprotein and its interaction with fibrinogen, Physiologist 10:78, 1967.

Ashbaugh, D. G., Bigelow, D. B., Petty, T. L., and Levine, B. E.: Acute respiratory distress in adults, Lancet 2:320, 1967.

Aviado, D. M.: Cardiovascular effects of some commonly used pressor amines, Anesthesiology 20:71, 1959.

Ballentine, T. V. N., Zuschneid, W., and Clowes, G. H. A., Jr.: Pulmonary vasoconstriction in hypovolemic low flow states, Physiologist 10:118, 1967.

Bates, D. V.: Import of radioactive gas studies of the lung on surgery and postoperative care, Bull. Am. Coll. Surgeons 54:355, 1969.

Bayley, T., Clements, J. A., and Osbahr, A. J.: Pulmonary and circulatory effects of fibrinopeptides, Circulation Res. 21:469, 1967.

Berman, I. R., and Ducker, T. B.: Changes in pulmonary, somatic, and splanchnic perfusion with increased intracranial pressure, Surg. Gynec. & Obst. 128:8, 1969.

Border, J. R., Tibbetts, J. C., and Schenk, W. G.: Hypoxic hyperventilation and acute respiratory failure in the severely stressed patient: Massive pulmonary arteriovenous shunts, Surgery 64:710, 1968.

Braun, K., and Stern, S.: Functional significance of the pulmonary venous system, Am. J. Cardiology 20:56, 1967.

Chu, J., Clements, J. A., Cotton, E. K., Klaus, M. H., Sweet, A. Y., and Tooley, W. H.: Neonatal pulmonary ischemia. Part I., Clinical and physiological studies, Pediatrics (Supp.) 40:709, 1967.

Clements, J. A.: Surface phenomena in relation to pulmonary function, Physiologist 5:11, 1962.

Clowes, G. H. A., Jr., Zuschneid, W., Turner, M., Blackburn, G., Rubin, J., Toala, P., and Green, G.: Observations on the pathogenesis of the pneumonitis associated with severe infections in other parts of the body, Ann. Surg. 167:630, 1968.

Cottrell, T. S., Levine, R., Senior, R. M., Wiener, J., Spiro, D., Fishman, A. P.: Electron microscopic alterations at the alveolar level in pulmonary edema, Circulation Res. 21:783, 1967.

Cournand, A., Motley, H. L., Werko, L., and Richards, D. W., Jr.: Physiological studies of the effects of intermittent positive pressure breathing on cardiac output in man, Am. J. Physiol. 152:162, 1948.

Daly, J. J.: Venoarterial shunting in obstructive pulmonary disease, New England J. Med. 278:952, 1968.

Doty, D. B., Moseley, R. V., Pruitt, B. A., and Randolph, J. G.: Hemodynamic consequences of respiratory insufficiency following trauma, J. Thoracic & Cardiovas. Surg. 58:374, 1969.

Gerst, P. H., Rattenborg, C., and Holaday, D. A.: The effects of hemorrhage on pulmonary circulation and respiratory gas exchange, J. Clin. Invest. 38:524, 1959.

Goldring, R. M., Turino, G. M., Cohen, G., Jameson, A. G., Bass, B. G., and Fishman, A. P.: The catecholamines in the pulmonary arterial pressor response to acute hypoxia, J. Clin. Invest. 41:1211, 1962.

Guyton, A. C., and Lindsey, A. W.: Effect of elevated left atrial pressure and decreased plasma protein concentration on the development of pulmonary edema, Circulation Res. 7:649, 1959.

Hamilton, R. W., Jr., Hustead, R. F., and Peltier, L. F.: Fat embolism: The effect of particulate embolism on lung surfactant, Surgery 56:53, 1964.

Henry, J. N., McArdle, A. H., Scott, H. J., and Gurd, F. N.: A study of the acute and chronic respiratory pathophysiology of hemorrhagic shock, J. Thoracic & Cardiovas. Surg. 54:666, 1967.

Hyman, A. L.: The effects of bradykinin on the pulmonary veins, J. Pharm. & Exper. Therap. 161:78, 1968.

Janoff, A., and Zeligs, J. D.: Vascular injury and lysis of basement membrane in vitro by neutral protease of human leukocytes, Science 161:702, 1968.

Keller, C. A., Schramel, R. J., Hyman, A. L., and Creech, O., Jr.: The cause of congestive lesions of the lung, J. Thoracic & Cardiovas. Surg. 53:743, 1967.

Kelman, G. R., Nunn, J. F., Prys-Roberts, C., and Greenbaum, R.: The influence of cardiac output on arterial oxygenation: A theoretical study, Brit. J. Anaesth. 39:450, 1967.

Kistler, G. S., Caldwell, P. R. B., and Weibel, E. R.: Development of fine structural damage to alveolar and capillary lining cells in oxygen-poisoned rat lungs, J. Cell Biol. 32:605, 1967.

Laurenzi, G. A., Yin, S., and Huarneri, J. M.: Adverse effect of oxygen on tracheal mucus flow, New England J. Med. 279:333, 1968.

Lee, A. B., and Kinney, J. M.: Ventilatory management of the pulmonary burn, Ann. New York Acad. Sc. 150:738, 1968.

Low, F. N., and Daniels, C. W.: Electron microscopy of the rat lung, Anat. Rec. 113: 437, 1952.

MacKenzie, G. J.: Circulatory and respiratory studies in myocardial infarction in cardiogenic shock, Lancet 2:7364, 1964.

McKay, D. G., Margaretten, W., and Csarossy, I.: An electron microscope study of endotoxin shock in rhesus monkeys, Surg. Gynec. & Obst. 125:825, 1967.

Nash, G., Blennerhassett, I. B., and Pontoppidan, H.: Pulmonary lesions with oxygen therapy and artificial ventilation, New England J. Med. 276:368, 1967.

Nies, A. S., Forsyth, R. P., Williams, H. E., and Melmon, K. L.: Contribution of kinins to endotoxin shock in unanesthetized rhesus monkeys, Circulation Res. 22:155, 1968.

Okinaka, A. J.: The pattern of breathing after operation, Surg. Gynec. & Obst. 125:785, 1967.

Pattle, R. E.: Properties, functions and origin of alveolar lining layer, Nature 175:1125, 1955.

Salvatore, A. J., Sullivan, S. F., and Popper, E. M.: Postoperative hypoventilation and hypoxemia in man after hyperventilation, New England J. Med. 280:467, 1969.

Sarnoff, S. J.: Some Physiologic Considerations in the Genesis of Acute Pulmonary Edema, in Wright, R. A., and Voith, I. (eds.) Pulmonary Circulation (New York: Grune & Stratton, Inc., 1959), pp. 273-282.

Shook, C. D., MacMillan, B. G., and Altemeier, W. A.: Pulmonary complications of the burn patient, Arch. Surg. 97:215, 1968.

Sladen, A., Laver, M. B., and Pontoppidan, H.: Pulmonary complications and water retention in prolonged mechanical ventilation, New England J. Med. 279:448, 1968.

Steim, J. M., Redding, R. A., Hauck, C. T., and Stein, M.: Isolation and characterization of lung surfactant, Biochem. & Biophys. Res. Commun. 34:434, 1969.

Stone, H. H., Rhame, D. W., Corbitt, J. D., Given, K. S., and Martin, J. D., Jr.: Respiratory burns: A correlation of clinical and laboratory results, Ann. Surg. 165:157, 1967.

Sugg, W. L., Craver, W. D., Webb, W. R., and Ecker, R. R.: Pressure changes in the dog lung secondary to hemorrhagic shock: Protective effects of pulmonary reimplantation, Ann. Surg. 169:592, 1969.

Sugg, W. L., Webb, W. R., and Ecker, R. R.: Prevention of lesions of the lung secondary to hemorrhagic shock, Surg. Gynec. & Obst. 127:1005.

Sugg, W. L., Webb, W. R., Nakae, S., Theodorides, T., Gupts, D. N., and Cook, W. A.: Congestive atelectasis: An experimental study, Ann. Surg. 168:234, 1968.

Sukhnandan, R., and Thal, A. P.: Effect of endotoxin and vasoactive agents on dibenzyline pre-treated lungs, Surgery 58:185, 1965.

Teplitz, C.: The ultrastructural basis for pulmonary pathophysiology following trauma, J. Trauma 8:700, 1968.

Tilney, N. L., and Hester, W. J.: Physiologic and histologic changes in the lungs of patients dying after prolonged cardiopulmonary bypass: An inquiry into the nature of post-perfusion lung, Ann. Surg. 166:759, 1967.

Tomlin, P. J., Howarth, F. H., and Robinson, J. S.: Postoperative atelectasis and laryngeal incompetence, Lancet 1:1402, 1968.

Vandenberg, R. A., Nolan, A. C., Reed, J. H., Jr., and Wood, E. H.: Regional pulmonary arterial-venous shunting caused by gravitational and inertial forces, J. Appl. Physiol. 25:516, 1968.

Veith, F. J., Deysine, M., Nehlsen, S. L., Panossian, A., and Hagstrom, J. W. C.: Pulmonary changes common to isolated lung perfusion, venovenous bypass and total cardiopulmonary bypass, Surg. Gynec. & Obst. 125:1047, 1967.

Veith, F. J., Hagstrom, J. W. C., Panossian, A., Nehlsen, S. L., and Wilson, J. W.: Pulmonary microcirculatory response to shock, transfusion, and pump-oxygenator procedures: A unified mechanism underlying pulmonary damage, Surgery 64:95, 1968.

Webb, W. R., and Cook, W. A.: Pulmonary changes in hemorrhagic shock, Surgery 64: 85, 1968.

Weibel, E. R., and Gil, J.: Electron microscopic demonstration of extracellular duplex lining layer of alveoli, Resp. Physiol. 4:42, 1968.

Wertzberger, J. J., and Peltier, L. F.: Fat embolism: The importance of arterial hypoxia, Surgery 63:626, 1968.

West, J. B.: Regional differences in gas exchange in the lung of erect man, J. Appl. Physiol. 17:893, 1962.

Willwerth, B. M., Crawford, F. A., Young, W. G., Jr., and Sealy, W. C.: The role of functional demand on the development of pulmonary lesions during hemorrhagic shock, J. Thoracic & Cardiovas. Surg. 54:658, 1967.

PATHOPHYSIOLOGY OF THE HEART

Bing, R. J.: Cardiac metabolism, Physiol. Rev. 45:171-213, 1965.

Bourassa, M., Campean, L., Bois, M., and Rico, O.: Myocardial lactate metabolism at rest and during exercise in ischemic heart disease, Am. J. Cardiol. 23:771, 1969.

Braunwald, E., and Frahm, C. J.: Studies on Starling's law of the heart, Circulation 24: 633, 1961.

Burton, A. C.: *Physiology and Biophysics of the Circulation* (Chicago: Year Book Medical Publishers, 1965).

Cho, Y. W.: Myocardial metabolic changes during acute hemorrhage, Angiology 16: 532, 1965.

Davson, H., and Eggleton, M. G. (eds.): *Starling and Evans' Principles of Human Physiology* (13th ed.; Philadelphia: Lea & Febiger, 1962).

Dodge, H. T., and Baxley, W.: Hemodynamic aspects of heart failure, Am. J. Cardiol. 22:24, 1968.

Gorlin, R., and Sonnenblick, E.: Regulation of performance of the heart, Am. J. Cardiol. 22:16, 1968.

Herman, M., and Gorlin, R.: Implications of left ventricular asynergy, Am. J. Cardiol. 23:538, 1969.

MacKenzie, G. J.: Circulatory and respiratory studies in myocardial infarction in cardiogenic shock, Lancet 2:7364, 1964.

McGregor, M., and Fam, W. M.: Regulation of coronary blood flow, Bull. New York Acad. Med. 42:940, 1966.

Marano, A. J.: Hemodynamic effects of ouabain in experimental acute myocardial infarction with shock, Am. J. Cardiol. 17:327, 1966.

Mason, D.: Usefulness and limitations of rate of rise of intraventricular pressure (dp/dt) in the evaluation of myocardial contractility in man, Am. J. Cardiol. 23:516, 1969.

Mosher, P.: Control of coronary blood flow by an autoregulatory mechanism, Circulation Res. 14:250, 1964.

Pool, P., and Braunwald, E.: Fundamental mechanisms in congestive heart failure, Am. J. Cardiol. 22:7, 1968.

Ross, J.: The assessment of myocardial performance in man by hemodynamic and cineangiographic techniques, Am. J. Cardiol. 23:511, 1969.

Sampson, J. J., and Hutchinson, J. C.: Heart failure in myocardial infarction, Prog. in Cardiovas. Disease 10:129, 1967.

Solace, R. T., and Downing, F.: Effects of *E. coli* endotoxemia on ventricular performance, Am. J. Physiol. 211:307, 1966.

Soroff, H. S.: Physiologic support of heart action, New England J. Med. 280:693, 1969.

Udhoji, V. N., Weil, N. H., Sambhi, M. P., and Rosoff, L.: Hemodynamic studies on clinical shock associated with infarction, Am. J. Med. 34:461, 1963.

Weissler, A. N.: The heart in heart failure, Ann. Int. Med. 69:929, 1968.

Weissler, A., Harris, W., and Schoenfield, C.: Bedside techniques for the evaluation of ventricular function in man, Am. J. Cardiol. 23:577, 1969.

LIVER

Ballinger, W. F., Vollenweider, H., and Montgomery, E. H.: The response of the canine liver to anaerobic metabolism induced by hemorrhagic shock, Surg. Gynec. & Obst. 112:19, 1961.

Cori, C. F., and Cori, G. T.: Glycogen formation in the liver from D- and L- lactic acid, J. Biol. Chem. 81:389, 1929.

Fine, J.: The Liver in Traumatic Shock, in Brauer, R. W. (ed.) *Liver Function* (Washington, D.C.: American Institute of Biological Sciences, 1958), p. 586.

Schimassek, H.: Lactate metabolism in the isolated perfused rat liver, Ann. New York Acad. Sc. 119:1013, 1965.

Schimassek, H.: Perfusion of isolated rat liver with a semisynthetic medium and control of liver function, Life Sc. 2:629, 1962.

Swenson, O., Grana, L., Inouye, T., and Donnellan, W. L.: Immediate and long-term effects of acute hepatic ischemia, Arch. Surg. 95:451, 1967.

Tait, I. B., and Eiseman, B.: Perfusion dynamics for extracorporeal hepatic assist, Arch. Surg. 93:131, 1966.

Torrance, H. B.: The control of the hepatic arterial circulation, J. Physiol. 158:39, 1961.

Vang, J. O., and Drapanas, T.: Metabolism of lactic acid and keto acids by the isolated perfused calf liver, Ann. Surg. 163:545, 1966.

CENTRAL NERVOUS SYSTEM

Stone, H. H., Donnelly, C. C., MacKrell, T. N., Brandstater, B. J., and Nemir, P., Jr.: The Effect of Acute Hemorrhagic Shock on Cerebral Circulation and Metabolism of Man, in Mills, L. C., and Moyer, J. H. (eds.) *Shock and Hypotension* (New York: Grune & Stratton, Inc., 1965).

ADRENAL GLAND

Special references

Ahlquist, R. P.: A study of the adrenotropic receptors, Am. J. Physiol. 153:586, 1948.

Beisel, W. R., and Rapoport, M. I.: Adrenocortical function and infectious illness, New England J. Med. 280:541 and 596, 1969.

Butcher, R. W.: Cyclic 3', 5'-AMP and the lipolytic effects of hormones on adipose tissue, Pharmacol. Rev. 18:237, 1966.

DeDuve, C.: The lysosome, Scient. Am. 208:64, 1963.

Fanestil, D. D.: Mechanism of action of aldosterone, Ann. Rev. Med. 20:223, 1969.

Hanison, T. S., Chawla, R. C., and Wojtalik, R. S.: Steroidal influences on catecholamines, New England J. Med. 279:136, 1968.

Havel, R. J., and Goldfien, A.: Role of sympathetic nervous system in metabolism of free fatty acids, J. Lipid Res. 1:102, 1959.

Herman, A. H., Mack, E. A., and Egdahl, R. H.: Adrenal cortical secretion following prolonged hemorrhagic shock, Surg. Forum 20:5, 1969.

Hokfelt, B., Bygdeman, S., and Sekkenes, J.: The Participation of the Adrenal Glands in Endotoxin Shock, in Bock, K. D. (ed.) *Shock: Pathogenesis and Therapy*, Ciba Internat. Symp. (Berlin: Springer-Verlag, 1962), p. 151.

Hume, D. M., and Nelson, D. H.: Adrenal cortical function in surgical shock, Surg. Forum 5:568, 1955.

Manger, W. M., Bollman, J. L., Maher, F. T., and Berkson, J.: Plasma concentration of epinephrine and norepinephrine in hemorrhagic and anaphylactic shock, Am. J. Physiol. 190:310, 1957.

Melby, J. C., Egdahl, R. H., and Spink, W. W.: Secretion and metabolism of cortisol after injection of endotoxin, J. Lab. & Clin. Med. 56:50, 1960.

Melby, J. C., and Spink, W. W.: Comparative studies on adrenal cortical function and cortisol metabolism in healthy adults and in patients with shock due to infection, J. Clin. Invest. 37:1791, 1958.

Murad, F., Chi, Y. M., Rall, T. W., and Sutherland, E. W.: Adenyl cyclase III. The effect of catecholamines and choline esters on the formation of adenosine-3', 5' phosphate by preparations from cardiac muscle and liver, J. Biol. Chem. 237:1233, 1962.

Robinson, G. A., Butcher, R. W., Oye, I., Morgan, H. E., and Sutherland, E. W.: The effect of epinephrine on adenosine-3', 5'-phosphate levels in the isolated perfused rat heart, Molec. Pharmacol. 1:168, 1965.

Robinson, G. A., Butcher, R. W., and Sutherland, E. W.: Adenyl cyclase as an adrenergic receptor, Ann. New York Acad. Sc. 139:703, 1967.

Sayers, G., and Solomon, N.: Work performance of rat heart-lung preparation: Standardization and influence of corticosteroids, Endocrinology 66:719, 1960.

Schumer, W.: Dexamethasone in oligemic shock, Arch. Surg. 98:259, 1969.

Sutherland, E. W.: Effect of hyperglycemic factor of pancreas and of epinephrine on glycogenolysis, Recent Prog. Hormone Res. 5:441, 1950.

Sutherland, E. W., and Rall, T. W.: Relation of adenosine-3', 5' phosphate and phosphorylase to action of catecholamines and other hormones, Pharmacol. Rev. 12:265, 1960.

Sutherland, E. W., and Robinson, G. A.: The role of cyclic 3', 5'-AMP in responses to catecholamines and other hormones, Pharmacol. Rev. 18:145, 1966.

Vander, A. J.: Control of renin release, Physiol. Rev. 47:359, 1967.

General references

Forsham, P. H.: Part I, The Adrenal Cortex, in Williams, R. H. (ed.) *Textbook of Endocrinology* (Philadelphia: W. B. Saunders Company, 1968), pp. 287-376.

Melmon, K. L.: Part II, Catecholamines and the Adrenal Medulla, in Williams, R. H. (ed.) *Textbook of Endocrinology* (Philadelphia, W. B. Saunders Company, 1968), pp. 379-400.

Tepperman, J.: *Metabolic and Endocrine Physiology* (2nd ed., Chicago: Year Book Medical Publishers, 1968), Chaps. 7 and 8.

Travis, R. H., and Sayer, G.: Adrenocorticotropic Hormone; Adrenocortical Steroids and Their Synthetic Analogs, in Goodman, L. S., and Gilman, A. (eds.) *The Pharmacological Basis of Therapeutics* (3d ed., New York: The Macmillan Company, 1960), pp. 1608-1648.

KIDNEY

Aukland, K., and Wolgast, M.: Effect of hemorrhage and retransfusion on intrarenal distribution of blood flow in dogs, J. Clin. Invest. 47:488, 1968.

Aukland, K.: Kidney Circulation During Hemorrhagic Hypotension, in Shepro, D., and Fulton, G. P. (eds.) *Microcirculation as Related to Shock* (New York: Academic Press, Inc., 1968).

Berliner, R. W.: Renal mechanism for potassium excretion, Harvey Lect. 55:141, 1959-1960.

Brown, E. B., Jr., and Goott, B.: Intracellular hydrogen ion changes and potassium movement, Am. J. Physiol. 204:765, 1963.

Charyton, C., and Purtilo, D.: Renal failure after epsilon-amino caproic acid therapy, New England J. Med. 280:1102, 1969.

Cuppage, F. E., and Tate, A.: Repair of the nephron following injury with mercuric chloride, Am. J. Path. 51:405, 1967.

Cuppage, F. E., Neagoy, D. R., and Tate, A.: Repair of the nephron following temporary occlusion of the renal pedicle, Lab. Invest. 17:660, 1967.

Earley, L. E., and Daugharty, T. M.: Sodium metabolism, New England J. Med. 281: 72, 1969.

Fenn, W. O., and Cobb, D. M.: Evidence for a potassium shift from plasma to muscles in response to an increased carbon dioxide tension, Am. J. Physiol. 112:41, 1935.

Goetz, K. L., Hermreck, A. S., and Trank, J. W.: Contribution of atrial receptors to diuresis following plasma expansion in conscious dogs, Fed. Proc. 28:584, 1969.

Gertz, K. H., Mangos, J. A., Braun, G., and Paget, H. D.: On the glomerular tubular balance in the rat kidney, Pflüger's Arch. ges. Physiol. 285:360, 1965.

Gombos, E. A., Lee, T. A., Salinas, J., and Mitrovic, M.: Renal response to pyrogen in normotensive and hypertensive man, Circulation 36:555, 1967.

Grimby, G.: Renal clearances at rest and during physical exercise after injection of bacterial pyrogen, J. Appl. Physiol. 20:137, 1965.

Hager, E. B., Hampers, C. L., and Merrill, J. P.: Acute renal insufficiency: The spectrum, Ann. Surg. 168:224, 1968.

Hardaway, R. M.: *Syndromes of Disseminated Intravascular Coagulation with Special Reference to Shock and Hemorrhage* (Springfield, Ill.: Charles C Thomas, Publisher, 1966).

Hermreck, A. S., and Thal, A. P.: Mechanisms for the high circulatory requirements in sepsis and septic shock, Ann. Surg. 170:677, 1969.

Koppel, M. H., Coburn, J. W., Matlock, M. M., Goldstein, H., Boyle, J. D., and Rubini, M. E.: Transplantation of cadaveric kidneys from patients with hepatorenal syndrome, New England J. Med. 280:1369, 1969.

Lauson, H. D., Bradley, S. E., and Cournand, A.: The renal circulation in shock, J. Clin. Invest. 23:381, 1944.

Mailloux, L., Swartz, C. D., Capizzi, R., Kim, K. E., Onesti, G., Ramivez, O., and Brest, A. N.: Acute renal failure after low-molecular weight dextran administration, New England J. Med. 277:1113, 1967.

McNay, J. L., and Goldberg, L. I.: Comparison of the effects of dopamine, isoproterenol, norepinephrine and bradykinin on canine renal and femoral blood flow, J. Pharmacol. & Exper. Therap. 151:23, 1966.

Oliver, J.: Correlations of structure and function and mechanisms of recovery in acute tubular necrosis, Am. J. Med. 15:535, 1953.

Oliver, J., MacDowell, M., and Tracy, A.: The pathogenesis of acute renal failure associated with traumatic and toxic injury: Renal ischemia, nephrotoxic damage and the ischemic episode, J. Clin. Invest. 30:1307, 1951.

Pitts, R. F.: *Physiology of the Kidney and Body Fluids* (2nd ed., Chicago: Year Book Medical Publishers, 1968).

Powers, S. R., Jr., Kiley, J. E., and Boba, A.: Renal Failure in Surgical Patients, in *Current Problems in Surgery* (Chicago: Year Book Medical Publishers, Nov., 1964).

Schmidt, P. J., and Holland, P. V.: Pathogenesis of the acute renal failure associated with incompatible transfusion, Lancet 2:1169, 1967.

Schwartz, W. B., and Relman, A. S.: Effects of electrolyte disorders on renal structure and function, New England J. Med. 276:383 and 452, 1967.

Scott, J. B., Emanuel, D. A., and Haddy, F. J.: Effect of potassium on renal vascular resistance and urine flow rate, Am. J. Physiol. 197:305, 1969.

Selkurt, E. E.: Renal Blood Flow and Renal Clearances during Hemorrhage and Hemor-

rhagic Shock, in Bock, K. D. (ed.) *Shock: Pathogenesis and Therapy* (Ciba Internat. Symp.) (Berlin: Springer-Verlag, 1962), p. 445.
Smith, H. W.: Lectures on the Kidney. University Extension Division, University of Kansas, Lawrence, Kansas, 1943.
Strauss, M. B., and Welt, L. G.: *Diseases of the Kidney* (Boston: Little, Brown & Company, 1963).
Topceglu, C., and Stahl, W. M.: Effect of bile infusion on the dog kidney, New England J. Med. 274:760, 1966.
Trueta, J., Barclay, A. E., Daniel, P. M., Franklin, K. J., and Prichard, M. M. L.: *Studies of the Renal Circulation* (Springfield, Ill.: Charles C Thomas, Publisher, 1947).

COAGULATION

Corrigan, J. J., Ray, W. L., and May, N.: Changes in the blood coagulation system associated with septicemia, New England J. Med. 279:851, 1968.
Hardaway, R. M.: *Syndromes of Disseminated Intravascular Coagulation* (Springfield, Ill.: Charles C Thomas, Publisher, 1966).
Jennings, P. B., Simmons, R. L., Sleeman, H. K., and Hardaway, R. M.: Hemodynamic, biochemical and coagulation alterations in endotoxin shock: Modification by induced tolerance in the dog, Ann. Surg. 167:204, 1968.
Kowalski, E.: Fibrinogen derivatives and their biologic activities, Seminars in Hematology 5:45, 1968.
McKay, D. G.: *Disseminated Intravascular Coagulation* (New York: Hoeber Medical Div., Harper & Row, 1965).
McKay, D. G.: Disseminated intravascular coagulation, Proc. Roy. Soc. Med. 61:1129, 1968.
McKay, D. G., and Margaretten, W.: Disseminated intravascular coagulation in virus diseases, Arch. Int. Med. 120:129, 1967.
McKay, D. G., Margaretten, W., and Csavossy, I.: An electron microscope study of the effects of bacterial endotoxin on the blood-vascular system, Lab. Invest. 15:1815, 1966.
McKay, D. G., Margaretten, W., and Csavossy, I.: An electron microscope study of endotoxin shock in rhesus monkeys, Surg. Gynec. & Obst. 125:825, 1967.
Merskey, C., Kleiner, G. J., and Johnson, A. J.: Quantitative estimation of split products of fibrinogen in human serum. Relation to diagnosis and treatment, Blood 28:1, 1966.
Merskey, C., Johnson, H. J., Kleiner, G. J., and Wohl, H.: The defibrination syndrome: Clinical features and laboratory diagnosis, Brit. J. Haemat. 13:528, 1967.
Seaman, A. J., Lutcher, L., Moffat, C. A., and Hueber, B. E.: Induced intravascular thromboembolic phenomena, Arch. Int. Med. 119:600, 1967.
Sohal, R. S., Sun, S. C., Colcolough, H. L., and Burch, G. E.: Heat stroke, Arch. Int. Med. 122:43, 1968.
Sirridge, M. S.: *Laboratory Evaluation of Hemostasis* (Philadelphia: Lea & Febiger, 1967).
Teger-Nilsson, A. C.: Studies on tissue thromboplastin, thrombin and fibrinopeptides in intravascular coagulation, Acta physiol. Scandinav., Supp. 319, 1968.
Thal, A. P. (ed.): Symposium on the role of intravascular coagulation in the immediate and late care of the severely injured person, J. Trauma, 9:645, 1969.

RETICULOENDOTHELIAL SYSTEM

Altura, B. M., and Hershey, S. G.: Use of reticuloendothelial phagocytic function as an index in shock therapy, Bull. New York Acad. Med. 43:259, 1967.
Fine, J., Palmerio, C., and Rutenburg, S.: New developments in therapy of refractory traumatic shock, Arch. Surg. 96:163, 1968.

Hershey, S. G., and Altura, B. M.: Effect of pretreatment with aggregate albumin on reticuloendothelial system activity and survival after experimental shock, Proc. Soc. Exper. Biol. & Med. 122:1195, 1966.

Noble, R. L., and Collip, J. B.: Quantitative method for production of experimental traumatic shock without hemorrhage in unanesthetized animals, Quart. J. Exper. Physiol. 31:187, 1942.

Ollodart, R. M., and Mansberger, A. R.: Effect of hemorrhage and reinfusion on bacterial clearance in the dog, Surg. Forum 16:76, 1965.

Ollodart, R. M.: Immunobacterial defense mechanisms in the human being during shock, Surg. Forum 14:21, 1963.

Palmerio, C., Aetterstrom, B., Shammash, J., Euchbaum, E., Frank, E., and Fine, J.: Denervation of the abdominal viscera for the treatment of traumatic shock, New England J. Med. 269:709, 1963.

Rittenbury, M. S., and Egdahl, R. H.: The effect of total pancreatectomy on experimental hemorrhagic pancreatitis, Fed. Proc. 19:190, 1960.

Rutenburg, S. H., Rutenburg, A. M., Smith, E. E., and Fine, J.: On the nature of tolerance of endotoxin, Proc. Soc. Exper. Biol. & Med. 118:620, 1965.

Rutenburg, S. H., Smith, E. E., Rutenburg, A. M., and Fine, J.: Degradation of endotoxin by splenic extracts, Antimicrobial Agents and Chemother. pp. 142-147, May, 1961.

Thal, A. P.: Surgical Physiology of the Exocrine Pancreas, in Davis, J. H., *Current Concepts of Surgery* (New York: McGraw-Hill Book Company, 1965).

Zweifach, B. W.: Contribution of reticulo-endothelial system to development of tolerance to experimental shock, Ann. New York Acad. Sc. 88:203, 1960.

Zweifach, B. W., and Hershey, S. G.: Protective mechanisms in shock, Ann. New York Acad. Sc. 66:1010, 1957.

4

Biochemical Alterations in Shock

Anoxia not only stops the machinery, it wrecks it.
HALDANE

Energy Metabolism in Shock

IF CELLS ARE TO SURVIVE and carry out their many functions, they must be able to release energy from the glucose molecule. This process is carried out by a series of minute steps, each releasing hydrogen from organic compounds and storing free energy in the high energy phosphate molecule, adenosinetriphosphate (ATP), from which it can be released readily. This release of energy from glucose by dehydrogenation is the opposite of photosynthesis, in which water and carbon dioxide unite to capture the energy supplied by the sun. The formation and storage of ATP takes place in the highly organized mitochondria of the cell; the complex respiratory change required to release this energy is dependent on oxygen for the removal of the released hydrogen in the form of water. Figure 4-1, in simplified form, illustrates the many reactions required to release energy from glucose.

The 6-carbon sugar is broken down into two 3-carbon pyruvic acid molecules with the release of hydrogen and a small amount of ATP. Under aerobic conditions this hydrogen is disposed of by combining with oxygen in the electron transport system with the formation of additional ATP. The oxidative decarboxylation of pyruvic acid transforms this 3-carbon molecule into the 2-carbon molecule acetic acid with release of carbon dioxide.

Acetic acid enters the Krebs cycle as acetyl coenzyme A. During the cycle, four further dehydrogenations take place with the liberation of energy in the form of ATP and the release of carbon dioxide. The hydrogen atoms released during the Krebs cycle do not combine immediately with oxygen; they first combine stepwise with a series of hydrogen acceptors and finally with oxygen to form water. The advantage of this long respiratory chain lies in the gradual liberation of energy stored as ATP

175

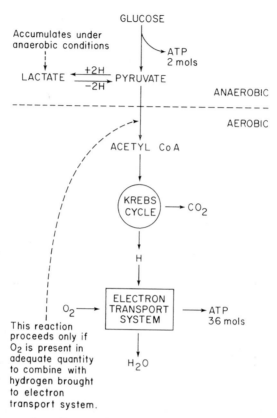

GLUCOSE

Accumulates under
anaerobic conditions → ATP
2 mols

LACTATE $\xrightarrow[-2H]{+2H}$ PYRUVATE

ANAEROBIC

- -

AEROBIC

ACETYL Co A

KREBS CYCLE → CO_2

H

O_2 → ELECTRON TRANSPORT SYSTEM → ATP 36 mols

This reaction proceeds only if O_2 is present in adequate quantity to combine with hydrogen brought to electron transport system.

H_2O

Fig. 4–1.—Energy for cell metabolism is derived from 6-carbon sugars. In anaerobic conditions present in poorly perfused tissues during shock, little O_2 is available to the electron transport system for disposing of hydrogen as water. As a result, lactic acid accumulates, the Krebs cycle is depressed, and little energy can be extracted from anaerobic breakdown of the glucose molecule. (From Thal, A. P., and Wilson, R. F.: Shock, in *Current Problems in Surgery* [Chicago: Year Book Medical Publishers, Sept., 1965].)

with a minimum waste of energy as heat. The ATP that is formed is necessary for virtually all the activities of the cell (Fig. 4-2).

In shock the final hydrogen acceptor, oxygen, is deficient; as a result, the hydrogen acceptors of the respiratory chain become saturated with accumulating hydrogen. Energy transformation in the Krebs cycle is seriously interfered with, and lactic acid can no longer be dehydrogenated into pyruvic acid. The main energy source remaining is in the anaerobic phase of glucose breakdown, which provides but a poor yield of ATP. With the fall in the energy available to the cell, its vital functions deterio-

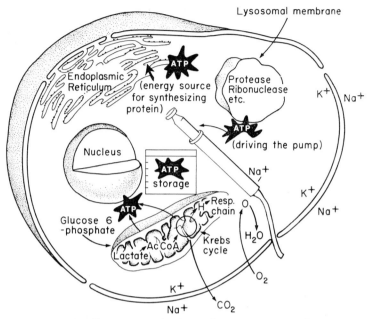

Fig. 4–2.—Normal cell. Energy in the form of ATP is necessary for protein and enzyme synthesis, maintenance of the sodium pump and reproduction of the cell. (From Thal, A. P., and Wilson, R. F.: Shock, in *Current Problems in Surgery* [Chicago: Year Book Medical Publishers, Sept., 1965].)

rate (Fig. 4-3). The important gradients necessary to retain potassium within the cell and sodium in the extracellular fluid can no longer be maintained. Sodium leaks into the cell and the level of potassium in the blood rises progressively. Energy is no longer available for the synthesis of protein and the vital enzymes necessary to maintain life. Finally, a step is reached when the structural elements of the cell break down; restoration of circulation at this late stage is without avail.

Ultrastructural Changes in Shock

Within the past few years, the work of DeDuve has focused attention on a small subcellular particle, the lysosome. By disruption of cells and differential ultracentrifugation, it is possible to concentrate these microscopic droplets containing powerful hydrolytic enzymes, including proteases, esterases, and phosphatases. Under normal circumstances these enzymes appear to play an important role in the intracellular digestive process. When the cell is damaged by the hypoxia of shock, the lysosomal

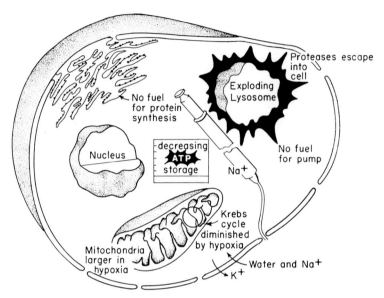

Fig. 4–3.—Shock (hypoxic) cell. Hypoxia reduces production of energy as ATP. When stored ATP is depleted, little energy is available for protein and enzyme synthesis and maintenance of the sodium pump. The lysosomal membrane loses its integrity and powerful proteases escape into the cell. (From Thal, A. P., and Wilson, R. F.: Shock, in *Current Problems in Surgery* [Chicago: Year Book Medical Publishers, Sept., 1965].)

membrane breaks down and these powerful agents are released intracellularly, destroying the fine and complex structure of the cell. These intracellular enzymes have been detected in the circulating blood after shock injury, and they possibly initiate the proteolytic state and alterations of the coagulation mechanism seen in advanced shock. Of considerable interest is the finding by Janoff that animals made tolerant to drum shock by graded injury have more stable lysosomes. Of further interest from the therapeutic viewpoint is Weissman's finding that treatment with steroids stabilizes the lysosome membrane and prevents release of lysosomal enzymes.

Acid-Base Regulation

Metabolic acidosis due to poor tissue perfusion has long been known to be a concomitant of shock. More recently, other types of acid-base disturbances have been found to accompany certain stages of shock. It is pertinent therefore to review the general subject of acid-base regulation.

The body's first line of defense against invading acid or base is the presence of buffers in body fluids. A buffer is defined as a substance which, in solution, will reduce the change in pH that would be produced by the addition of strong acid or strong base. The usual buffers are mixtures of weak acids and their salts, or weak bases and their salts. In the body we are concerned with buffering (1) H_2CO_3, formed by hydration of carbon dioxide; or its conjugate base, HCO_3^-, and (2) noncarbonic acids, so-called fixed acids, or their conjugate bases. The principal buffer of the body serving to blunt the pH change produced by an increase in the concentration of carbonic acid is the hemoglobin buffer pair, KHb/HHb. The principal buffer pair acting to reduce the pH change produced by invasion of acids or bases other than carbonic is the HCO_3^-/H_2CO_3 buffer pair itself.

The quantitative relationship between pH, H_2CO_3, and HCO_3^- concentrations is expressed in the Henderson-Hasselbalch equation:

$$pH = pK'_1 + \log \frac{[HCO_3^-]}{[H_2CO_3]}$$

Since $H_2CO_3 = s\ P_{CO_2}$, the expression may be rewritten:

$$pH = pK'_1 + \log \frac{[HCO_3^-]}{s\ P_{CO_2}}$$

At 38° C, s has the value of 0.03 in plasma when concentrations are expressed in millimoles per liter (mM/liter) and pK'_1 has the value 6.10. The normal value for HCO_3^- in arterial plasma is 24 mM per liter and the normal value for P_{CO_2} is 40 mm Hg. Therefore, the equation with normal values is:

$$pH = 6.10 + \log \frac{24}{0.03 \times 40} = 6.10 + 1.3 = 7.40$$

It should be pointed out that the Henderson-Hasselbalch equation applies to blood plasma and not to whole blood. Since the pH of whole blood is the pH of plasma and the P_{CO_2} of whole blood and plasma are identical, however, these two variables may be determined directly on whole blood and used in the equation to calculate bicarbonate concentration of plasma. The Henderson-Hasselbalch equation makes it clear that blood pH depends on the ratio of bicarbonate concentration and CO_2 tension. Evidently we would have normal pH if plasma bicarbonate were 12 mM per liter and P_{CO_2} were 20 mm Hg, or if bicarbonate were 36 and P_{CO_2} were 60.

It is helpful to visualize the interrelationships among the three variables of the Henderson-Hasselbalch equation by graphic representation. Any two of these three variables can be plotted against each other with the third appearing as a series of constant values, or all three variables can be plotted against each other on triaxial paper. One of the more successful teaching approaches is that presented by Peters and Van Slyke and employed very effectively by Davenport in his monograph, *ABC of Acid Base Chemistry*. In this approach, pH is plotted against bicarbonate concentration with CO_2 tensions shown as a series of isobars (Fig. 4-4); this figure is simply a graphic representation of the Henderson-Hasselbalch equation. It gives no information whatever about the behavior of blood in or out of the body. If we take a sample of oxygenated blood having a hemoglobin concentration of 15 gm% and divide it into three aliquots, equilibrate the first with a P_{CO_2} of 20, the second with a P_{CO_2} of 40, the third with a P_{CO_2} of 60, and then determine the pH of each aliquot, the points illustrated in Figure 4-5 will obtain. A straight line through these points constitutes the so-called normal CO_2 buffer curve, or normal CO_2 buffer slope of true plasma. Since this is simply a CO_2 titration of blood, for which Hb is the principal buffer, the slope of this line is primarily a function of the Hb concentration.

If we repeat this experiment, but in the second instance equilibrate the blood with mixtures of gas having the same CO_2 tensions but containing nitrogen instead of oxygen, we will obtain a second set of points describing

Fig. 4–4.—A graphic representation of the relationship among the three variables of the Henderson-Hasselbalch equation. This graph is commonly called the pH-HCO$_3^-$ diagram.

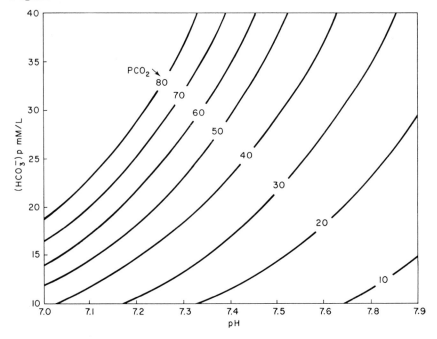

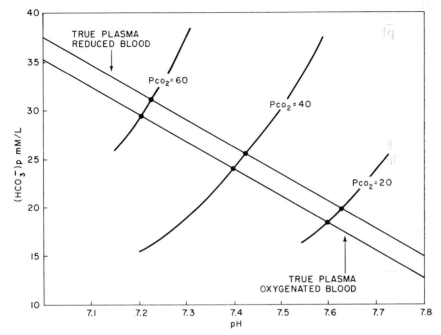

Fig. 4–5.—In vitro CO_2 buffer curves of reduced and oxygenated true plasma.

a line parallel to, but lying above, the line obtained with oxygenated Hb. That reduced Hb carries more CO_2 at the same pH is again evidence that reduced Hb is a weaker acid than oxygenated Hb. For each millimole of oxygen liberated from Hb, 0.7 mM of H^+ is taken up from solution and thus 0.7 mM of CO_2 can be carried with no change in pH.

The equation for the slope of the CO_2 buffer line of true plasma is given by the equation:

$$\frac{\Delta[HCO_3^-]_p}{\Delta\,pH} = -\,[2.5\,(Hb)_B + 10\,(Pr)_B]$$

in which $(Hb)_B$ is hemoglobin in millimoles per liter of blood water, $(Pr)_B$ is plasma protein concentration expressed in the same units, and $(HCO_3^-)_p$ is bicarbonate concentration in millimoles per liter of plasma water. For blood of normal hemoglobin and protein concentration, the slope is approximately 30 mM of HCO_3^- per liter of plasma per pH unit. Units of the slope of the line in these terms are designated "slykes" (abbreviated sl) in honor of Dr. D. D. Van Slyke, one of the major contributors to our understanding of acid-base chemistry. The equation indicates that plasma proteins are also buffers for carbonic acid; however, quantitatively Hb ordinarily accounts for 85% of the buffering. It is significant that both buffers are contained in vascular fluid and are absent, or present to only a very minor extent, in other extracellular fluids. Since plasma HCO_3^- is in ready-diffusion equilibrium with interstitial fluid, any change in plasma bicarbonate concentration resulting from a change in CO_2 tension is quickly shared with most of the remainder of the extracellular fluid. This means that the in vivo CO_2 blood buffer line has a much lower slope than blood in vitro. The equation for the in vivo CO_2 buffer slope is:

$$\frac{\Delta[HCO_3^-]_p}{\Delta pH} = - \left\{ \frac{V_B}{Ve} [2.5\,(Hb)_B + 10\,(Pr)_B] + \frac{Ve - V_B}{Ve} [10\,(Pr)_I] \right\}$$

in which V_B is volume of blood water, Ve is volume of extracellular fluid water, and $(Pr)_I$ is protein concentration in interstitial fluid water. Normal values give an in vivo slope of approximately 12 sl. That is, the in vitro slope of approximately 30 sl has been diluted by a factor of 2.5. Again, a principal determinant of the slope of this line is the Hb concentration of blood. Figure 4-6 demonstrates the change in slope of the in vivo CO_2 buffer line produced by changes in Hb concentration. If $\pm$ 1 mM per liter in plasma HCO_3^- is accepted as normal variation around the mean value, a band 2 mM per liter in width may be drawn for the normal slope (Fig.

Fig. 4–6.—In vivo CO_2 buffer curves of true oxygenated plasma taken from bloods of varying hemoglobin concentrations.

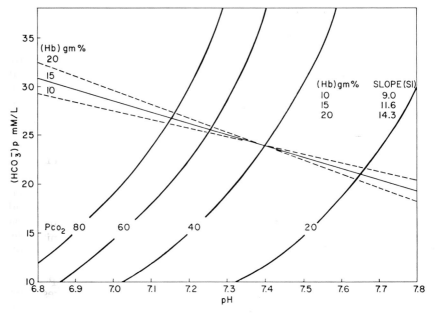

4-7). This band includes the buffer slopes for Hb concentrations between 5 and 20 gm% over the range of Pco_2 values from 20 to 80 mm Hg, and thus the variation in buffer slope due to variations in hemoglobin concentration over these ranges may be largely ignored.

By using the pH bicarbonate diagram as exhibited in Figure 4-7, one can represent all the possible variations in the three variables of the Henderson-Hasselbalch equation. For example, an increase in CO_2 tension titrates the Hb buffers of the blood, increases the bicarbonate concentration, and moves the point up the normal CO_2 buffer slope to the left, reducing blood pH. This is respiratory acidosis. Although the bicarbonate concentration was increased by Hb buffering, it was not increased in proportion to the increase in CO_2 tension and the pH fell. For those who prefer to think in terms of the equation rather than a graph, respiratory acidosis is the situation in which the primary change is an increase in CO_2 tension (denominator of the fraction) with a proportionately smaller increase in HCO_3^- (numerator of the fraction) and a decrease in the value of the fraction.

Reducing the CO_2 tension would titrate the Hb buffers in the opposite

Fig. 4–7.—A useful diagram for clinical evaluation of the acid-base status of a patient. The in vivo buffer slope is that of true plasma from blood of normal hemoglobin concentration. The dashed lines are 1 mM/L of (HCO_3^-)p above and below the normal buffer line.

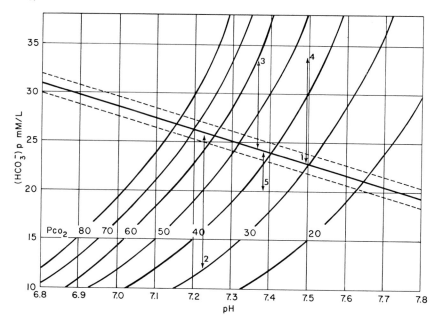

direction, move the point down the buffer slope to the right, and increase the pH. This is respiratory alkalosis. Primary alterations in CO_2 tensions are spoken of as respiratory changes, since the CO_2 tension of alveolar air and arterial blood is governed primarily by the effectiveness of alveolar ventilation.

Invasion of an acid stronger than carbonic would convert bicarbonate to H_2CO_3, and if there was no change in Pco_2, the blood would be titrated down the Pco_2 isobar, which swings to the left as it moves down, and the pH would fall. This is metabolic acidosis. It is represented in the Henderson-Hasselbalch equation as a decrease in the numerator of the fraction with no change in the denominator. Addition of strong base with constant Pco_2 results in the formation of additional bicarbonate, titrating the blood up the Pco_2 isobar and resulting in an increase in blood pH. This is metabolic alkalosis.

The four primary uncompensated acid-base disturbances are:

1. Respiratory acidosis. Represented graphically by any point on the

Fig. 4–8.—Primary acid-base abnormalities and partially compensated states depicted on the pH-HCO_3^- diagram. (1) Respiratory acidosis, (2) partially compensated respiratory acidosis, (3) respiratory alkalosis, (4) partially compensated respiratory alkalosis, (5) metabolic acidosis, (6) partially compensated metabolic acidosis, (7) metabolic alkalosis, (8) partially compensated metabolic alkalosis.

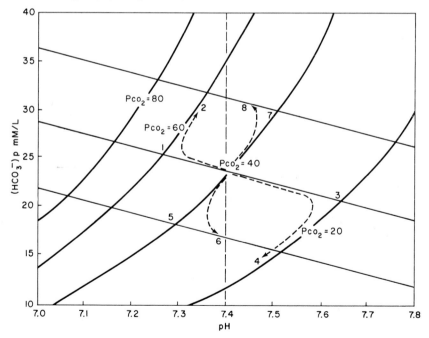

normal buffer line left of the normal point (Fig. 4-8, point 1); character-ized numerically by increased P_{CO_2}, slightly increased HCO_3^-, and de-creased pH. This condition is produced by increased CO_2 tension resulting from inadequate ventilation of the lungs.

2. Respiratory alkalosis. Represented graphically by any point on the normal buffer line to the right of the normal point (Fig. 4-8, point 3); characterized numerically by decreased P_{CO_2}, slightly decreased HCO_3^-, and increased pH. Respiratory alkalosis results from hyperventilation. This condition is frequently present in the shock patient.

3. Metabolic acidosis. Represented graphically by any point on the $P_{CO_2} = 40$ isobar below the normal buffer line (Fig. 4-8, point 5); charac-terized numerically by decreased HCO_3^-, normal P_{CO_2}, and decreased pH. This condition in the shock patient is likely to be due to increased blood lactic acid resulting from poor tissue perfusion. Ordinarily, this condition will be accompanied by some degree of reduced CO_2 tension—a compen-satory change as outlined in the following section.

4. Metabolic alkalosis. Represented graphically by any point on the $P_{CO_2} = 40$ isobar above the normal buffer line (Fig. 4-8, point 7); charac-terized numerically by increased HCO_3^-, normal P_{CO_2}, and increased pH. This condition could be the result of losing HCl by vomiting, or it could result from the infusion of excess bicarbonate solution.

COMPENSATORY CHANGES

When any of the four primary acid-base disturbances exists in the body for longer than a few minutes, compensatory mechanisms are set into effect, resulting in secondary changes that tend to restore blood pH toward normal. In the case of primary metabolic disturbances, the com-pensatory changes occur relatively quickly; in the case of primary respira-tory changes, compensation is brought into effect more slowly.

RESPIRATORY ACIDOSIS

When the primary disturbance is CO_2 retention, restoration of pH toward normal can be effected only by an increase of bicarbonate concen-tration; this is accomplished by the kidneys. With maintained elevated CO_2 tension there is increased reabsorption of bicarbonate by the renal tubules and plasma bicarbonate increases, largely at the expense of reduc-tion of chloride. If the CO_2 tension is not above 60 mm Hg and is main-tained for days or weeks, the compensation may be nearly complete, with pH restored to near normal. With CO_2 retention as the primary distur-bance and elevation of bicarbonate as the compensatory mechanism, we speak of a compensated or partially compensated respiratory acidosis. It is not correct to speak of this condition as respiratory acidosis and metabolic alkalosis. Metabolic alkalosis is another type of primary disturbance and is not a compensating mechanism. A partially compensated respiratory acidosis is shown as position 2 in Figure 4-8.

Respiratory Alkalosis

Compensation for respiratory alkalosis requires a reduction in HCO_3^- concentration. If the hyperventilation producing respiratory alkalosis continues over a long period, as might be the case with the patient on an improperly adjusted respirator, the kidneys will lose bicarbonate by decreasing reabsorption and thus decrease the concentration of bicarbonate in the plasma. The pH would be restored toward normal and a state of compensated, or partially compensated, respiratory alkalosis would result. Position 4 in Figure 4-8 illustrates this condition. Again, it is not correct to call this condition respiratory alkalosis and metabolic acidosis.

Metabolic Acidosis

To compensate for the low pH of metabolic acidosis, reduction in CO_2 tension is required. Since respiratory chemoreceptors are sensitive to increased hydrogen ion concentration, respiration is increased almost immediately following the decrease in pH in metabolic acidosis, and an increase in ventilation follows. This situation is illustrated by position 6 in Figure 4-8. Clinically we would expect to find some reduction in CO_2 tension accompanying any metabolic acidosis unless the patient was not responsive to elevated hydrogen ion concentration.

Metabolic Alkalosis

Metabolic alkalosis can be compensated only by an increase in CO_2 tension. With the decrease in hydrogen ion concentration, decreased stimulation of the respiratory chemoreceptors takes place and some decrease in ventilation follows. Although some compensation is found in metabolic alkalosis, both experimentally and clinically, the compensation is rarely, if ever, complete. In experimental metabolic alkalosis, produced either acutely by infusion of $NaHCO_3$ or chronically by removal of gastric hydrochloric acid, partial compensation as evidenced by an increase in CO_2 tension was regularly found. In no case, however, was the compensation complete. It would hardly be expected that body economy would allow restoration of pH at the expense of diminished ventilation with resulting inadequate delivery of oxygen to tissues. Position 8 in Figure 4-8 illustrates a partially compensated metabolic alkalosis.

USE OF THE DIAGRAM

The pH–HCO_3^- diagram can be divided into four quadrants separated by the $Pco_2 = 40$ isobar and the normal buffer line (Fig. 4-9). The upper left and lower right quadrants are the areas of compensation in which the initial pH of any primary disturbance is moved back toward the pH 7.40 line. The lower left and upper right quadrants are the quadrants in which acid-base aberrations are compounded. In the left quadrant both metabolic and respiratory acidosis are present, and in the right quadrant both types of alkalosis are found.

The deviation of Pa_{CO_2} above or below the normal value of 40 mm Hg measures the respiratory component in an acid-base disturbance. In order to quantitate the nonrespiratory component [ΔHCO_3^-], it is necessary to know the slope of the CO_2 buffer curve. A simple illustration will make

Fig. 4–9.—The pH-HCO_3^- diagram divided into 4 labeled quadrants to indicate the acid-base designation of a blood sample giving values that place it in one of the quadrants.

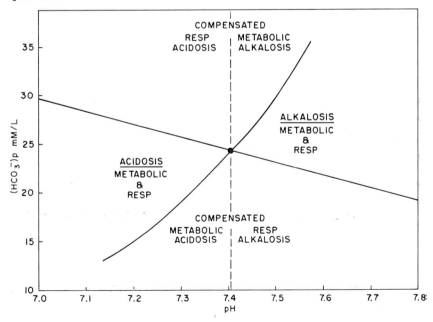

this clear. Suppose, for example, that an arterial blood sample drawn from a patient has a Pco_2 of 80 mm Hg, a pH of 7.21, and a bicarbonate of 31 mM per liter. Immediately, these questions arise: "Is the bicarbonate of 31 mM per liter the value that would be produced by the buffering and distribution resulting from increasing the Pco_2 from 40 to 80 mm Hg?" "Have compensatory mechanisms increased bicarbonate concentration or has metabolic acidosis reduced the bicarbonate below the cencentration which would have been produced by the Pco_2 increase alone?" By placing a point on Figure 4-7 at $Pco_2 = 80$ and $(HCO_3^-)p = 31$, we can see immediately that the HCO_3^- value is approximately 5 mM per liter higher than would have been produced by the respiratory change alone. As the diagram demonstrates, the plasma bicarbonate value to be expected at any given CO_2 tension depends on the pH. Thus, a plasma bicarbonate concentration of 24 mM per liter is normal at pH 7.40; distinctly low at pH 7.10, and high at pH 7.70. A sufficiently accurate estimate of the non-respiratory component can be obtained by using Figure 4-7 and simply measuring the deviation of the plasma bicarbonate value from the value that would be expected at that pH.

In the following examples the $\Delta(HCO_3^-)p$ has been estimated by plotting the values on such a diagram.

	pH	Pco_2	(HCO_3^-)	ΔHCO_3^-
1	7.51	30	23	0
2	7.22	30	11.8	−15
3	7.37	60	33.6	+9
4	7.50	45	34	+11
5	7.38	35	20	−4

Acid-Base Derangements in Shock

It is now clear that the acid-base status of the post-traumatic patient is not always one of simple metabolic acidosis due to inadequate tissue perfusion. In a group of 66 severely wounded soldiers who were in hemorrhagic shock when hospitalized, Cloutier et al. reported that 13 had low pH, low plasma bicarbonate, and normal Pco_2. Mean arterial plasma values in these patients were pH 7.15, HCO_3^- 15.9 mM per liter, and Pco_2 42.1 mm Hg. This is simple uncomplicated metabolic acidosis. It is surprising that there was no increase in ventilation in response to the low pH. It was assumed that these patients were so severely injured and had lost blood rapidly to the point at which they were not responsive to the acidosis as a respiratory stimulus.

In the same study 45 patients had pH values between 7.31 and 7.49 with average Pco_2 of 33.2 and HCO_3^- of 22 mM per liter. These patients had a mild metabolic acidosis which was, on the average, compensated by a slight degree of hyperventilation. The remaining 8 patients were frankly alkalotic with blood pH greater than 7.5, Pco_2 of 30, and bicarbonate of 28.6 mM per liter. These patients demonstrated both respiratory and metabolic alkalosis.

Moore and co-workers divide the response of the post-traumatic patient who is experiencing pulmonary insufficiency into four stages. In the immediate post-shock state (phase I) and after stabilization of the cardiovascular state, the patient exhibits simple respiratory alkalosis. In this phase the lactic acid increase which developed during the poor perfusion state has been metabolized and only a slight lactacidemia, if any, is present. In phase II, respiratory alkalosis continues with low Pco_2 and elevated pH, and only in phase III with advancing pulmonary insufficiency is Pco_2 elevated slightly above normal and blood pH less than 7.40. In phase IV, the preterminal state, Pco_2 is elevated, pH is very low, and a combination of respiratory and metabolic acidosis is present.

Hyperventilation hypocapnia is such a common finding after an episode of shock that it merits comment. Several different mechanisms may be operating to produce hyperventilation under these conditions. In the patient who is still responsive, the metabolic acidosis of the initial shock phase would result in increased ventilation. After stabilization of the cardiovascular state with restoration of adequate tissue perfusion and metabolism of the excess lactic acid, it might be expected that the hyperventilation would subside. If the low Pco_2 has been maintained for several hours, however, it is quite possible that cerebrospinal fluid bicarbonate concentration may have been lowered to the degree that any elevation of CO_2 tension toward normal will produce an increased hydrogen ion concentration in the cerebrospinal fluid with a resulting continued stimulus for increased breathing. A second factor that may operate to increase ventilation in these patients is low arterial blood oxygen tension. Again, if the hyperventilation has been continued for several hours, elevation of oxygen tension above 100 mm Hg may not result in a decrease in ventilation to its normal value. In cases of head injury, direct stimulus of respiratory centers may be producing the hyperventilation.

Figure 3-26 illustrates a situation in which hyperventilation had been present for some 30 hours, after which the patient did not tolerate elevations of CO_2 tension to levels that were still below the levels she had exhibited before the hyperventilation began.

REFERENCES

ENERGY METABOLISM IN SHOCK

Brin, M.: The synthesis and metabolism of lactic acid isomers, Ann. New York Acad. Sc. 119:942, 1965.

Dahl, N. A., and Balfour, W. M.: Prolonged anoxic survival due to preexposure to anoxia: Brain ATP and lactate changes, Fed. Proc. 22:2823, 1963.

Drury, D. R., and Wick, A. N.: Chemistry and metabolism of L (+) and D (−) lactic acids, Ann. New York Acad. Sc. 119:1061, 1965.

Hartmann, A. F., and Senn, M. J. E.: Studies in the metabolism of sodium r-lactate: I. Response of normal human subjects to the intravenous injection of sodium r-lactate, J. Clin. Invest. 11:327, 1932.

Huckabee, W. E.: Relationships of pyruvate and lactate during anaerobic metabolism: I. Effects of infusion of pyruvate or glucose and of hyperventilation, J. Clin. Invest. 37:244, 1958.

Huckabee, W. E.: Abnormal resting blood lactate: II. Lactic acidosis, Am. J. Med. 30: 840, 1961.

LePage, G. A.: Biological energy transformations during shock as shown by tissue analyses, Am. J. Physiol. 146:267, 1946.

Olson, R. E.: "Excess lactate" and anaerobiosis, Ann. Int. Med. 59:960, 1963.

Trinkle, J. K., Rush, B. F., and Eiseman, B.: Lactate metabolism following hemorrhage, Surg. Forum 18:1, 1967.

ULTRASTRUCTURAL CHANGES

deDuve, C.: Lysosomes: A New Group of Cytoplasmic Particles, in *Subcellular Particles* (New York: Ronald Press Company, 1959).

Hift, H., and Strawitz, J. G.: Irreversible hemorrhagic shock in dogs: Problem of onset of irreversibility, Am. J. Physiol. 200:269, 1961.

Janoff, A., Weissmann, G., Zweifach, B. W., and Thomas, L.: Pathogenesis of experimental shock. IV. Studies on lysosomes in normal and tolerant animals subjected to lethal trauma and endotoxemia, J. Exper. Med. 116:451, 1962.

Weissmann, G., and Thomas, L.: Studies on lysosomes: I. Effects of endotoxin, endotoxin tolerance, and cortisone on release of enzymes from granular fraction of rabbit fever, J. Exper. Med. 116:433, 1962.

ACID-BASE REGULATION

Beisel, W. R., and Rapoport, M. I.: Adrenocortical function and infectious illness, New England J. Med. 280:541, 596, 1969.

Brackett, N. C., Cohen, J. J., and Schwartz, W. B.: Carbon dioxide titration curve of normal man, New England J. Med. 272:6, 1965.

Brown, E. B., and Clancy, R. L.: In vivo and in vitro CO_2 blood buffer curves, J. Appl. Physiol. 20:885, 1965.

Brown, E. B., and Michel, C.: Whole body CO_2 exchange, Proc. Internat. Union Physiol. Sc. 6:185, 1968.

Cloutier, C. T., Lowery, B. D., and Carey, L. C.: Acid-base disturbances in hemorrhagic shock, Arch. Surg. 98:551, 1969.

Davenport, H. W.: *The ABC of Acid-Base Chemistry* (Chicago: The University of Chicago Press, 1958).

Moore, F. D., Lyons, J. H., Pierce, E. C., Morgan, A. P., Jr., Drinker, P. A., MacArthur, J. D., and Dammin, G. J. (eds.): *Post-Traumatic Pulmonary Insufficiency* (Philadelphia: W. B. Saunders Company, 1969).

Peters, J. P., and Van Slyke, D. D.: Hemoglobin and oxygen; carbonic acid and acid-base balance, in *Quantitative Clinical Chemistry,* Vol. 1, *Interpretations* (Baltimore: Williams & Wilkins, 1931), Chaps. 12 and 18.

Reeves, J. L., and Brown, E. B., Jr.: Respiratory compensation to metabolic alkalosis in dogs: Influence of high oxygen concentration, J. Appl. Physiol. 13:179, 1958.

Siggaard-Andersen, O.: *The Acid-Base Status of the Blood* (Copenhagen: Munksgaard, 1964).

Winters, R. W., Engel, K., and Dell, R. B.: *Acid-Base Physiology in Medicine* (Cleveland: The London Company, and Copenhagen: Radiometer A/S, 1968).

Woodbury, J. W.: Regulation of pH, in Ruch, T. C., and Patton, H. D. (eds.): *Physiology and Biophysics* (Philadelphia: W. B. Saunders Company, 1966), Chap. 46.

5

Important Measurements and Useful Calculations in Monitoring

Clinical Observation

IN THE CARE of the patient in shock, a continuous record of the clinical, hemodynamic, and chemical measurements will help to identify the type of shock, define its severity, and measure the efficacy of therapy.

Hypotension, while commonly regarded as the prime requisite for the diagnosis of shock, may actually be a late sign. Often the initial reaction to injury is vasoconstriction, which may mask a considerable fall in cardiac output before hypotension is manifest. Early recognition of the signs of increased sympathetic activity provides an important basis for the clinical diagnosis of shock. The experienced clinician notes the anxious face, the pale, mottled, clammy skin and the cool, sweating extremities, the collapsed veins of the dorsum of the hand, the rapid thready pulse, and the heavy breathing. The patient's history may be of prime importance in pointing to the origin of the illness. After the physical examination, chest x-ray, and routine laboratory examinations have been carried out, the following clinical variables are recorded at frequent intervals:

State of consciousness: restless, anxious, agitated, depressed
Skin: temperature, moistness, color, and turgor
Mucous membranes: color, moistness
Nail beds: color, capillary refill
Peripheral veins: collapsed or distended
Neck veins: collapsed or distended
Pulse: rate and quality
Respiration: rate and depth
Urine output: hourly

Hemodynamic Measurements

The arterial blood pressure alone is a poor indication of the severity of shock. Some patients with a normal or even a raised blood pressure due to excessive vasoconstriction are on the verge of disaster, whereas patients with generalized vasodilation may readily tolerate rather severe hypotension. An example of this is seen following cervical cord section. The management of the shock episode is usually based upon frequent measurements of central venous pressure (CVP), blood pressure, and pulse rate. The graphic recording of these values every 15 minutes, or oftener if needed, gives a general picture of the changes and trends in the patient's condition and reflects the response to treatment. In general, the shock patient has a narrow pulse pressure and tachycardia. After effective therapy, a widening of the pulse pressure and a fall in pulse rate are signs of hemodynamic improvement.

Progress toward recovery or deterioration is best signaled hemodynamically by considering together the response of the CVP, arterial pressure, and urinary output to treatment. More complicated measurements, such as cardiac output or calculated stroke volume and total peripheral resistance, allow a more precise appraisal of the patient's cardiovascular response. The equipment for such measurements is now becoming more generally available, but careful clinical observation alone and simple measurements often provide sufficient information to form a rough estimate of these values.

CENTRAL VENOUS PRESSURE

In all forms of shock the physician must be assured, above all, that the atrial filling pressure is adequate to provide an effective cardiac output. This essential information is gained by direct measurement of the CVP. In addition, inspection of the veins of the dorsum of the hand or foot gives information regarding contraction or expansion of the peripheral venous reservoir provided the extremities are kept warm.

PITFALLS IN THE TECHNIQUE OF MEASURING AND IN INTERPRETING CENTRAL VENOUS PRESSURE

To accomplish the object of this procedure, the tip of a large bore catheter must be placed within the superior vena cava or right atrium (Fig. 5-1). Often these catheters, placed blindly through an arm vein, end up in unexpected sites: curling up the jugular vein near the base of the skull, passing across the innominate vein to the opposite arm, or extending down the inferior vena cava below the diaphragm. In addition, impaction or clotting of the tip may occur at any site. Accordingly, satisfactory placement must be checked thoroughly and a zero point marked on the wall of the patient's chest before measurement is made. Free flow of solution indicates that the

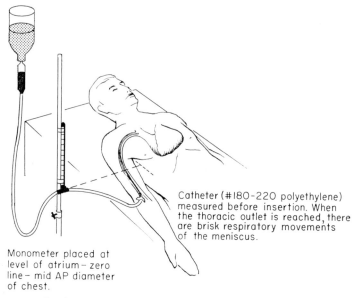

Catheter (#180-220 polyethylene) measured before insertion. When the thoracic outlet is reached, there are brisk respiratory movements of the meniscus.

Monometer placed at level of atrium – zero line – mid AP diameter of chest.

Fig. 5–1.—A basilic or brachial vein cut down at the elbow is performed and a large polyethylene catheter is passed as far as the superior vena cava or until wide excursions in central venous pressure occur with each breath. Zero reference point for measurements is the middle of the anteroposterior diameter of the chest. Central venous pressure can also be measured by direct puncture into the subclavian vein under and parallel to the first portion of the clavicle. (From Thal, A. P., and Wilson, R. F.: Shock, in *Current Problems in Surgery* [Chicago: Year Book Medical Publishers, Sept., 1965].)

tip is not impacted, and wide respiratory excursion assures that the tip is within the thoracic cavity. A final check is evident when the chest x-ray is examined.

Interpretation of CVP measurements is made in conjunction with other clinical and hemodynamic responses, and the value is seldom considered as an isolated guide to therapy. It reflects the filling pressure at which the right ventricle is operating. A low-level (less than 2 cm) CVP indicates an inadequate right atrial filling pressure, hence, hypovolemia; a high level (over 15 cm) indicates heart failure. Between these extremes, other information and even a test of volume loading is usually necessary for a meaningful interpretation of the CVP. When the diagnosis of hypovolemia is in doubt, a clinical and hemodynamic response to rapid volume loading of 500 ml of blood or colloid solution within a 20 minute period is often valuable. This form of therapy may be fraught with hazard if the patient is not closely observed for signs of cardiac failure and pulmonary congestion. These signs are manifested by a rise of left atrial pressure which precedes, often by minutes or hours, the rise in CVP. Accordingly, symptoms of dyspnea with the physical signs of pulmonary congestion are urgent indications for stopping the infusion. Conversely, an improvement in the patient's clinical condition, a lessening of skin vasoconstriction, and improvement in hourly urine output and in arterial blood pressure without signs of overloading are indications for continuing and increasing the infusion. This cardiovascular response to fluid load undoubtedly is the single most valuable diagnostic tool in differentiating hypovolemic from cardiogenic shock.

Central venous pressure is a resultant of several factors acting together. These factors include the competence of the right ventricle, the volume of blood within the central veins, the intrathoracic pressure, and the venous tone. It is clear then that artifacts in the interpretation of CVP are likely to occur in the patient on vasoconstrictor drugs which increase venous tone or on positive-pressure ventilation which produces an increase in intrathoracic pressure. The assumption that CVP reflects left ventricular filling pressure cannot be relied upon; gross discrepancies may be found in pulmonary embolism when the CVP is high and the left ventricular filling pressure low. Similar changes may be seen in the respiratory distress syndrome; resistance to blood flow through the lungs may be increased due to the extensive parenchymal pulmonary lesions.

The same discrepancies also may occur in patients with acute myocardial infarction who are receiving vasopressor treatment or beta adrenergic stimulating drugs. Again, as pointed out previously, with frank left ventricular failure, the rise in CVP may be delayed as long as the right ventricle remains competent.

Chemical Measurements

Measurements of arterial pH, Pco_2, and Po_2 are so important in the care of the critically ill patient that every major hospital should provide this service around the clock. As stated previously, the typical acid-base change in advanced shock is metabolic acidosis demonstrated by a falling plasma bicarbonate, compensatory hypocapnea, and venous desaturation. The HCO_3^- deficit indicates the degree of cellular hypoxia, which can be measured more precisely by the determination of serum lactate. This measurement, however, is not generally available in most hospitals.

Repeated measurements of venous saturation in samples drawn from a constant site, preferably close to the right atrium, offer a valuable measure of cellular hypoxia. Serum sodium levels indicate trends toward cellular overhydration or dehydration. Elevated potassium values may dictate the need for dialysis. Many other determinations, including that of blood volume, can also be done, but are of relatively less value in shock since they are difficult to interpret unless extreme deficits are present. One reason for this difficulty is the altered capacity of the vascular system in the shock patient. A dynamic relationship, such as the response of the venous pressure to loading, provides more useful information.

Central venous blood hemoglobin saturation cannot be assumed to approximate mixed blood venous saturation in the patient in shock. The studies of Shineman et al. illustrate a poor correlation ($r = 0.55$) between central venous blood saturation and mixed venous blood saturation, but an excellent correlation between high right atrial blood hemoglobin ($r = 0.97$) and mixed venous blood hemoglobin saturation. In shock, comparison of central venous blood hemoglobin saturation with mixed venous blood hemoglobin saturation reveals a higher value for the former. This finding probably relates to the maintenance of blood flow in the brain producing a higher central venous blood hemoglobin saturation in the presence of a low saturation in the inferior vena cava because of low flow in its area of drainage.

PULMONARY GAS EXCHANGE

One of the most significant recent developments in the care of shock patients has been the recognition of the severity of the lung dysfunction which often precedes the change in the chest x-ray by several days. Ventilator assistance is often necessary, and under these circumstances the following measurements are required for optimal support:

Tidal volume: obtained from spirometer of ventilator
Ventilatory rate
Peak airway pressure
$F_{I_{O_2}}$ (O_2 concentration of inspired air): readily determined with the Beckman paramagnetic O_2 analyzer
Arterial P_{CO_2}, P_{O_2}

Simple calculations from these data give minute volume and an indication of total chest compliance. More sophisticated but important equations reveal the physiologic dead space and venous admixture. Measurement of arterial P_{O_2}, when $F_{I_{O_2}}$ is unknown, blinds the clinician to the extent of lung damage. For example, an arterial P_{O_2} of 80 mm Hg in room air reveals satisfactory gas exchange, whereas a P_{O_2} of 120 mm Hg at an inspired O_2 of 80% shows severe ventilation perfusion imbalance.

A simple and valuable guide to the degree of shunting may be obtained by measuring the arterial Po_2 after the patient has breathed 100% oxygen for 15 minutes. Under these circumstances, the alveolar Po_2 = barometric pressure − (water vapor pressure + alveolar CO_2 partial pressure [assumed to equal arterial Pco_2]) = 760 − (47 + 40) = 673 mm Hg. The normal A-aDo_2 is approximately 40 mm Hg.

As the pulmonary venous admixture increases, the A-aDo_2 widens and, conversely, response to therapy is indicated by a narrowing of this difference. Charting of these values provides an excellent measure of the therapy (see Figs. 5-3 and 5-4).

More complicated measurements and calculations give information of great help in providing optimal care for the patient. While these values were formerly obtainable only in the research investigative unit, currently they are becoming available in the clinical care area.

Determination of Blood Flow through an Organ

Blood flow through an organ can be estimated by the Fick principle if three variables are known. These variables are (1) rate of addition to or removal from the blood of any measurable substance (S) by the organ, (2) Concentration of S in blood flowing into the organ, (S)a, and (3) Concentration of S in blood flowing from the organ, (S)v.

The rate at which blood is delivering S into the organ is the product of rate of blood flow into the organ ($\dot{Q}$in), and (S)a

$$\dot{S}in = \dot{Q}in(S)a$$

Similarly, the rate at which S is leaving the organ is

$$\dot{S}out = \dot{Q}out(S)v$$

Normally $\dot{Q}out = \dot{Q}in = \dot{Q}$
If S is added to the blood by the organ

$$\dot{Q}(S)v = \dot{Q}(S)a + \dot{V}s \qquad (1)$$

in which $\dot{V}s$ is the rate at which S is added to the blood by the organ.

$$\dot{Q} = \frac{\dot{V}s}{(S)v - (S)a} \qquad (2)$$

When the indicator substance is being removed from the blood by the organ, i.e., (S)v < (S)a, the signs in the denominator are reversed and $\dot{V}s$ becomes the rate of removal of S from the blood.

Cardiac Output

Oxygen fick technique.—When equation (2) is applied to the measurement of pulmonary blood flow with oxygen as the indicator substance, it is called the Oxygen Fick equation.

$$\dot{Q} = \frac{\dot{V}_{O_2}}{(O_2)a - (O_2)\bar{v}} \qquad (3)$$

Example: If the rate of oxygen uptake is 240 ml per minute and mixed venous and arterial blood O_2 concentrations are 14 vol% and 20 vol% respectively, cardiac output is

$$\dot{Q} = \frac{240 \text{ ml/min}}{0.20 \text{ ml/ml} - 0.14 \text{ ml/ml}} = \frac{240 \text{ ml/min}}{0.06 \text{ ml/ml}} = 4{,}000 \text{ ml/min}$$

Normally pulmonary blood flow is equal to cardiac output, and C.O. is usually substituted for $\dot{Q}$ in equation (3). In order to have an adequate sample of blood (mixed venous blood) for determination of O_2 concentration of blood flowing into the lungs a catheter must be threaded into the pulmonary artery. The "aorta" sample may be obtained from any artery.

DYE DILUTION TECHNIQUE.—In the dye dilution technique, instead of relying on the organ to add a substance to the blood, a known quantity of a dye is injected into the blood flowing into the organ, and its concentration is measured in the blood draining the organ. The principle utilized is that of determining the volume of dilution of a known quantity of dye injected into the blood and simultaneously determining the time required for this volume to pass a point in the circulation.

The volume of dilution will be

$$Y = \frac{D}{\bar{C}}$$

in which

Y = Volume in which D is diluted
D = Quantity of dye injected
$\bar{C}$ = Mean concentration of dye in blood

Thus if 10 mg of dye is injected and the mean concentration in the blood in which it is diluted is 5 mg per liter, the volume of dilution is 2 liters

$$Y = \frac{10 \text{ mg}}{5 \text{ mg/liter}} = 2 \text{ liters}$$

If this volume of dyed blood passes a point in the circulation in 20 seconds, blood flow is

$$2 \times \frac{60}{20} = 6 \text{ liters per minute}$$

The general expression is

$$\dot{Q} = \frac{D \times 60}{\bar{C}t}$$

where t is the time in seconds for first passage of the dye.

Mean concentration of the dye in the blood is determined by recording the concentration as a continuous variable from first appearance until the dye reappears the second time by recirculation, measuring the area (A) under the properly corrected curve, and dividing by the time.

$$\overline{C} = \frac{A}{t}$$

Then
$$\dot{Q} = \frac{D \times 60}{\dfrac{A \times t}{t}} = \frac{D \times 60}{A} \tag{5}$$

Various methods have been used for measuring the area under the curve, and instruments are available that make this measurement, compute the flow, $\dot{Q}$, and present a digital readout of the value immediately upon completion of drawing the blood through the instrument.

When the dye is injected into a central vein and the sample is drawn from an artery, pulmonary blood flow or cardiac output is measured.

THE SHUNT EQUATION.—Consider the situation in which part of the pulmonary blood flow (cardiac output) is perfusing well-ventilated alveoli and the remainder is perfusing nonventilated alveoli (Fig. 5-2). Total pulmonary blood flow ($\dot{Q}T$) may be calculated by the Fick equation as follows:

$$\dot{Q}T = \frac{\dot{V}O_2}{Ca_{O_2} - C\bar{v}_{O_2}} \tag{1}$$

in which $\dot{V}O_2$ is rate of oxygen uptake from the lungs in cubic centimeters per minute (ml per min.), Ca_{O_2} and $C\bar{v}_{O_2}$ are oxygen concentration of arterial blood and mixed venous blood respectively, expressed as cubic centimeters per one hundred milliliter (cc per 100 ml) of blood. $\dot{Q}T$ has

Fig. 5–2.—The concept of venous admixture used in the shunt equation.

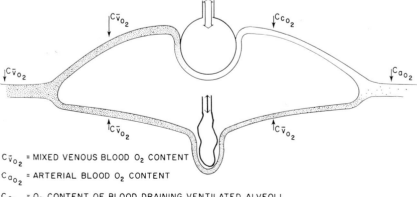

$C\bar{v}_{O_2}$ = MIXED VENOUS BLOOD O_2 CONTENT

Ca_{O_2} = ARTERIAL BLOOD O_2 CONTENT

Cc_{O_2} = O_2 CONTENT OF BLOOD DRAINING VENTILATED ALVEOLI

the same dimensions as $\dot{V}_{O_2}$.

Similarly the flow through ventilated alveoli, ($\dot{Q}_A$), is

$$\dot{Q}_A = \frac{\dot{V}_{O_2}}{C_{C_{O_2}} - C\bar{v}_{O_2}} \tag{2}$$

in which $C_{C_{O_2}}$ is O_2 concentration of blood that has perfused ventilated alveoli (2). The fraction of total flow perfusing ventilated alveoli is

$$\frac{\dot{Q}_A}{\dot{Q}_T} = \frac{C_{a_{O_2}} - C\bar{v}_{O_2}}{C_{C_{O_2}} - C\bar{v}_{O_2}} \tag{3}$$

This equation states that the value of the fraction approaches 1 (all blood perfusing ventilated alveoli; no shunt) as $C_{a_{O_2}}$ approaches $C_{C_{O_2}}$. From this point on O_2 concentrations will be expressed as vol%. Since the fraction $\dot{Q}_s/\dot{Q}_T$ is dimensionless, any unit of concentration may be used so long as it is used consistently, and vol% is more convenient than cc per 100 ml.

More commonly the shunt flow, i.e., flow through unventilated alveoli ($\dot{Q}_s$), is calculated as a fraction of total flow. This fraction ($\dot{Q}_s/\dot{Q}_T$) is $1 - \frac{\dot{Q}_A}{\dot{Q}_T}$. Therefore

$$\frac{\dot{Q}_s}{\dot{Q}_T} = 1 - \left[\frac{C_{a_{O_2}} - C\bar{v}_{O_2}}{C_{C_{O_2}} - C\bar{v}_{O_2}} \right] = \left[\frac{C_{C_{O_2}} - C_{a_{O_2}}}{C_{C_{O_2}} - C\bar{v}_{O_2}} \right] \tag{4}$$

This equation indicates that the fraction of blood shunted approaches zero as $C_{a_{O_2}}$ approaches $C_{C_{O_2}}$.

The values for all three variables in this equation are rarely, if ever, available; however, the equation is useful if certain conditions and assumptions are observed.

The oxygen concentration of any blood sample is the sum of O_2 combined with hemoglobin plus dissolved O_2.

Vol% O_2 combined with Hb = $1.34 \times$ (Hb) $\times$ % saturation

in which (Hb) is gm% and the constant 1.34 is cc of O_2 combined with 1 gm Hb when the Hb is 100% saturated with O_2.

Vol% O_2 dissolved = 0.003 P_{O_2}

in which 0.003 is the solubility coefficient of O_2 in blood at 38°C expressed as vol% per mm Hg.

Total O_2 concentration (vol%) = $(1.34 \times Hb \times \% \text{ saturation}) + .003$ P_{O_2} (5)

Thus if an arterial blood with a hemoglobin concentration of 15 gm% is 90% saturated at a $P_{A_{O_2}}$ of 70 mm Hg, its O_2 content is

$C_{a_{O_2}} = (1.34 \times 15 \times .9) + (.003 \times 70)$
$\quad\quad = 18.09 + 0.21$
$\quad\quad = 18.3$ vol%

Substituting equation (5) for each of the values in (4) we have

$$\frac{\dot{Q}s}{\dot{Q}T} = \frac{\{[1.34\,(Hb)\,\%\,sat.\,c] + .003\,Pc_{O_2}\} - \{[1.34\,(Hb)\,\%\,sat.\,a] + .003\,Pa_{O_2}\}}{\{[1.34\,(Hb)\,\%\,sat.\,c] + .003\,Pc_{O_2}\} - \{[1.34\,(Hb)\,\%\,sat.\,\bar{v}] + .003\,P\bar{v}_{O_2}\}} \tag{6}$$

If we assume that the blood perfusing well-ventilated alveoli has the same O_2 tension as alveolar air, PA_{O_2} may be substituted for Pc_{O_2}. If we make our measurement only after the patient has breathed 100% O_2 for 15 minutes we may assume 100% saturation of blood perfusing ventilated alveoli. Now the first term of the fraction becomes

$$1.34(Hb) + .003\,PA_{O_2}$$

If, under the same conditions, the oxygen tension of arterial blood (determined with an O_2 electrode) is 150 mm Hg or higher, arterial blood is also 100% saturated and the equation may be rewritten

$$\frac{\dot{Q}s}{\dot{Q}T} = \frac{1.34(Hb) + .003\,PA_{O_2} - 1.34(Hb) + .003\,Pa_{O_2}}{1.34(Hb) + .003\,PA_{O_2} - [1.34(Hb)\,\%\,sat.\,\bar{v}] + .003\,P\bar{v}_{O_2}} \tag{7}$$

$$= \frac{.003\,(PA_{O_2} - Pa_{O_2})}{Cc_{O_2} - C\bar{v}_{O_2}}. \tag{8}$$

When c and a are both 100% saturated

$$Cc_{O_2} = Ca_{O_2} + .003\,(PA_{O_2} - Pa_{O_2}) \tag{9}$$

Substituting (9) in (8)

$$\frac{\dot{Q}s}{\dot{Q}T} = \frac{.003\,(PA_{O_2} - Pa_{O_2})}{(Ca_{O_2} - C\bar{v}_{O_2}) + .003\,(PA_{O_2} - Pa_{O_2})} \tag{10}$$

(Remember that equations 7 through 10 are valid *only* when Pa_{O_2} is high enough to insure 100% oxygen saturation of arterial blood. Equation 6 does not have these restrictions.)

Equation 10 makes it clear that under the conditions outlined above and with a constant arterial venous O_2 difference ($Ca_{O_2} - C\bar{v}_{O_2}$), changes in $\dot{Q}s/\dot{Q}T$ will be reflected directly in changes in $PA_{O_2} - Pa_{O_2}$. When the patient is breathing any mixture of O_2 and N_2,

$$PA_{O_2} = \text{Barometric pressure (B)} - PA_{N_2} - PA_{CO_2} - PA_{H_2O} \tag{11}$$

Pa_{CO_2} is assumed to be the same as PA_{CO_2}. When the patient has been breathing 100% oxygen for 15 minutes, PA_{N_2} is assumed to be zero. Under these conditions then,

$$PA_{O_2} = B - Pa_{CO_2} - PA_{H_2O} \tag{12}$$

Example: Calculate fractional shunt from the following data (patient has breathed 100% oxygen for 15 minutes):

$$B = 738 \text{ mm Hg}$$
$$Pa_{CO_2} = 32 \text{ mm Hg}$$
$$PA_{H_2O} = 50 \text{ mm Hg (patient temperature} = 38° \text{ C)}$$
$$Pa_{O_2} = 180 \text{ mm Hg}$$
$$P\bar{v}_{O_2} = 35 \text{ mm Hg}$$
$$\% \text{ sat. } \bar{v} = 70$$
$$Hb = 13.5 \text{ gm}\%$$
$$\overline{PA_{O_2}} = 738 - 32 - 50 = 656 \text{ mm Hg}$$

From equation 7

$$\frac{\dot{Q}s}{\dot{Q}T} = \frac{.003\,(656-180)}{[(1.34 \times 13.5) + (.003 \times 656)] - [(1.34 \times 13.5 \times .7) + (.003 \times 35)]}$$

$$= \frac{1.43}{7.29} = 20\% \text{ shunt}$$

If a mixed venous blood sample had not been available and a normal value of 6 vol% had been assumed for $Ca_{O_2} - C\bar{v}_{O_2}$ the fraction would have been

$$\frac{\dot{Q}s}{\dot{Q}T} = \frac{1.43}{6 + 1.43} = 19\% \text{ shunt}$$

In other words, a reasonably good estimate of shunt can be made by looking at the calculated PA_{O_2} minus the determined Pa_{O_2} when the patient is breathing 100% oxygen. With normal resting O_2 utilization (normal metabolic rate) and normal cardiac output, ($Ca_{O_2} - C\bar{v}_{O_2} = 5$ to 6 vol%) there will be about 5% shunt for each 100 mm Hg A-ao_2 tension difference.

Frequently in the intensive care ward central venous and arterial catheters are left in place. If the % oxygen in the inspired air is known, an estimate of shunt can be made without having the patient breathe 100% oxygen.

Example:

Patient breathing 40% oxygen

$$B = 743 \text{ mm Hg}$$
$$Pa_{CO_2} = 36 \text{ mm Hg}$$
$$PA_{H_2O} = 50 \text{ mm Hg}$$
$$Pa_{O_2} = 65 \text{ mm Hg}$$
$$\% \text{ sat. a} = 90$$
$$P\bar{v}_{O_2} = 32 \text{ mm Hg}$$
$$\% \text{ sat. } \bar{v} = 60$$
$$Hb = 10 \text{ gm}\%$$
$$\overline{PA_{N_2}} \simeq .6\,(743 - 50) = 416$$
$$PA_{O_2} \simeq 743 - 36 - 50 - 416 = 240 \text{ mm Hg}$$

From equation 6

$$\frac{\dot{Q}s}{\dot{Q}_T} = \frac{[(1.34 \times 10) + (.003 \times 240)] - [(1.34 \times 10 \times .9) + (.003 \times 65)]}{[(1.34 \times 10) + (.003 \times 240)] - [(1.34 \times 10 \times .6) + (.003 \times 32)]}$$

$$= \frac{14.12 - 12.26}{14.12 - 8.1} = \frac{1.86}{6.0} = 31\%$$

DEAD SPACE EQUATION.—The air we exhale consists of two fractions. The first fraction has not participated in gas exchange, and its composition is identical with that of inhaled air. This air has come from anatomic dead space plus ventilated but nonperfused alveoli. The second fraction has participated in gas exchange and has the composition of alveolar air.

The first fraction is dead space volume, (V_D). The second fraction is alveolar volume, (V_A), and together they make up the tidal volume, (V_T).

$$V_T = V_D + V_A \qquad (1)$$

Dead space volume may be calculated as follows:
For any gas in the exhaled air

$$V_T F_E = V_D F_I + V_A F_A \qquad (2)$$

Substituting the value of V_A from (1) in (2)

$$V_T F_E = V_D F_I + (V_T - V_D) F_A \qquad (3)$$

Solving for V_D

$$V_D = V_T \left(\frac{F_A - F_E}{F_A - F_I} \right) \qquad (4)$$

If CO_2 is used as the reference gas

$$V_D = V_T \left(\frac{F_{A_{CO_2}} - F_{E_{CO_2}}}{F_{A_{CO_2}} - F_{I_{CO_2}}} \right) \qquad (5)$$

If the patient is breathing air or any other mixture containing no CO_2, ($F_{I_{CO_2}} = 0$) and

$$V_D = V_T \frac{F_{A_{CO_2}} - F_{E_{CO_2}}}{F_{A_{CO_2}}} \qquad (6)$$

Since

$$F_{CO_2} = \frac{P_{CO_2}}{B - P_{H_2O}},$$

$$V_D = V_T \frac{P_{A_{CO_2}} - P_{E_{CO_2}}}{P_{A_{CO_2}}} \qquad (7)$$

If an alveolar gas sample (end tidal) and mixed expired air are analyzed chemically for CO_2, equation (6) is used. If CO_2 meters, recording directly in P_{CO_2}, measure $P_{A_{CO_2}}$ and $P_{E_{CO_2}}$, equation (7) is used. If $P_{a_{CO_2}}$ is being measured, the assumption may be made that $P_{a_{CO_2}} = P_{A_{CO_2}}$ and the equation may be rewritten

$$V_D = V_T \frac{P_{a_{CO_2}} - P_{E_{CO_2}}}{P_{a_{CO_2}}} \tag{8}$$

Fig. 5–3.—Intensive care unit monitoring charts for pulmonary gas exchange.

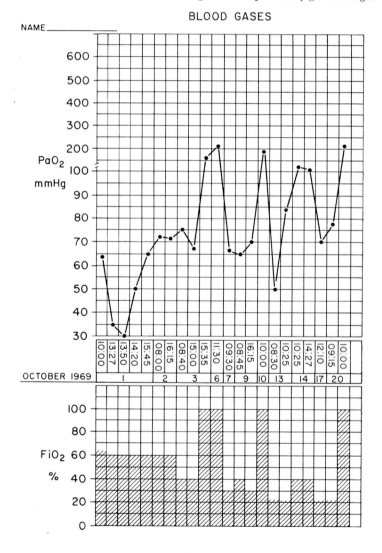

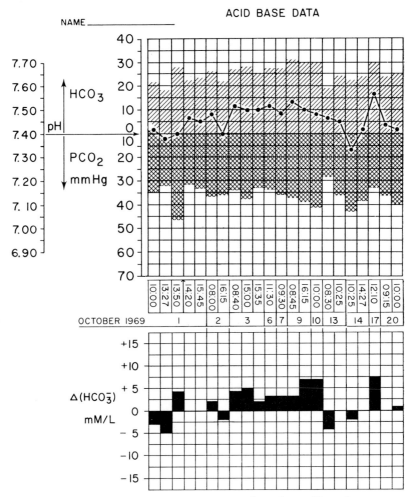

Fig. 5–4.—Intensive care unit monitoring charts for acid base data.

REFERENCES

Borow, M., and Escaro, R.: The reliability of central venous pressure monitoring and errors in its interpretation, Surg. Gynec. & Obst. 127:1288, 1968.

Klein, L. A., and Ketcham, A. S.: Monitoring the central venous pressure, Surg. Gynec. & Obst. 124:120, 1967.

Phillips, S. J.: Technique of percutaneous subclavian vein catheterization, Surg. Gynec. & Obst. 127:1079, 1968.

Rapaport, E., and Scheinman, M.: Rationale and limitations of hemodynamic measurements in patients with acute myocardial infarction, Mod. Concepts Cardiovas. Dis. 38:55, 1969.

6

The Patterns of Shock

WHILE EARLY HYPOVOLEMIC or cardiogenic shock has a clear-cut pattern and a fairly predictable response to therapy, the ultimate outcome is often determined by the subsequent failure of vital organs as a result of initial damage during the shock episode or by the encroachment of pre-existing disease. This sequence of events in shock is illustrated in Figure 6-1. In hemorrhagic or traumatic shock, pre-existing vital organ function is often normal, whereas in cardiogenic and septic shock the existence of a chronic disease process already may have encroached upon the function of one or several vital organs. The study of McAbe and Jackson points dramatically to the importance of host factors in determining recovery from sepsis. Consequently, in defining the depth of shock and the prognosis in a given case, it becomes necessary to have measurements of the reserve function of vital organs and to recognize the signs of impending organ failure (Chapter 7).

Fig. 6–1.—The natural history of shock and the factors determining survival. (From Thal, A. P., and Kinney, J. M.: Prog. Cardiovas. Dis. 9:527, 1967. Used by permission of Grune & Stratton, Inc.)

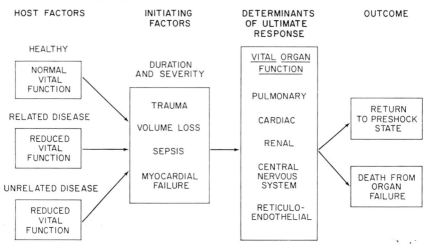

CARDIOGENIC SHOCK

Pure cardiogenic shock is most commonly the result of myocardial infarction. The diagnosis may be established by a typical history and electrocardiographic evidence of myocardial ischemia. The chest x-ray may show pulmonary edema with or without cardiac enlargement. Elevated levels of transaminase in the absence of pulmonary, skeletal muscle, or liver damage are also of value in establishing the diagnosis. Patients generally show evidences of severe peripheral vascular constriction. The skin has a mottled cyanotic appearance and is cold and clammy; the blood pressure is usually low and, if there is concomitant right-sided cardiac failure, the venous pressure may be high. In the differential diagnosis of cardiac shock, massive pulmonary embolism and septic shock should be considered. In an aged patient, this may be extremely difficult. Pyrexia and leukocytosis may be part of the picture of myocardial infarction and render its separation from sepsis difficult. In pulmonary embolism the dyspnea is often out of proportion to the pain and hypotension, and the chest x-ray shows no signs of congestion. With myocardial infarction the dyspnea, especially in the early stages, reflects pulmonary vascular congestion. When the differential diagnosis cannot be made in any other way, forward pulmonary angiograms or lung-scanning techniques may be diagnostic for massive pulmonary embolism.

Sequential measurement of central venous pressure (CVP) provides one of the valuable guides in therapy. Cohn has recently compared (CVP) measurements with left ventricular end-diastolic pressure measurements in patients in shock. In general, CVP measurements agree with left ventricular end-diastolic pressures. The exception to this statement has been dealt with in Chapter 5. Cohn demonstrated that left ventricular end-diastolic pressure was elevated in all patients with shock following myocardial infarction, even when the CVP was normal. On the other hand, in pulmonary embolism, CVP was always elevated whereas left ventricular end-diastolic pressure was usually normal. Therefore, left ventricular end-diastolic pressure could be used to differentiate myocardial infarction and pulmonary embolism shock, but this measurement is not practical for clinical use. After infusion of plasma expanders or isoproterenol therapy, changes in CVP generally reflect similar changes in left ventricular end-diastolic pressure. After administration of norepinephrine and dopamine, however, CVP may be altered in such a way that significant increases in left ventricular end-diastolic pressure may occur while CVP remains unchanged.

Recently, serious ventilation-perfusion defects have also been recognized in the lungs of patients who have suffered myocardial infarction.

$\overset{\circ}{V}_A/\overset{\circ}{Q}$ CHANGES IN CARDIOGENIC SHOCK

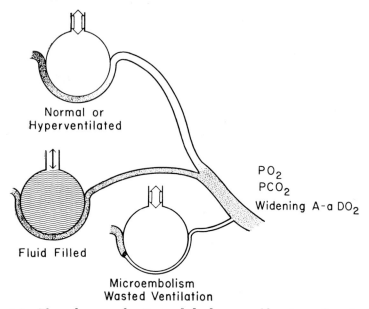

Fig. 6–2.—The pulmonary shunting and deadspace problem in cardiogenic shock. Treatment is designed to support pulmonary gas exchange by increasing the number of functioning alveolar units.

The A-aDO$_2$ increases, and full saturation of arterial hemoglobin may be secured only by assisted ventilation at increased oxygen concentrations. Results of the reports in Table 6-1 reflect some initial measurements of cardiac output in cardiogenic shock.

When the fall in cardiac output occurs gradually over a long period, as in chronic heart disease, a low cardiac output may be tolerated at rest. In

TABLE 6-1.—INITIAL MEASUREMENTS OF CARDIAC OUTPUT
IN CARDIOGENIC SHOCK

AUTHOR	NUMBER OF PATIENTS	MEAN CARDIAC INDEX L/MIN/M^2	MEAN TOTAL PERIPHERAL RESISTANCE DYNE-SEC/CM^5
Freis	3	1.8	2080
Smith	7	1.6	1840
Gilbert	7	1.0	3040
Gammill	14	2.9	1760
Broch	17	2.0	——
MacKenzie	6	1.7	——
Thal	7	1.8	1750

TABLE 6-2.—HEMODYNAMIC VALUES RESULTING FROM
CONSTANT ISOPROTERENOL INFUSION

HR	CO (L/MIN)	TPR (DYNES-SEC/CM^5)	BP (MM HG)	CVP (CM H$_2$O)	
0	1.5	3470	70/60	10.0	
1	1.6	5050	110/96	7.0	Isoproterenol drip
2	1.7	4695	106/94	7.0	
3	1.2	6333	104/90	8.0	
4	1.7	4092	106/80	7.0	
5	1.8	4043	106/80	9.0	

shock, however, the insult is sudden, the stroke volume plunges, and circulatory readjustments are made by diversion of blood flow to vital areas. In essence, the hemodynamic changes in cardiogenic shock are manifest by low cardiac output, low stroke volume, high peripheral resistance, and often an increase in venous pressure. This state is tolerated for only relatively short periods, and the mortality rate in patients demonstrating shock after myocardial infarction is high, varying between 70 and 100% in various series. An approach to the treatment of this condition is given in Chapter 7.

CASE HISTORY.—*Cardiogenic Shock*

This 65-year-old male was admitted to the ICU because of severe substernal chest discomfort associated with nausea, sweating, and numbness in both arms. His admission diagnosis was acute myocardial infarction. Following admission, he developed severe hypotension, sweating, and pallor. Moist rales could be heard in all lung fields. Heart tones were extremely distant, and a prominent gallop rhythm was present. The electrocardiogram revealed atrial fibrillation, old apical myocardial infarction, and a recent anterolateral myocardial infarction with occasional ventricular premature contractions (VPC). Chest x-ray revealed marked cardiomegaly and evidence of hilar congestion. Over the next 72 hours, the patient was supported by constant isoproterenol infusion. He gradually became refractory to this medication and expired quietly. The hemodynamic values reflected low cardiac output and high total peripheral resistance. These values were not significantly altered by infusion of isoproterenol (see Table 6-2).

HYPOVOLEMIC SHOCK

Loss of blood or other body fluids in quantities sufficient to reduce venous return is one of the common causes of shock encountered by the surgeon. Fluid loss may be obvious, as in external bleeding or after hemorrhage from the gastrointestinal tract, or it may be less easily appreciated when it evaporates from the skin after burns or infiltrates extensively in and around areas of severe trauma. In response to the falling blood pressure and the diminishing intravascular volume, all the mechanisms designed to restore blood pressure and conserve body water come into play, as shown by tachycardia, vasoconstriction, and oliguria. The blood pressure is initially sustained, but with failure of compensation it falls. The CVP and cardiac output are low.

Several studies, including those of Cournand, Hopkins, and Simeone, as well as our own, show cardiac indices ranging from 1 to 2 liters/min/M^2, and total peripheral resistance from 1500 to 3000 dyne-sec/cm^5. Final confirmation of the hypovolemic state is obtained by a favorable response to the infusion of intravenous fluid. Blood pressure and cardiac output rise while CVP fluctuates within the normal range. The urine output increases, and the skin, which was formerly cold, clammy, and mottled, becomes warm and dry as sympathetic tone relaxes.

Damage to the heart and kidneys occurs during the hypotensive period. Less well recognized is the damage to the reticuloendothelial system and the heightened susceptibility to infection which follows hypovolemic shock. As a result, the initial problem of hypovolemia may give way to one of sepsis. Several days after severe trauma, when fluid volume has been restored and arterial pressure is normal, the impaired ability to resist bacterial infection becomes manifest. All the features of the hypermetabolic septic state then supervene and the patient dies of multiple organ failure.

Septic Shock

In the majority of patients with septic shock, the underlying disease process is of such serious nature that there is already a severe degree of impairment in vital organ function before the onset of shock. Moreover, it is not uncommon for such patients to experience all the hyperdynamic signs of sepsis for days or even weeks before the shock episode occurs, but it is still not clear what factors tip the balance from sepsis into septic shock. The importance of the underlying disease process in determining the outcome is demonstrated by the study of McAbe and Jackson and more recently by that of Fried and Vosty. In studying 270 patients with gram-negative bacteremia, the latter investigators showed that the mortality rate of patients with a rapidly fatal underlying disease was 86%, with an ultimately fatal disease it was 46%, and with nonfatal disease it was 16%. Prior therapy with adrenal corticosteroids was associated with a significantly higher mortality rate among patients with an ultimately fatal disease. Septic shock is rare in children and is seen most commonly in old men and in young women after postpartum or postabortion complications.

Among the serious conditions that predispose to septic shock are diabetes and cirrhosis, leukemia and carcinoma, immunosuppressive therapy, biliary tract obstruction due to neoplasm or stones, prostatism with pyelo--

nephritis, ulcerative colitis, complicated forms of diabetes, postabortal and postpartum sepsis, and a variety of surgical conditions where extensive operation has been performed for malignancy, particularly in the regions of the esophagus and the pancreas. Leaking anastomoses with peritonitis and subphrenic abscess often are causes, and the mortality rate is extremely high. The sepsis associated with burns, now almost invariably due to gram-negative organisms, becomes important during the second and third week after extensive body burns. Coupled with the hemodynamic and metabolic demands imposed by the sepsis itself is the excessive fluid and heat loss through the burn eschar bringing about a chronic state of heightened caloric expenditure. Shock is especially likely to follow endoscopic procedures of the infected urinary tract. Host factors are clearly of the highest importance since only half the patients who experience gram-negative septicemia develop shock.

The clinical picture of septic shock in a typical case may be characterized by chills, fever, and leukocytosis. Initially, the skin may be warm and flushed and the patient quite responsive in spite of the hypotension. The urine output may be satisfactory. There is usually a marked tachycardia. Suddenly, the blood pressure drops, the patient becomes oliguric, and the skin may become cold and clammy, although in some instances of low-resistance–septic shock, a warm, dry skin may persist. The CVP is usually slightly reduced or normal, the blood pressure is variable, but usually reduced, the hematocrit is usually within normal range, and the white blood count may reflect sepsis. On the other hand, with a recent insult or in an aged patient, the white count may not be of value in making the diagnosis of sepsis. Blood volume is usually within the normal range, although occasionally there is a reduction in plasma volume. Nevertheless, these patients often respond favorably to fluid administration. In the hypotension associated with sepsis, there may be a quite remarkable hyperventilation with arterial hypocarbia and hypoxemia.

Early studies in septic shock were made by Gilbert. The cardiac index

TABLE 6-3.—REPORTED MEASUREMENTS OF CARDIAC OUTPUT AND CALCULATED
TOTAL PERIPHERAL RESISTANCE IN CLINICAL SEPTIC SHOCK

AUTHOR	NUMBER OF PATIENTS	MEAN CARDIAC INDEX L/MIN/M²	MEAN TOTAL PERIPHERAL RESISTANCE DYNE-SEC/CM⁵
Gilbert	4	3.6	low
Udhoji	4	1.4	2110
Hopkins	12	2.4	1660
MacLean	2	2.7	870
Thal et al.	20	3.5	680

in four of the patients was 3.6 liters/min/M² with a "low" total peripheral resistance. In contrast to Gilbert's study was that of Weil and his associates who reported that the average cardiac index in bacteremic shock in his studies on four patients was 1.4 liters/min/M² and the average resistance was 2305 dyne-sec/cm⁵.

MacLean reported on 20 patients in shock. Of these, 2 seemed to be in septic shock without hypovolemia. The average cardiac index for these 2 patients was 2.7 liters/min/M², and the total peripheral resistance was 870 dyne-sec/cm⁵. Hopkins *et al.* reported on 24 patients in shock of whom 12 had sepsis. Seven of these had a total peripheral resistance which could be considered normal or low, but three others had a total peripheral resistance greater than 2000 dyne-sec/cm⁵.

Our measurements in pure septic shock, in which hypovolemia and cardiac failure could be excluded, show a generally similar pattern of response. Ten of the 13 cases with sepsis had a cardiac index of 2.4 liters/min/M² or higher and five of these had cardiac indices above 3.75 liters/min/M². Similarly, when total peripheral resistance was calculated, 12 of the 13 patients with pure septic shock had a total peripheral resistance less than 1000 and 5 had a total peripheral resistance less than 500 dyne-sec/cm⁵. From our studies, it would appear that the cardiac output in sepsis is higher than in other forms of shock and that total peripheral resistance is correspondingly lower.

An important hemodynamic problem that frequently develops in patients with septic shock is myocardial failure. By plotting left ventricular work against CVP, abnormal left ventricular function can be demonstrated with surprising frequency in patients who are in septic shock. Siegal has recently stressed this problem by demonstrating that an attempt at volume expansion may result in further elevation of filling pressures rather than in an augmentation of cardiac output, indicating that the heart is already on the flat portion of Starling's curve. The explanation for this depressed myocardial function is not clear. In many patients, evidence of myocardial failure developed only after the patients had been in a high output state for several days. Presumably the mechanism of heart failure in this instance was depletion of myocardial catecholamines from the sustained hyperdynamic state. The possibility that endotoxemia itself causes a depressant effect on cardiac performance has been raised by some and denied by others. Recent studies have also incriminated a polypeptide (myocardial-depressant factor) as the cause of heart failure in patients with septic shock.

Impending heart failure is recognized by a steadily falling cardiac output in the presence of a rising CVP, indicating the need for myocardial support. In sepsis the use of a beta adrenergic stimulating drug such as isoproterenol poses certain problems because of the existing tachycardia and low vascular resistance. The prognosis in septic shock is significantly related to the initial cardiac output determination and to the seriousness of the underlying disease process. In our experience, the mortality rate for patients with an initial cardiac index less than 2.5 liters/min/M² was 75%, whereas the mortality rate for patients with an initial cardiac index greater than 2.5 was only 15%. The p value correlating survival with cardiac index was less than .02. It is possible that the poor prognosis in a patient with a low cardiac output indicates severe underlying heart disease or hypovolemia and that this type of patient is simply unable to meet the demand for a raised cardiac output necessitated by the vasodilated state of sepsis.

Knowledge regarding the hemodynamic response of humans to endotoxin derives from the relatively few measurements made by renal physiologists using contaminated inulin and typhoid vaccine in the study of renal hyperemia. This work, by Homer Smith, has clearly shown that sublethal amounts of bacterial pyrogens in man produce a delayed peripheral vasodilatation and a rise in cardiac output. The mechanism by which sepsis causes shock is unclear, and it appears likely that several different responses to sepsis are seen in man. Generalizations from data obtained in endotoxin shock in dogs can be applied to man only with some risk of error since the hemodynamic and morphologic changes are so grossly dissimilar.

The septic animal model, as distinct from the endotoxic model, resolves some of the seemingly contradictory data in man. Clearly, sepsis in man and animal has a number of reproducible effects. The oxygen consumption rises, cardiac output increases, and total peripheral resistance falls. The large rise in cardiac output appears to result from the fall in vascular resistance rather than from the relatively small increase in oxygen consumption. There is clearly a considerable increase in flow to the area of sepsis, the kidneys, and abdominal viscera. Flow to the skin and muscle is variable and is more closely associated with heat regulation. These fascinating changes in blood flow distribution appear to follow the release of a vasodilator substance from the area of sepsis. Under the stress of severe peripheral vasodilation the heart comes under strong sympathetic stimulation and must pump more blood to maintain blood pressure. When plasma volume is diminished by fluid sequestration within the area of inflammation, or when cardiac failure fails to maintain the raised output, low cardiac output and high vascular resistance may develop. The hemodynamic picture in septic man, as in the animal model, is characterized by wide fluctuation in hemodynamic measurements. These measurements must be made repeatedly to characterize the response at any given time and to

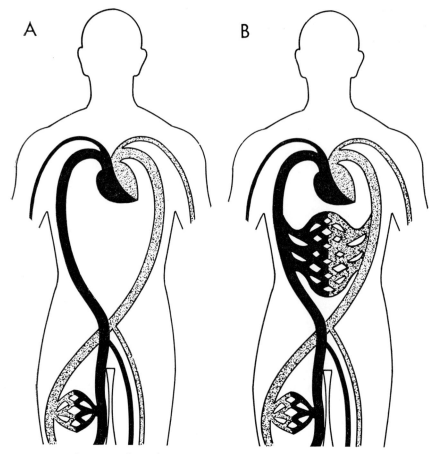

Fig. 6–3.—Concepts of circulatory response to sepsis. These drawings display a local area of severe sepsis (in the right thigh for the purpose of illustration). An earlier concept (A) suggested that the hyperdynamic circulatory response was accounted for by heightened flow through the area of sepsis. Current experimental work (B) supports the contention that the high cardiac output is a response to lowered resistance and to increased flow in the splanchnic viscera and kidneys, as well as the area of sepsis. Release of a vasodilator substance may be responsible for this altered vascular reactivity.

measure the response to therapy. In particular, the presence of hypovolemia or cardiac failure should be identified by the measurement of arterial and venous pressure during fluid loading.

The origins of pure septic shock are far from clear, but careful analysis shows that two special clinical categories of septic shock may be identified when either hypovolemia or cardiac failure becomes the dominant feature of the illness. Ultimate recovery is often limited by lung damage or renal failure. Massive gastrointestinal hemorrhage with disseminated intravascular coagulation often complicates the advanced case.

As distinct from cardiac and hypovolemic shock, the element of regional vasodilation that appears to exist in many patients with septic shock presents interesting implications, for if tissue perfusion were normally distributed, one would expect that signs of cellular hypoxia would not be present. In fact, this did not prove to be true since several of our patients had severe metabolic acidosis. There are several possibilities to account for this phenomenon: nutritive blood flow may be diverted to the inflamed region, where considerable A-V shunting occurs; or the blood flow may be unevenly distributed, some areas such as skin and muscle being hypoperfused, while others more influenced by septic vasodilator substances have an enhanced blood flow. Finally, the possibility exists that bacterial products acting directly on the cell impair oxidative phosphorylation regardless of blood perfusion. The toxic effects of endotoxin on the polymorphonuclear leukocyte are now well established, and it seems possible that direct effects on other cells account for some of the phenomena of shock. The chemical mediators released by endotoxins, such as histamine, the vasoactive polypeptides or, more probably, the endogenous pyrogens released from damaged leukocytes, may possibly be implicated in the vasodilator response to sepsis.

Neurogenic Shock

Complete transection or severe injury to the spinal cord to the degree that the edema causes functional interruption results in a state referred to as neurogenic shock. The interruption of anatomic function causes a loss in vasomotor tone and vasodilatation and hypotension from loss of peripheral vascular resistance. The use of the term shock for this condition is misleading since it bears little relationship to the more common forms of shock. Patients with spinal shock who receive adequate ventilatory support customarily remain well oriented, dry and warm, have good filling of peripheral veins, and produce satisfactory urine outputs, but septic complications are apt to develop. The loss of autonomic control of cutaneous blood vessels may be severe enough to render the patient poikilothermic, the body temperature tending to rise or fall passively, depending upon ambient conditions of temperature and humidity. The hyperpyrexia so commonly described in these patients is usually a late phenomenon resulting from sepsis. Clinical findings of hypovolemic shock do not occur after head injury unless there is considerable external bleeding and, if present, strongly suggest some associated injury.

Shock Associated with Fractures of the Pelvis

Fat embolism, renal failure, and shock due to massive retroperitoneal hemorrhage are complications to be feared in patients who suffer severe pelvic fracture. Usually the fractures leading to these complications involve the pubic rami and are often associated with central dislocations of the hip. Lung injury resulting from shock, fat embolism, and intravascular coagulation may also be seen in these patients. Approximately 40% of patients with pelvic fracture show clinical signs of shock due to hemorrhage. Initially, then, the problem is one of control of hemorrhage. Unfortunately, the bleeding from the shattered fragments of pelvic bone and the torn highly vascular soft tissues is extremely difficult to control.

Various maneuvers have been tried, including ligation of the hypogastric artery and even ligation of a common iliac artery on one side, but the collateral blood supply in this region is so rich that bleeding is rarely controlled by these approaches. The anatomic location and the extent of the hemorrhage can often be gauged by displacement of the bladder seen on the cystogram. There are often important associated injuries, particularly to the bladder and urethra. Fracture of the pelvis is often associated with head, chest, and abdominal injuries, including ruptured spleen, kidney, liver, and bowel. Deaths among these patients are often the result of delayed or inadequate treatment of the extensive blood loss. Tragically, other injuries so often associated with a fractured pelvis divert the surgeon's attention from the major life-threatening problem of continuing hemorrhage while facial lacerations and long bone and jaw fractures receive minute care. The retroperitoneal bleeding is usually protracted, insidious, and only partially contained by the soft tissue so that the extent may not be appreciated until severe compensatory vasoconstriction has been present for many hours. In common with the management of other severe injuries, attention must be focused primarily on the life-threatening injury in the patient with pelvic fracture, and not until an adequate blood volume has been established and the patient's condition becomes stable should attention be diverted to other lesser injuries. Twenty-four to 48 hours after injury, ventilatory difficulties may signal the development of pulmonary fat embolism.

Fat Embolism

The major life-threatening effect of fat embolism is diffuse lung damage which limits effective gas exchange. Shock is seldom a concomitant of this illness until the terminal stages of consolidation of the lung lead to intractable hypoxia and right-sided heart failure. Pathologically, there is an increase in the amount of neutral fat in the lung, but the actual lung damage is brought about by free fatty acids released by hydrolysis within the lung. Fat embolism may be associated with thromboembolism. The diagnosis is made by the history, which in the vast majority of patients involves fracture of one or more of the long bones in the lower extremities, but it may be seen after rib fractures or even after severe soft tissue injury. Petechial hemorrhages, often found in the anterior axillary fold or in the subconjunctival area, help to establish the diagnosis. There is characteristically a thrombocytopenia and a raised serum lipase level. The thrombocytopenia is seen at the time the petechiae become evident, and the diagnosis may be established by the finding of fat droplets in the urine.

It is not clear whether all the fat found in the lungs emanates from fractured bone. In fact, as Clowes has shown, some fatty material may often be found in the lungs of dogs dying of hypovolemic shock. That catecholamines mobilize fatty acids is well known and this, too, may have some bearing on the common lesion found in this variety of the respiratory distress syndrome. The extreme toxicity of these fatty acids on the lung has been clearly established by Peltier. Under the electron microscope, there is a marked vesiculation and thickening of the capillary endothelium and alveolar wall. In addition, depletion or inactivation of lung surfactant may contribute to the spreading atelectasis noted in these patients. The x-ray finding of diffuse infiltration of the lung parenchyma usually follows overt evidence of interference with pulmonary gas exchange by several days. The whole clinical and radiologic picture is nonspecific and common to the many etiologies of the respiratory distress syndrome.

When shock is seen soon after fracture, it is almost invariably due to hemorrhage and hypovolemia, occasionally to massive pulmonary embolism, but rarely to fat embolism. Although fat may be found in the lungs of these patients, it seems doubtful that it is significant during the early stages of most cases of traumatic shock.

The prophylactic treatment of fractures by immediate immobilization is of the highest importance. When the lesion is established in the lung, the need for respiratory support follows the usual guidelines to be discussed later. Specific treatment by use of heparin, steroids, and intravenous alcohol is still under study, whereas the prevention of shock by adequate volume replacement and the use of tracheostomy and ventilatory support, when indicated, have clearly shown their value by tiding the severely injured lung over the insult of fat embolism. Nevertheless, the lung lesion may be so severe that adequate oxygen exchange cannot be maintained even when the inspired oxygen concentration is increased to 100%. The progressively widening difference between alveolar and arterial oxygen tension characterizes a group of cases for which, at the moment, there is no effective means of therapy. It seems clear that in this group of patients long-term extracorporeal oxygenation is the hope for the future.

PULMONARY EMBOLISM

Pulmonary embolism is a common and an oft-undiagnosed cause of shock. Fitts' study of the cause of death after hip fracture in the elderly patient revealed a 38% incidence at autopsy of fatal pulmonary embolism whereas in comparable cases, in which autopsy was not performed, pulmonary embolism was thought to be a cause of death in only 2%. Study of the microcirculation (draining an area of low blood flow or after trauma) demonstrates extensive formation of microaggregates of white cells, platelets, and red cells. Pulmonary microembolism must therefore be considered as an almost constant occurrence in all patients in shock. As shown earlier, the development of extensive pulmonary microembolism results in an ever-increasing physiologic dead space. Several conditions predispose toward pulmonary embolism, including recent operation, protracted bed rest, congestive heart failure, fracture or trauma to the lower extremities, or injury or neoplasm of the pancreas. The two major physiologic effects of acute pulmonary embolism occur when more than 60% of the pulmonary vasculature is obstructed. This results in a pressure load on the right ventricle and culminates in failure. The second physiologic event occurs as a result of the failure to perfuse a large ventilated segment of the lung; in effect, wasted or dead-space ventilation.

The patient may complain of marked dyspnea and some substernal pain; there may be considerable anxiety and the event terminated within a few minutes or after several hours by cardiovascular collapse. On physical examination, a loud pulmonic second sound, parasternal heave, distended neck veins, gallop rhythm, and a tender, enlarged liver may be revealed. Tachycardia, tachypnea, cyanosis, and hypotension often complete the picture. Chest x-ray may show an enlarged right ventricle and widened pulmonary artery segments with unilateral embolism. There may be hyperlucence of the whole or part of a lung. Acute right ventricular strain with right axis deviation and the S-1, Q-3, T-3 pattern is the typical EKG pattern in about 60% of these cases. This occurs only in the presence of acute failure of the right ventricle. The shock associated with massive pulmonary embolism usually follows a period of acute cor pulmonale, suggested by the symptoms and signs previously discussed. The CVP or, better still, the right ventricular systolic and end-diastolic pressures, are generally raised and the CVP usually exceeds 15 cm of water. DelGuercio has utilized a long catheter placed, by flow guidance into the right ventricle, to identify the high right ventricular systolic pressure seen charac-

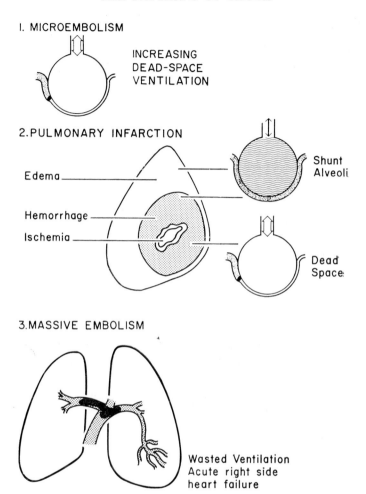

I. MICROEMBOLISM

INCREASING
DEAD-SPACE
VENTILATION

2.PULMONARY INFARCTION

Edema

Hemorrhage

Ischemia

Shunt
Alveoli

Dead
Space

3.MASSIVE EMBOLISM

Wasted Ventilation
Acute right side
heart failure

Fig. 6–4.—Anatomy of pulmonary embolism.

teristically in pulmonary embolism. The major diagnostic problem involves differentiation from massive myocardial infarction with shock and cardiac failure. These two conditions may be differentiated tentatively, but special examinations are needed to confirm the diagnosis.

A presumptive diagnosis may be made by the iodinated 131 serum albumin macroaggregate lung-scanning technique which can be performed in even the most critically ill patients and completed in less than 2 hours. Some investigators have even performed lung scanning at the bedside. A normal scan excludes massive pulmonary embolism. Selective pulmonary angiography is the definitive diagnostic test for pulmonary embolism and also allows an estimation of the extent of pulmonary vascular obstruction (see Fig. 6-5). The object of treatment is to provide cardiac and ventilatory support while treatment with anticoagulants and, possibly, thrombolysins such as urokinase is undertaken.

For treating the hypotension, intravenous infusion of isoproterenol hydrochloride, 4 mg diluted in 1 liter of 5% dextrose solution, is helpful. The object is to provide inotropic support while treatment with anticoagulants and possibly thrombolysins (urokinase) is undertaken. Careful monitoring of heart rate, blood pressure, and CVP is necessary since isoproterenol may produce ventricular tachycardia. Persistent hypotension, after adequate therapy with isoproterenol or, failing that, metaraminol, is the chief indication for the operation of embolectomy, but the majority of patients are best handled without operation.

Heparin is administered intravenously in doses of approximately 10,000 units every 4 hours controlled by measurements of coagulation time. In addition, the use of a fibrinolytic agent, urokinase, is currently under investigation and initial studies appear promising. Ventilatory support is given according to standard principles guided by measurements of blood gases.

Fig. 6–5.—Pulmonary angiogram showing embolic masses in the right pulmonary artery and upper lobe branches on the left and reduced perfusion of over two thirds of the lung.

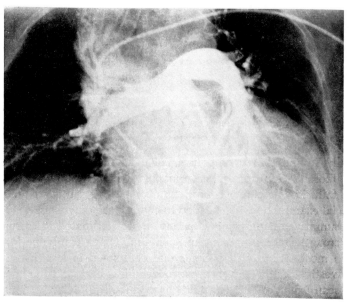

TABLE 6-4.—DIFFERENTIAL DIAGNOSIS

	MASSIVE PULMONARY EMBOLISM	MASSIVE MYOCARDIAL INFARCTION
Onset	Sudden with dyspnea predominating	Sudden with pain predominating
Neck vein	Markedly distended	Distended
Auscultation of lungs	Dry	Wet
Chest x-ray	Lung fields hyperlucent PA segment enlarged	Congested or Pulmonary edema

Embolectomy is reserved for patients failing to respond to the supportive measures outlined and is best undertaken when partial support can be given by means of a mobile heart-lung machine connected through the femoral vessels. With this type of support, the patient can be maintained during pulmonary angiography and the induction of anesthesia. If embolectomy must be carried out, ligation of the inferior vena cava should be undertaken at the same time. Donaldson's review of patients with massive fatal pulmonary embolism suggests that 70–80% of these patients die within 2 hours of the onset of symptoms. Contrary to previous assumptions Miller has shown that pulmonary valve closure is not accentuated in the

Fig. 6–6.—Electrocardiogram prior to pulmonary embolism.

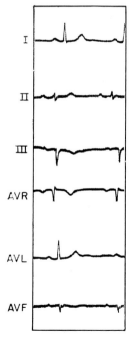

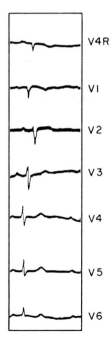

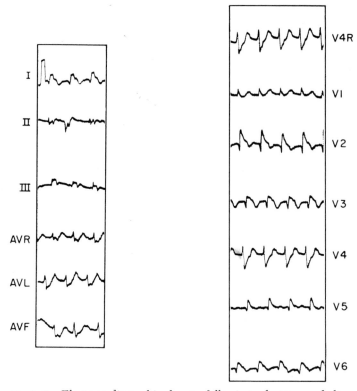

Fig. 6–7.—Electrocardiographic changes following pulmonary embolism.

majority of cases. The x-ray study was of very limited value in making the diagnosis and, even cardiac catheterization, in the face of massive embolism, revealed some patients in whom right atrial and right ventricular end-diastolic pressures were normal. Because of this inconsistency, Miller feels that pulmonary arteriography is mandatory for making the diagnosis.

CASE HISTORY.—*Massive Pulmonary Embolism*

This 58-year-old woman suffered sudden unexplained cardiovascular collapse the day following a hysterectomy. Initially, she was extremely cyanotic and her extremities were cold and clammy. Blood pressure and pulse were unobtainable. She was successfully resuscitated with external cardiac massage and IV epinephrine. Her electrocardiogram following resuscitation showed clear-cut changes with sinus tachycardia, right bundle branch block, and right axis deviation. (Figs. 6-6 and 6-7). It was felt that these changes were compatible with acute pulmonary embolus. Cardiac catheterization was performed and revealed pulmonary hypertension (PA pressure 45/25) and right heart failure (RA pressure 16 mm Hg). Pulmonary arteriogram revealed multiple filling defects in the pulmonary artery and lack of perfusion to much of the right lung field (Fig. 6-5). Since blood pressure could not be maintained, operation was carried out. Marked clinical improvement in the patient was achieved following surgical removal of multiple large pulmonary emboli.

SHOCK ASSOCIATED WITH BARBITURATE INTOXICATION

A shocklike picture is frequently seen following suicidal doses of barbiturates, but the mechanism is poorly understood. Weil and others have demonstrated that a relative deficit in the plasma volume frequently occurs in these patients and that this relative hypovolemia is the primary alteration. The average plasma volume in 15 patients in shock following barbiturates was 34 ml per kilogram compared to an average normal value of 42 ml per kilogram. Central venous pressure was usually low and a significantly lower cardiac output and elevated total peripheral resistance were found in these patients. More importantly, following volume expansion, the cardiac index responded appropriately in all patients so that a relatively normal plasma volume was associated with a return to a normal cardiac index. At times, this required the administration of up to 6 liters of fluid over a 12-hour period. Cardiac output may also be increased when vasopressor drugs are used in amounts that increase the mean arterial pressure to approximately 90 mm Hg. With further elevations of arterial pressure, the response is generally unfavorable in that the cardiac output decreases and peripheral vascular resistance increases even further. Aggressive replacement of fluid volume with monitoring of CVP and ventilatory support by means of a nasotracheal tube and volume ventilator are the treatments of choice in this condition.

POSTABORTIVE AND POSTPARTUM SEPSIS AS A CAUSE OF SHOCK

Studdiford and Douglas, in their classic paper in 1956, showed that in septic shock associated with abortion or postpartum sepsis hysterectomy could be a lifesaving procedure. The microorganisms involved are usually gram-negative, often coliforms and sometimes the anaerobic clostridia. The special features of this illness are the association with pregnancy and the unique responses of the pregnant woman to overwhelming sepsis.

McKay and others have shown that the pregnant animal develops a generalized Shwartzman reaction in response to a single injection of endotoxin, indicating that the reticuloendothelial system, under these circumstances, is more readily blocked and endotoxin less readily inactivated. Also, immune gamma globulins fail to cross the placental membrane and are not produced by the conceptus, which is extremely vulnerable to *E. coli* intrauterine infection, especially after injury. The infection antedates the development of hypotension by several days. In the advanced case, renal damage may be a dominant feature. Our studies indicate that these patients show the classical form of high cardiac output, low vascular resistance shock which apparently is the result of vasodilator substances released from interaction between bacteria and tissues of the host. There is a special tendency to septic pulmonary embolism and an extensive thrombophlebitis extending up the uterine veins.

Therapy is directed toward early evacuation of uterine contents, massive broad-spectrum antibiotic therapy, support of red cell mass and plasma volume (these patients are often anemic as a result of hemorrhage from the uterus as well as hemolysis), and ventilatory support if indicated by blood gases or labored respiration. If the patient fails to respond promptly to this treatment, there should be no hesitation in removing the uterus and ligating the ovarian veins at a high level. Postoperatively, careful monitoring should be undertaken, using the guidelines of CVP, arterial pressure, urine output, and repeated measurements of blood gases and body weight. Plasma and blood are the standbys of fluid therapy. Bacterial cultures should be available and will direct the course of antibiotic therapy. Ventilatory support may be necessary. The administration of large doses of steroids has been recommended by some investigators, but documentation of their value remains to be established. Certainly, steroids are not a substitute for the proved measures already discussed.

SHOCK FOLLOWING PANCREATITIS

While fulminating pancreatitis is occasionally seen in childhood, the majority of cases occur in the older age group. Alcoholism, cholelithiasis, and diabetes constitute the common predisposing illnesses. Currently, the disease is also occasionally seen after treatment with immunosuppressive drugs. Postoperative pancreatitis is especially likely to occur after extensive manipulation of the biliary tract or ampulla of Vater or after gastric surgery, particularly after distal gastric resections. A well-known culprit is the long-armed T-tube placed across the ampulla. Extensive pancreatic necrosis also follows blunt trauma to the abdomen. While it is currently not possible to link these diverse disease states into a common etiologic pattern, the effects of pancreatic injury can be explained fairly readily.

The disease follows two general patterns. The first constitutes the edematous form commonly seen in alcoholics and is characterized by severe epigastric pain often radiating to the back or one of the upper quadrants. There is little systemic response, aside from a mild rise in temperature and a slight tachycardia. The illness often lasts from a few hours to a few days and remits spontaneously or after treatment with nasogastric suction and intravenous fluids. A rare but often lethal form of the disease, acute necrotizing pancreatitis, may have an abrupt onset which is characterized by agonizing abdominal pain, ascites, ileus, and profound shock. The dramatic nature of this illness has led to the concept that it is associated with a unique hemodynamic response. In the majority of instances this is certainly untrue and the hypotension responds well to correction of fluid and electrolyte defects. In the massive necrotizing form, however, there does indeed appear to be an unusual form of shock, characterized by changes in capillary permeability within the pancreas and its environs. There is an enormous outpouring of protein-rich ascitic fluid and marked retroperitoneal edema, while the paralyzed bowel gives the clinical features of severe ileus. As a result of the plasma loss, the hemoglobin climbs in a manner reminiscent of the severe surface burn. The pain may be extreme, and hypotension and oliguria complete the picture. The underlying problem seems to center about the release from the damaged pancreas of agents capable of altering capillary permeability. Proteolytic reactions are initiated early in the course of the disease, leading to the conversion of bradykininogen to the active polypeptide bradykinin. Histamine and other vasoactive substances are set free, and there is a tremendous outpouring of fluid into the peritoneal cavity together with a loss of protein-rich fluid in and around the pancreas. The various substances released from the damaged pancreas increase fluid loss across the capillary membrane and may be involved in precipitating intravascular microaggregation of platelets, red cells, or fibrin thrombi. The net effect is an impaired tissue perfusion, local plasma loss, red cell aggregation and sequestration, leading to a fall in venous return and a fall in cardiac output.

TREATMENT.—The elevation of the blood and urinary levels of pancreatic enzymes associated with the typical history and physical signs of pancreatitis make the diagnosis likely. Raised enzyme levels after duodenal perforation, torsion of the afferent loop of a Billroth II gastric reconstruction, or impaction of a gallstone in the ampulla of Vater may present a diagnostic problem which can be solved only by exploration. Conversely, severe pancreatic necrosis is occasionally seen in the absence of hyperamylasemia.

Treatment is designed both to prevent further stimulation of the pancreas, using nasogastric siphonage, and to support venous return and renal function by the appropriate administration of fluids. These patients may require enormous quantities of plasma and saline. The hematocrit can be used as a guideline to plasma replacement. Broad-spectrum antibiotics should be used liberally because of the hazards of secondary infection and pancreatic suppuration. In severe cases with ascites, peritoneal dialysis has occasionally been used with success.

Certain potentially lethal complications of pancreatitis should be anticipated, the most significant complication being massive upper gastrointestinal hemorrhage. A significant number of patients who survive the initial shock of pancreatic necrosis die within the first 10 days of massive upper gastric intestinal hemorrhage from superficial erosions of the stomach and duodenum. Consequently, acid neutralizing agents should be dripped into the stomach through the nasogastric tube. In spite of such treatment severe gastric hemorrhage may occur, suggesting that this is not purely an acid-peptic phenomenon. Pulmonary complications are extremely common. Ventilation is impaired due to the marked abdominal distention, and extensive microatelectasis is likely to occur. Mediastinal and pleural effusions are not rare. Blood gases must be carefully monitored and ventilatory support given where needed. Acute pancreatitis may produce disseminated intravascular coagulation, initially resulting in local thrombosis and pulmonary microembolism, and ending in an incoagulable state. Also, oliguria and anuria are likely to follow the severe shock seen in acute pancreatitis.

The basics of treatment are similar to those applied in other forms of hypovolemic shock. In pancreatitis, however, the severity of the fluid loss is often not appreciated until the illness is in an advanced state. Careful monitoring of CVP, arterial blood pressure, urine output, and blood gases is mandatory in caring for these critically ill patients.

REFERENCES

CARDIOGENIC SHOCK

Broch, O. J., Humerfelt, S., Haarstad, J., and Mybre, J. R.: Hemodynamic studies in acute myocardial infarction, Am. Heart J. 57:522, 1959.

Cohn, J. N.: Myocardial infarction shock revisited, Am. Heart J. 74:1, 1967.

Dietzman, R. H., and Lillehei, R. C.: The treatment of cardiogenic shock. V. The use of corticosteroids in the treatment of cardiogenic shock, Am. Heart J., 75:274, 1968.

Freis, E. D., Schnaper, H. W., Johnson, R. L., Schreimer, G. E.: Hemodynamic alterations in acute myocardial infarction: I. Cardiac output, mean arterial pressure, total peripheral resistance, "central" and total blood volumes, venous pressure and average circulation time, J. Clin. Invest. 31:131, 1952.

Gammill, J. F., Applegarth, J. J., Reed, C. E., Fernald, J. D., and Antenucci, A. J.: Hemodynamic changes following acute myocardial infarction using the dye injection method for cardiac output determination, Ann. Int. Med. 43:100, 1955.

Gilbert, R. P., Goldberg, M., and Griffin, J.: Circulatory changes in acute myocardial infarction, Circulation 9:847, 1954.

Kuhn, L. A., Kline, H. J., Marano, A. J., Jr., Hamby, R. I., Cestero, J., Cohn, L. J., Weinrauch, H., and Berger, M.: Mechanical increase of vascular resistance in experimental myocardial infarction with shock, Circulation Res. 19:1086, 1966.

McCabe, W. R., and Jackson, G. G.: Gram-negative bacteremia I and II, Arch. Int. Med. 110:847, 1963.

MacKenzie, G. J., Taylor, S. H., Flenley, D. C., McDonald, A. H., Staunton, H. P., and Donald, K. W.: Circulatory and respiratory studies in myocardial infarction and cardiogenic shock, Lancet 2:825, 1964.
Nielsen, B. L., and Marner, I. L.: Shock in acute myocardial infarction, Acta. Med. Scand. 175:65, 1964.
Smith, W. W., Wikler, N. S., and Fox, A. C.: Hemodynamic studies of patients with myocardial infarction, Circulation 9:352, 1954.

HYPOVOLEMIC SHOCK

Hopkins, R. W., Sabaga, G., Penn, I., and Simeone, F. A.: Hemodynamic aspects of hemorrhagic and septic shock, J.A.M.A. 191:127, 1965.
Lillehei, R. C., Longerbeam, J. K., Block, J. H., and Manax, W. G.: The nature of irreversible shock: Experimental and clinical observations, Ann. Surg. 160:682, 1964.
Lowery, B. D., Clutier, C. T., and Carey, L. C.: Blood gas determinations in the severely wounded in hemorrhagic shock, Arch. Surg. 99:330, 1969.
Schumer, W.: Dexamethasone in oligemic shock, Arch. Surg. 98:259, 1969.
Thal, A. P., and Wilson, R. F.: Shock Resulting from Fluid Loss, in Weil, M. H., and Shubin, H. (eds.): Diagnosis and Treatment of Shock (Baltimore: Williams & Wilkins Company, 1967).

SEPTIC SHOCK

Albrecht, M., and Clowes, G. H. A.: The increase of circulatory requirements in the presence of inflammation, Surgery 56:158, 1964.
Bennett, I. L., Finland, M., Hamburger, M., Kass, L., Lepper, M., and Waisbren, B. A.: The effectiveness of hydrocortisone in the management of severe infection, J.A.M.A. 183:462, 1963.
Broder, G., and Weil, M. H.: Excess lactate: An index of reversibility of shock in human patients, Science 143:1457, 1964.
Clowes, G., Vucinic, N., and Weidner, N.: Circulatory and metabolic alterations associated with survival or death in peritonitis, Ann. Surg. 163:866, 1966.
Cohn, I., Jr.: Bacterial factors in shock, J. Louisiana M. Soc. 119:3, 1967.
Cohn, J. D., Greenspan, M., Goldstein, C. R., Gudwin, A. L., Siegel, J. H., and Del-Guercio, L. R. M.: Arteriovenous shunting in high cardiac output shock syndromes, Surg. Gynec. & Obst. 127:282, 1968.
DelGuercio, L. R. M., Cohn, J. D., Greenspan, M., Feins, N. R., and Kornitzer, G.: Pulmonary and Systemic Arteriovenous Shunting in Clinical Septic Shock (Third International Conference on Hyperbaric Medicine) (Washington, D.C.: National Academy of Sciences, 1966), pp. 337-342.
Feigelson, P., and Feigelson, M.: Studies on the Mechanism of Cortisone Actions, in Litweck, G., and Kritchewski, D. (eds.): Actions of Hormones on Molecular Processes (New York: John Wiley & Sons, Inc., 1964), pp. 218-233.
Fine, J.: The Bacterial Factor in Traumatic Shock (Springfield, Ill.: Charles C Thomas, Publisher, 1954).
Freid, M. A., and Vosti, K. L.: The importance of underlying disease in patients with gram-negative bacteremia, Arch. Int. Med. 121:418, 1968.
Fukuda, T., Okuma, H., and Hata, N.: Epinephrine shock: Its relation to plasma epinephrine level and the mechanism of its protection by gluco-corticoid, Jap. J. Physiol. 17:746, 1967.
Gallin, J. I., Kaye, D., and O'Leary, W. M.: Serum lipids in infection, New England J. Med. 281:1082, 1969.
Gilbert, R. P., Honing, K. P., Griffin, J. A., Becker, R. J., and Adelson, B. H.: Hemodynamics of shock due to infection, Stanford M. Bull. 13:239, 1955.
Henderson, A. H., Most, A. S., and Sonnenblick, E. H.: Depression of contractility in rat heart muscle by free fatty acids during hypoxia, Lancet 2:825, 1969.

Hermreck, A. S., and Thal, A. P.: Mechanisms for the high circulatory requirements in sepsis and septic shock, Ann. Surg. 170:677, #4, 1969.

MacLean, L. D., Duff, J. H., Scott, H. M., and Peretiz, D. I.: Treatment of shock in man based on hemodynamic diagnosis, Surg. Gynec. & Obst. 120:1, 1965.

MacLean, L. D., Mulligan, W. G., MacLean, A. P. H., and Duff, J. H.: Patterns of septic shock in man: A detailed study of 56 patients, Ann. Surg. 166:543, 1967.

Oji, N., and Shreeve, W. W.: Gluconeogenesis from 14c- and 3H-labeled substrates in normal and cortisone-treated rats, Endocrinology 78:765, 1966.

Siegal, J. H., Greenspan, H., DelGuercio, L.: Abnormal vascular tone, defective oxygen transport and myocardial failure in human septic shock, Ann. Surg. 165:504, 1967.

Simmons, D. H., Nicoloff, J., and Guze, L. B.: Hyperventilation and respiratory alkalosis as signs of gram-negative bacteremia, J.A.M.A. 174:2196, 1960.

Smith, H. W.: Lectures on the Kidney (Lawrence, Kans.: University Extension Division, University of Kansas, 1943).

Udhoji, V. N., and Weil, N. H.: Hemodynamic and metabolic studies on shock associated with bacteremia, Ann. Int. Med. 62:966, 1965.

Udhoji, V. N., Weil, M. H., Sambhi, M. P., and Rosoff, L.: Hemodynamic studies on clinical shock associated with infection, Am. J. Med. 34:461, 1963.

Waisbren, B. A.: An essay regarding pathogenesis and treatment of shock due to bacteremia with special reference to "gram-negative" shock, Progr. Cardiov. Dis. 10:123, 1967.

Waisbren, B. A.: Gram-negative shock and endotoxin shock, Am. J. Med. 36:819, 1964.

Weil, M. H.: The cardiovascular effects of corticosteroids, Circulation 25:718, 1962.

Weil, M. H., Shubin, H., and Biddle, M.: Shock caused by gram-negative microorganisms: Analysis of 169 cases, Ann. Int. Med. 60:384, 1964.

Wilson, R. F., Thal, A. P., Kindling, P. H., Grifka, T., and Ackerman, E.: Hemodynamic measurements in septic shock, Arch. Surg. 91:121, 1965.

Fractured Pelvis

Fitts, W. T., Jr.: Thromboembolism: The clinical picture, J. Trauma 9:661, 1969.

Miller, W. E.: Massive hemorrhage in fractures of the pelvis, South. M. J. 56:933, 1963.

Peltier, L. F.: Complications associated with fractures of the pelvis, J. Bone & Joint Surg. 47-A(5):1060, 1965.

Perry, J. F., Jr., and McClellan, R. J.: Autopsy findings in 127 patients following fatal traffic accidents, Surg. Gynec. & Obst. 119:586, 1964.

Fat Embolism

Ashbaugh, D. G., and Petty, T. L.: Use of corticosteroids in the treatment of respiratory failure associated with massive fat embolism, Surg. Gynec. & Obst. 123:493, 1966.

Emson, H. E.: Fat embolism studies in 100 patients dying after injury, J. Clin. Path. 11:28, 1958.

Peltier, L. F.: The diagnosis of fat embolism, Surg. Gynec. & Obst. 131:371, 1965.

Peltier, L. F.: Fat embolism: A pulmonary disease, Surgery 62:756, 1967.

Peltier, L. F.: Fat embolism: The amount of fat in human long bones, Surgery 40:657, 1956.

Peltier, L. F.: Fat embolism: The toxic properties of neutral fat and free fatty acids, Surgery 40:665, 1956.

Peltier, L. F.: A few remarks on fat embolism, J. Trauma 8:812, 1968.

Barbiturate Poisoning

Berman, L. B., Jeghers, J., Schreiner, G. E., and Pallotta, A. J.: Hemodialysis, an effective therapy for acute barbiturate poisoning, J.A.M.A. 161:820, 1956.

SHOCK FOLLOWING PANCREATITIS

Gjessing, J.: Peritoneal dialysis in severe acute hemorrhagic pancreatitis, Acta chir. scandinav. 133:645, 1967.

Thal, A. P.: Surgical Physiology of the Exocrine Pancreas, in Davis, J. H. (ed.): *Current Concepts in Surgery* (New York: McGraw-Hill Book Company, Inc., 1965), pp. 217–246.

Wall, A. J.: Peritoneal dialysis in the treatment of severe acute pancreatitis, M. J. Australia 2:281, 1965.

SEPTIC ABORTION

Bartlett, R. H., and Yahia, C.: Management of septic chemical abortion with renal failure, New England J. Med. 281:747, 1969.

McKay, D. G.: *Disseminated Intravascular Coagulation: An Intermediary Mechanism of Disease* (New York: Hoeber Med. Div., Harper & Row, 1965).

Reid, D. E.: Assessment and management of the seriously ill patient following abortion, J.A.M.A. 199:805, 1967.

Studdiford, W. E., and Douglas, G. W.: Placental bacteremia: Significant finding in septic abortion accompanied by vascular collapse, Am. J. Obst. & Gynec. 71:842, 1956.

7

Treatment

The Prophylaxis of Shock

PREOPERATIVE PREPARATION.—In so heterogeneous a state as shock, treatment must be individualized and aimed at the support of the vital organ system under threat. More important than the proper treatment of established shock is the recognition of clinical states in which the threat of shock may be imminent and where proper action may avert it. The patient facing major surgery is constantly under threat of shock-inducing injury; this is particularly true when there is serious underlying cardiovascular, lung, liver, or renal disease. Several high-risk groups may be identified. Chronic cardiac patients operated upon in a hypokalemic and hyponatremic state due to prolonged diuretic therapy are liable to develop arrhythmias and ineffective cardiac action. Patients with bowel obstruction often vomit and aspirate during induction of anesthesia, and fluid and electrolytes may be seriously depleted by prolonged nasogastric suction. Anemias place additional demands upon the vascular system for blood gas transport.

Particularly important is the preoperative correction of underlying sepsis, especially in patients with prostatism and pyelonephritis who are about to undergo endoscopy. Pulmonary sepsis can be vastly improved by preoperative inhalation therapy, postural drainage, and antibiotic therapy. Urinary tract infection or pulmonary sepsis should be treated before undertaking an operation on other systems. Preoperative instruction in deep breathing is particularly important in the preparation of all patients having major surgery. Even patients with normal lungs can be managed with less risk of postoperative pulmonary complication if they have had training in deep ventilation and coughing by a chest physiotherapist before the operation. Drugs that depress the immune response, such as steroids or antimetabolites, are particularly hazardous in predisposing to postoperative sepsis and shock.

INTRAOPERATIVE CARE.—Careful planning of the surgical procedure to avoid unnecessary trauma, blood loss, and delay is mandatory. Septic

230

shock is particularly likely to follow manipulation of the biliary or urogenital areas when there is established suppurative disease. When this is encountered at operation or suspected preoperatively, broad-spectrum antibiotic coverage must be started before or during the operation. Operative blood loss is usually underestimated by the surgeon and overestimated by the anesthesiologist. Quantitation is important, and the weighing of sponges and measurement of blood in collection bottles provides a conservative estimate of actual blood loss. Estimated intraoperative losses of over 1,000 ml should be replaced by blood and balanced saline solution. Replacement should be carried out as the loss occurs and not delayed until signs of hypovolemia develop. Large-volume rapid blood replacement is damaging for many reasons, including impaction of microemboli in the lungs and excessive citrate loading leading to metabolic alkalosis.

Intraoperative measurement of central venous pressure and urinary flow are important adjuncts to measuring the adequacy of blood replacement. The surgeon has a unique opportunity to observe the state of the circulation. The color of the gut, pulsation in the marginal jejunal vessels, the color of the venous blood, and collapse or overfilling of the great veins attest to the adequacy of the peripheral circulation. This information should be integrated with the anesthesiologist's measurements of arterial and central venous pressure in arriving at decisions regarding supportive treatment. Attention should be paid to the patient's metabolic status. The mechanisms for thermal regulation (shivering and cutaneous vasoconstriction) are inhibited by general anesthesia and muscle relaxants. Heat loss from a long procedure in a cool operating room may be significant. Roe has demonstrated that in patients without demonstrable metabolic abnormalities there is a reduction in body temperature of 1–3°C during surgical procedures. He found that the duration of the operation, the use of muscle relaxants, and the age of the patient are closely related to the degree of hypothermia which develops. In the recovery room, as the effects of anesthesia wear off, there is an attempt to restore body temperature by shivering and cutaneous vasoconstriction, leading to increased O_2 demand. Roe also finds that when the fall in body temperature has exceeded 1°C, there is a tendency to overshoot in the first 24–48 hours, producing a febrile reaction. With the increase in O_2 consumption, relatively minor degrees of respiratory obstruction, pneumonia, or underlying cardiovascular disease may not be tolerated and increase the risk of collapse and death.

Cutaneous vasoconstriction and shivering are readily appreciated by the physician, and measures should be taken to reduce the loss of body heat during the operation and to provide warmth during recovery from the operation. Too often, immediately after the operation, the patient is placed in a cold environment with negligible skin coverage. By failing to control heat loss, an additional metabolic load is placed upon the postoperative patient.

POSTOPERATIVE CARE.—The common causes of shock during an operation and in the immediate postoperative period are hypovolemia and myocardial infarction. Cardiac tamponade is always suspected when, after open heart surgery, there is a progressive fall in cardiac output, a rising central venous pressure, and cessation of chest tube drainage. Careful observation of the postoperative patient may reveal evidence of intra-abdominal bleeding, as shown by nontympanitic abdominal distention, or intrathoracic bleeding. Postoperative distention, especially acute gastric distention, reduces venous return and may readily induce shock in the hypovolemic patient. Deflation of the stomach by nasogastric intubation results in striking improvement. Again, preventing heat loss avoids undue stress in already ill patients.

The Patient with Multiple Injuries

The basic tenets in the care of patients with multiple injuries are that life-threatening injuries take precedence and that over-all responsibility for care be vested in one person. The worst fate that can befall the patient with multiple injuries is that responsibility be shared by several specialists. This becomes all too evident in the operating room where team after team of specialists operate in sequence, each concerned only with his own field. A critically injured patient should be in the operating room long enough only to ensure proper care of life-threatening injury before he is returned to the intensive care unit for careful monitoring and cardiopulmonary support. Treatment of lacerations and many fractures may often be delayed for 24 hours after temporary dressing and immobilization to allow early care of the circulation and ventilation.

Burns

Burns present an especially interesting and challenging study in shock and sepsis. Initial therapy should follow the accepted procedures of fluid therapy, remembering that there is considerable heat loss by evaporation of water through the burn eschar and consequently a hypermetabolic state develops to maintain body temperature. These patients present a high risk when taken to the operating room for debridement. In addition to loss of thermal regulation with general anesthesia, as described earlier, there is additional evaporative heat loss both from the eschar and debrided area. When returned from surgery, they face a dual metabolic load of burn plus hypothermia and substantial risk of collapse and death. Often large areas of eschar—through which considerable water loss occurs—and bare skin are exposed directly to the low ambient temperature of the recovery room. Although the burn patient represents the most extreme metabolic demand because of sepsis and inability to control cutaneous water loss, the septic patient who also functions at a higher metabolic rate is also subject to many of the risks seen in the severely burned patient. Roe has demonstrated these phenomena in burn and septic patients in a most graphic manner.

Treatment of Established Shock

"To turn a swamp into a running brook."

Too often the diagnosis of shock brings forth an alarm reaction on the part of the physician. To this he responds by giving fluids, steroids, vasopressors, buffer agents, and any other recently touted nostrum. No significant measurements are made and if, by virtue of the natural homeostatic mechanisms, the patient survives, a triumph for some one or other drug is claimed. On the other hand, if the patient should die, shock is pronounced irreversible.

It is self-evident that no single method of treatment may be applied to all patients in shock since the clinical manifestations of shock are common responses to injuries of widely differing origin. For example: the shock associated with hemorrhage and that resulting from myocardial infarction are both characterized by impaired tissue perfusion and share the clinical features of hypotension (cold, clammy extremities and oliguria). The former, however, responds favorably to fluid administration whereas the same treatment for cardiogenic shock may be damaging.

The aim of therapy is to restore tissue perfusion, but in the various types of shock this is accomplished by different and sometimes opposing methods. Accordingly, the first step in treatment is to formulate an understanding of the underlying disease process and the particular hemodynamic problem which exists at the moment, then gauge success or failure of therapy by repeated measurements.

In advanced shock several organ systems may be damaged. Primary attention must always be focused upon cardiovascular and respiratory systems as well as the kidneys. On seeing a shock patient for the first time, the problem should be evaluated in an orderly manner so as to provide the crucial physiologic information necessary for treatment.

Initial Evaluation of the Shock Patient

Brief history while blood and urine samples are taken.—The central venous catheter inserted at this time may be used for blood sampling, infusions, and pressure measurements. The placement of a radial artery catheter allows repeated measurement of blood gases, arterial pressure, and cardiac output.

PHYSICAL EXAMINATION, RAPID BUT WITH SPECIAL ATTENTION TO:

1. Ventilation.—Estimation of effectiveness and the amount of respiratory work being performed. Auscultation of both sides of the chest.

2. Skin color, turgor, sweating.

3. Blood pressure, pulse rate, central venous pressure.

4. Abdominal examination: distention, tenderness, rigidity, fluid, or masses. Insertion of a nasogastric tube may provide useful information as well as improve venous return by reducing gastric distention.

5. Extremities: Fracture, soft tissue injury. Rough estimation of fluid loss into an injured limb.

6. Urine output—insertion of Foley catheter: hourly measurement, identification of myoglobin after crush injury.

7. Initial essential laboratory values; hematocrit, white blood count, blood and urine sugar, BUN, arterial blood pH, P_{CO_2}, P_{O_2}. Excess or deficit of bicarbonate and serum electrolytes.

8. Chest x-ray.

9. Blood culture.

The information now available should enable the clinician to form an intelligent understanding of altered function and, in particular, to identify the vital organ systems most clearly in need of support. In essence, therapy is directed toward vital organ support and is carried out in a titrative manner based on repeated measurement of response.

INITIAL TREATMENT

A brief résumé of the initial considerations in treatment follows; the specific details are given in the appropriate sections later in this chapter.

CARDIOVASCULAR SUPPORT

1. Venous return.—Efforts to increase venous return by fluid load are a primary concern unless there is clear evidence of left or right ventricular overload.

2. Control of myocardial force, rate and rhythm.—Impairment of ventricular ejection is judged by failure to support the circulation in spite of adequate venous return. Experience and judgment are needed to decide whether to drive the heart with betamimetic agents or glucagon, reduce rate and increase stroke volume with digitalis, reduce irritability with Pronestyl or lidocaine, or reduce peripheral resistance with vasodilator drugs. A detailed discussion of this important problem follows under the section Myocardial Support, later in this chapter.

3. Support of blood pressure.—The vital coronary and cerebral circulations require a mean blood pressure of at least 60 mm Hg. This must be maintained even if vasoconstrictor drugs are needed as a temporary expedient until more effective cardiovascular support can be given.

SUPPORT OF PULMONARY GAS EXCHANGE

1. Ventilation.—Clinical examination and measurements of arterial Po_2 and Pco_2 should immediately indicate the need for supplemental oxygen, nasotracheal intubation or tracheostomy, and assisted or controlled ventilation. The work of breathing may be so increased in shock that support should be considered even in the face of normal blood gases.

2. Oxygen transport.—The optimal hematocrit range lies between 35 and 40%. This measurement serves as a guide in deciding whether to replace with packed cells, whole blood or plasma.

FURTHER TREATMENT AND EVALUATION

By the time initial circulatory and ventilatory support have been given, the majority of patients who will ultimately recover will have already responded favorably. In more complicated cases, the cause of the shock should be evident at this point and specific measures such as the control of hemorrhage, drainage of abscesses, and the institution of antibiotic therapy will have been undertaken. In advanced cases, the development of severe metabolic acidosis, rising venous pressure, impaired pulmonary gas exchange, oliguria, stupor, and evidences of intravascular coagulation point to the likelihood of death.

It should be borne in mind that shock which starts out in one category may evolve into a complex of several forms. Sepsis, for example, may be complicated by cardiac failure. Hypovolemia may precipitate myocardial damage. These combined forms are more commonly seen in the aged patient, but unexpected myocardial damage may be encountered even in the young patient who has experienced protracted hypotension. Finally, after the successful treatment of shock, complications such as infection, gastrointestinal bleeding, pulmonary embolism, and arterial thrombosis may take the patient's life.

FLUID REPLACEMENT

Hypovolemia is the most commonly mistreated form of shock and yet it is the form most readily responsive to therapy. Hypovolemia is not only important in states in which fluid or blood loss is obvious but also may be a critical factor in the treatment of septic shock and the shock associated with barbiturate intoxication.

Formerly, many major operations were accompanied by oliguria and hypotension. In all likelihood, this problem arose out of a failure to appreciate the extent of the fluid and blood loss during an extensive operative procedure. Today, with the recognition of the large fluid loss that occurs, balanced saline solution and blood are given to make up the fluid deficit, and postoperative oliguria can be averted. Shires' contention that large extracellular fluid deficits (20–40%) follow trauma or hemorrhage has been challenged on methodologic grounds by Moore and Maloney. Nevertheless, the volume of saline given during operations continues to be out of proportion to the operative loss and, since the former restrictions on postoperative saline infusions have been lifted, a clear tendency toward flooding the patient during and after an operation has developed. This has been documented in Vietnam by Mills *et al.*, who showed a high incidence of fatal pulmonary edema in casualties treated with massive amounts of Ringer's lactate.

After obvious extensive injury, whether due to blood loss, trauma, burns, or peritonitis, guidelines must be drawn to indicate the rate and volume of fluid replacement as well as the choice of fluid. These judgments are based upon careful and repeated observations of the clinical signs and the hemodynamic and biochemical measurements discussed earlier. Reliance upon a single measurement is fraught with hazard. For example, it is not generally recognized that in the severely vasoconstricted state the venous pressure rises disproportionately in spite of relative hypovolemia, but with relaxation of the venous reservoir, as occurs after alpha adrenergic blockade, greatly increased volumes are well tolerated. The basic guide to fluid therapy in shock is the concept of titration coupled with repeated measurements.

VOLUME REQUIREMENTS.—The physician treating shock, regardless of its origin, must be assured above all that the atrial filling pressure is adequate to produce an effective cardiac output. This essential information is gained by clinical observation of the pressure in the veins of the neck or, better still, by measurement of central venous pressure (see Fig. 5-1). Unless the venous pressure is already above 10 cm of water, the effect of rapidly loading the circulation with 500–1,000 ml of fluid in 20 minutes is estimated. A rapid rise in venous pressure indicates that the heart is loaded to its capacity but, on the other hand, when there is a favorable response in arterial blood pressure without significant rise in venous pressure, a state of hypovolemia probably exists. This cardiovascular response to fluid load is the single most important measurement that can be made in the shock patient. If the venous pressure rises rapidly, the load must be discontinued forthwith.

Failure of the left side of the heart may be signaled by the onset of dyspnea and basal rales before the central venous pressure reflects the overload. The response of the venous pressure to fluid administration provides a dynamic gauge for measuring fluid replacement in shock. No rule of thumb for fluid replacement can possibly apply in the shock state, in which the capacitance of the circulation is constantly changing and myocardial function may be considerably impaired by a prolonged period of hypotension. The damaged heart may be capable of producing an adequate output only at a considerably raised atrial pressure. Often in advanced shock, blood pressure can be maintained only by increasingly large infusions of fluid. Responses of this type almost invariably end in pulmonary edema. In this situation efforts should be directed toward improving myocardial function rather than excessive fluid loading.

The volume of fluid which may be infused is also restricted by sympathetic venoconstriction which limits the capacity of the venous reservoir. The hematocrit serves only as a guide to indicate the need for red cells or a plasma expander. Once a satisfactory clinical response has been achieved, care must be taken to avoid overloading the patient even if the venous pressure remains on the low side. Daily measurements of body weight provide an important guide to volume replacement.

CHOICE OF FLUID REPLACEMENT.—The choice of fluid replacement depends on the nature of the loss. A fraction of the normal red cell mass will usually suffice for oxygen transport provided the compensatory increase in plasma volume is adequate to maintain a normal total blood volume and the heart is capable of increasing its output. The added burden of anemia should be avoided in the elderly patient or the individual with ischemic heart disease.

The shock-damaged heart appears to function best at a hematocrit level of 35–40%. The total extracellular fluid reservoir comprises about 20% of the body weight. Roughly one-fifth of this extracellular fluid volume is plasma and the remainder is interstitial fluid which resembles plasma but has a lower protein content. For emergency expansion of the extracellular fluid space, Ringer's lactate, which has an electrolyte content close to that of extracellular fluid, has gained popular acceptance.

Replacement with glucose water, free of electrolytes, carries the danger of inducing a hypo-osmolar state with attendant cellular edema. In burns, however, when the evaporative water loss may be enormous, large quantities of glucose water may be required. The types of fluid used for replacement in shock patients may be divided into three broad classes: blood, plasma expanders, and electrolyte solutions.

Blood.—A loss of 500 ml of blood in the normal individual is tolerated without marked signs of hypovolemia. Slow loss of even one liter may be attended by slight response; loss of a volume of blood greater than this, or rapid loss of a smaller volume, is usually followed by severe clinical and hemodynamic changes. As indicated above, the use of solutions without red cells to expand plasma volume will often bring about homeostasis, provided the bleeding has ceased and the heart is able to raise its output. When bleeding continues, replacement with blood is mandatory. Even here, however, the combined use of blood and electrolyte solutions such as Ringer's lactate appears to have merit.

Replacement with colloid-containing fluid is mandatory in maintaining plasma volume. With the narrowed caliber of the terminal vessels in shock and the tendency toward red cell aggregation, it is advantageous to reduce the viscosity of blood. Plasma expanders accomplish this by hemodilution. Once the blood volume has been expanded to the point at which there is an adequate atrial filling pressure, the necessity for red blood cell replacement can be judged by the hematocrit level. In a patient with a raised venous pressure associated with anemia, the use of packed red blood cells is indicated.

Plasma and plasma expanders.—In conditions in which there is excessive loss of plasma protein (especially in acute pancreatitis, peritonitis, or burns), the use of molecules large enough to be retained in the vascular space is mandatory. While plasma is the replacement of choice for these conditions, electrolyte solutions to which albumin is added are also valuable.

Plasmanate is a sterile solution of human plasma proteins obtained by cold ethanol fractionation (albumin, alpha and beta globulin). No blood-coagulating factors or immune globulins are included. The solution has the advantage of being heat-treated at 60°C to reduce the possibility of hepatitis. Its chief value is for albumin replacement and plasma expansion.

Commercial dextran (molecular weight 70,000) is a better volume expander than low-molecular-weight dextran (molecular weight 40,000) because it leaves the vascular space less readily. Both dextrans have been used to prevent thrombosis in small blood vessels, but there is conflicting evidence in regard to any specific value of low-molecular-weight dextran in shock. Either dextran used in volumes over 2 liters carries the hazard of bleeding.

Innumerable papers and hundreds of pages of advertising testify to the unique properties of low-molecular-weight dextran as a specific agent to improve microcirculatory flow, but careful review of this material by Repogle, Read, and others points to the lack of adequate control in the majority of data presented. The weight of this abundant testimony must now be questioned in the cold light of controlled experimentation. In vitro studies, using the most sensitive viscometers, demonstrate that all the dextrans increase the viscosity and yield shear stress, provided the hematocrit is maintained at a constant level. The mechanism is thought to be one of red-cell coating and intercellular bonding. The higher the molecular weight, the greater the tendency for red cell aggregation. While the lower molecular weight dextrans produce less viscosity effect, there is no convincing in vitro evidence to indicate a specific desludging action. When hemodilution is allowed to occur, the improvement in flow is quite comparable, no matter how the hemodilution is produced, and is related to the degree of hemodilution rather than to any specific microvascular effect of low-molecular-weight dextran.

There is considerable evidence to support the thesis that a moderate degree of hemodilution by any one of a number of plasma volume expanders will improve tissue perfusion and cardiac output. Low-molecular-weight dextran appears to be somewhat disadvantageous in this connection in that its intravascular position is maintained for a shorter period of time than with the commercial dextran. It is thus apparent that a moderate degree of hemodilution, regardless of the origin, reduces blood viscosity and yield shield stress by lowering red cell and fibrinogen concentration and by increasing the velocity of flow in the microcirculation.

Electrolyte solutions.—Expansion of the extracellular fluid space is an important part of the treatment of traumatic shock. It is not unusual in injuries where fluid is sequestered in the traumatized organs that fluids must be given until the patient gains an extra 3–4 kg of weight in order to maintain an adequate venous pressure. When homeostasis is established, this excess fluid is lost by diuresis.

In the patient without heart disease (especially after trauma), fluids containing sodium become of paramount importance in expanding the extracellular space. The specific value of Ringer's lactate solution is its stability and its function as a source of sodium when the lactate has been converted to bicarbonate. Since the ability of the liver to convert lactate to bicarbonate is reduced in severe shock, a question has been raised concerning the wisdom of administering Ringer's lactate solution in shock patients with severe metabolic acidosis. In the patient with advanced shock and metabolic acidosis, glucose water with the addition of sodium bicarbonate is preferable in correcting metabolic acidosis and expanding the extracellular volume. Isotonic sodium chloride may also be used for expansion of the extracellular space, but if a large volume is given without buffer, it may potentiate the acidosis of shock.

ACID-BASE CORRECTION

In shock, metabolic acidosis is a consequence of inadequate tissue perfusion and the resultant accumulation of the acid by-products of anaerobic metabolism. The basis of logical treatment is to correct this by restoring tissue perfusion, not simply by loading with buffer. Metabolic acidosis, however, may be so severe that other methods of improving cardiovascular function will fail. This position is often seen immediately after cardiac arrest in which immediate buffering with sodium bicarbonate aids resuscitation. Accordingly, correction of this defect may be necessary before optimal tissue perfusion can be secured. *Sodium bicarbonate* is the standby of buffer therapy. It provides expansion of the extracellular space and buffers the accumulating hydrogen ion producing carbonic acid which is volatilized in the lung.

The usual 50 ml ampule of 7% sodium bicarbonate contains approximately 45 mEq of bicarbonate. Hypertonic bicarbonate solution should be given slowly, and usually not more than two-thirds of the deficit is replaced in one injection without repeat measurements of blood gases. Fifty percent sodium bicarbonate in water is now available as a prepared solution containing 595 mEq per liter of sodium and an equal concentration of bicarbonate. Hitherto, because of problems in the commercial preparation and sterilization of bicarbonate, sodium lactate has dominated the treatment of metabolic acidosis. In the severe metabolic acidosis of shock with the evidence of failure to metabolize lactate, however, bicarbonate solutions are the buffers of choice since no intermediate metabolic action is required for conversion. In severe metabolic acidosis the amount of bicarbonate needed to buffer the extracellular space may be roughly determined using the following formula:

$$\text{Dosage (mEq)} = 0.2 \times \text{body weight (kg)} \times (27 \text{ mEq/L} - \text{serum bicarbonate mEq/L})$$

In severe acidosis, half the calculated dose is given initially; the dose is then adjusted according to pH determinations.

THAM—(Tris-hydroxymethyl aminomethane)

$$NH_2 - C \begin{array}{c} CH_2\,OH \\ -CH_2\,OH \\ CH_2\,OH \end{array}$$

According to Bronsted's classification, this substance is a weak base. In the presence of acid, the following reaction takes place:

$(CH_2\,OH)_3\text{-}\,C - NH_2 + HA \rightleftharpoons (CH_2\,OH)_3 - C - NH_3^+ + A^-$
A^- may be HCO_3^-, Cl^- or lactate$^-$

This substance is a powerful hydrogen ion acceptor and can be used in the treatment of either metabolic or respiratory acidosis. It has the additional advantage of crossing the cell membrane and counteracting intracellular acidosis. Because of its alkalinity (pH 12), it must be administered in fairly large volumes of fluid and, although it also functions as a diuretic, this extra volume may lead to a problem of overloading. It is a powerful respiratory depressant and may be dangerous unless mechanical ventilatory assistance is readily available. It is usually given slowly as a 0.3 molar solution which is obtained by dissolving 18 gm in 500 ml of diluent. With better understanding of the perfusion problem in shock, THAM is seldom used today.

Myocardial Support

CONTROL OF RATE.—The heart rate of a critically ill patient is frequently abnormal. Myocardial ischemia or disturbance of conduction may result in sinus bradycardia. Sinus tachycardia, with rates of 100–150 beats per minute, is commonly associated with fever and hypoxia. There is good physiologic evidence to suggest that variation in cardiac rates between 60 and 150 beats per minute does not alter cardiac output as long as there is sinus rhythm. Even at sinus rates well in excess of 150, there is little, if any, fall in cardiac output as a result of the tachycardia.

Several drugs are available to control heart rate. Sinus bradycardia with rates below 60 can frequently be corrected by the intravenous administration of atropine in doses of 1–2 mg. Intravenous isoproterenol in doses of 5–10 μg per minute will also correct sinus bradycardia. There is little advantage to be gained by an increase in cardiac rate in sinus bradycardia, however, since cardiac output does not usually fall unless the heart rate falls below 40 beats per minute.

Digitalis, dilantin, and propranolol are drugs that slow sinus tachycardia. Digitalis is frequently ineffective in slowing sinus tachycardia, and digitalis intoxication may result if the dosage given is one which will control the rate significantly. While dilantin generally has a slowing effect on heart rate, the sinus tachycardia of shock is but little influenced. Propranolol administered intravenously in doses of 2 mg will result in slowing of the heart rate. In this fashion, the sinus tachycardia can be abolished or controlled. But the negative inotropic effect of propranolol may be seriously detrimental to a patient in shock, especially if his cardiac output is already low. Therefore, there is little to be gained and a great deal to be lost from the administration of intravenous propranolol to critically ill patients with sinus tachycardia. Control of heart rate is usually best effected by improving the circumstances that led to the sinus tachycardia, that is, lowering of fever, draining of an abscess, correction of acidosis, treatment of hypoxia, and replacement of blood volume.

CONTROL OF ARRHYTHMIAS.—The hypoxic myocardium stimulated by endogenously released catecholamines is particularly susceptible to devel-

TABLE 7-1.—DIAGNOSIS OF COMMON CARDIAC ARRHYTHIMIAS

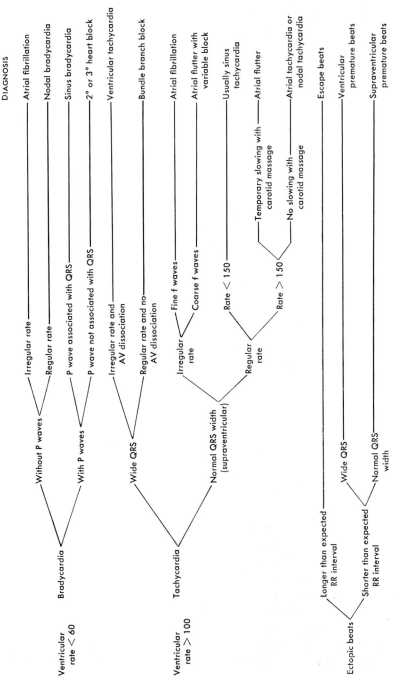

oping an arrhythmia which may diminish the efficiency of the heart and decrease cardiac output. Electrolyte disturbances, especially hyperkalemia and hypokalemia, alter the contractility of the myocardium and add to the risk of ventricular irritability and arrhythmias. Both metabolic acidosis and respiratory alkalosis tend to be detrimental to myocardial function, but most damaging of all is persistent hypotension causing a fall in coronary perfusion.

The proper treatment of cardiac arrhythmias requires their prompt and correct diagnosis (Table 7-1). In all cases, adequate ventilation and oxygenation must be ensured and the precipitating causes treated. Certain arrhythmias can be diagnosed by physical signs at the bedside. For example, auricular flutter is diagnosed by observing flutter waves in the jugular pulsations in the neck. Atrioventricular dissociation may be diagnosed by a varying intensity of the first heart sound and by cannon waves in the jugular venous pulse.

TABLE 7-2.—TREATMENT OF COMMON CARDIAC ARRHYTHMIAS

Ventricular fibrillation:
  Electric shock
  IV bretylium 300 mg
Bradycardia:
  Withhold digitalis
  IV atropine 0.5–1 mg, if rate is below 40
  Isuprel drip 5 μg per minute
  Transvenous pacemaker for 2°–3° heart block
Ventricular tachycardia:
  IV lidocaine 50–100 mg
  IV Pronestyl 100–200 mg
  IV bretylium 300 mg
  IV Dilantin 150 mg (with digitalis intoxication)
  Electrical cardioversion (not with digitalis intoxication)
  Pacing with transvenous pacemaker
Supraventricular tachycardia:
  IV Inderal 1–2 mg
  IV digoxin .75 mg (not nodal tachycardia if digitalis-induced)
  Electrical cardioversion
Escape beats:
  IV atropine 0.5–1 mg.
  Withhold digitalis
  Transvenous pacing
Ventricular prematurities:
  IV lidocaine drip 2 gm per 24 hr
  IV pronestyl 100 mg
  IV Inderal 1–2 mg
Supraventricular prematurities:
  May not require therapy
  IV digoxin 0.75 mg
  IV Inderal 1–2 mg

Most cardiac arrhythmias, however, require an electrocardiographic diagnosis. Occasionally, specific diagnostic measures may aid in the diagnosis of arrhythmias. For example, recording an electrocardiogram with carotid massage may enable one to observe previously undetected flutter waves. The gradual and slight slowing of heart rate with carotid massage may also permit differentiation of sinus tachycardia from an arrhythmia such as an atrial tachycardia.

Recently, we have made use of intra-atrial EKGs in order to diagnose more difficult arrhythmias in which P wave activity is not otherwise readily discernible. In this fashion, ventricular tachycardia can be distinguished from supraventricular tachycardia with aberrant conduction by noting the correlation of atrial activity with ventricular activity. Ventricular tachycardia is almost always associated with atrioventricular dissociation. In general, ventricular premature contractions and ventricular arrhythmias such as ventricular tachycardia are manifested by wide QRS complexes since depolarization is occurring outside the specialized conduction system. Most supraventricular arrhythmias, on the other hand, show a QRS complex of normal width. Occasionally, however, aberrant conduction may occur with a supraventricular tachycardia and this may mimic ventricular tachycardia.

The treatment of choice for most supraventricular tachycardias is rapid intravenous digitalization of the patient (Table 7-2). Most auricular tachycardias can be abolished by effective digitalization. Atrial fibrillation and atrial flutter respond to digitalization by increasing the degree of AV block and slowing the heart rate to a physiologic level. Since digitalis itself may cause arrhythmias, it is important not to give additional digitalis if the arrhythmia is digitalis-induced. Paroxysmal atrial tachycardia with block is one type of digitalis-induced arrhythmia.

The diagnosis of digitalis intoxication may pose a serious problem in shock. Recently, attention has been directed toward the diagnosis of digitalis intoxication with atrial fibrillation. Under these circumstances the RR interval tends to become regular, or a repetitive pattern is observed in the RR intervals. If the supraventricular arrhythmia is digitalis-induced, either no treatment or treatment with Dilantin or propranolol is indicated.

Ventricular irritability and ventricular arrhythmias can usually be treated effectively with quinidine and quinidine-like drugs. In recent years, intravenous lidocaine has gained wide popularity. This quinidine-like local anesthetic can be lifesaving in treating and preventing ventricular arrhythmias. When one observes frequent ventricular premature contractions in a critically ill patient, lidocaine may be administered by continuous intravenous drip, usually in doses of 1 to 2 gm per 24 hours. Occasionally, marked ventricular irritability or runs of ventricular tachycardia can be terminated by the administration of a single bolus of lidocaine. Fifty to one hundred mg of lidocaine is usually given intravenously for this purpose.

The main toxicity of lidocaine is its ability to cause CNS reactions, particularly grand and petit mal seizures. Propranolol (Inderal) is a beta-blocking drug which has some effectiveness in treating both supraventricular and ventricular arrhythmias. It can be given in doses up to 200 mg per 24 hours orally and can be given in doses up to 20 mg for 24 hours intravenously. In the critically ill patient, 1 to 2 mg of propranolol injected intravenously may rapidly terminate a supraventricular arrhythmia or decrease ventricular irritability.

Propranolol frequently fails to abolish supraventricular arrhythmias, but will almost always cause slowing of the heart rate, either by slowing the atrial pacemakers or by increasing the degree of A-V block. In a critically ill patient, it may cause asthma or may aggravate underlying respiratory insufficiency. Propranolol also has a tendency to decrease myocardial contractility and diminish cardiac output, which may be a serious limitation in a shock patient who already has limited myocardial function.

In recent years, dilantin has gained wide support as a drug effective in digitalis-induced arrhythmias. Dilantin will abolish other side effects of digitalis such as visual disturbances. Digitalis-induced arrhythmias such as paroxysmal atrial tachycardia (PAT) with block, bigeminy, and trigeminy are ideally treated with intravenous dilantin. Usually 100–150 mg of dilantin is administered intravenously over a period of several minutes and is repeated every 4–6 hours. Dilantin may produce adverse effects by causing an important diminution in cardiac contractility and cardiac output. When administered too rapidly, severe hypotension may occur. Both dilantin and propranolol tend to cause bradycardia and should be used cautiously in a patient with preexisting bradycardia or second or third degree heart block.

Recently another drug, bretylium tosylate, has gained widespread attention as an antiarrhythmia agent. Bretylium was initially used many years ago as an antihypertensive drug. Unlike lidocaine, quinidine, pronestyl, or dilantin, bretylium exerts antiarrhythmic effects without diminishing cardiac output and has been shown to stop ventricular fibrillation in a dog within several seconds after administration intravenously. It is particularly effective in diminishing ventricular irritability and in terminating refractory ventricular tachycardia. It has been used in patients who have been repeatedly defibrillated electrically. Bretylium should be seriously considered for use in a patient who has been defibrillated several times. The

SYNCHRONIZATION
OF
COUNTERSHOCK

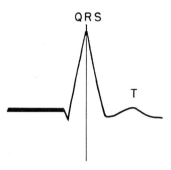

Fig. 7–1.—The synchronized artifact falls in the middle of the QRS complex.

most serious drawback to this drug is its tendency to produce nausea and hypotension. It is usually administered in doses of approximately 5 mg per kilogram every 12 hours intravenously or intramuscularly.

Electrical countershock has become a very reliable means of terminating many cardiac arrhythmias. It is indicated as the treatment of choice for all arrhythmias with tachycardia when digitalis intoxication can be excluded. When a direct-current synchronizer is available, auricular and ventricular tachycardias can be terminated safely by synchronizing the electrical depolarization within the QRS complex of the electrocardiogram. Depolarization can be carried out with minimal risk of inducing ventricular tachycardia or ventricular fibrillation. When a patient develops ventricular fibrillation, electrical defibrillation is the only reliable means of terminating the arrhythmia. Synchronized, direct-current cardioversion will abolish most arrhythmias, particularly when combined with quinidine, procaine amide, or lidocaine (Figs. 7-1, 7-2).

Fig. 7–2.—Electrocardiograms before and after cardioversion. Top strip shows atrial fibrillation. In the bottom strip, normal sinus rhythm has been restored.

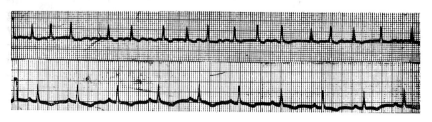

Electrical pacing has been used recently both to protect a patient who develops bradycardia or heart block and to prevent and treat ventricular tachycardias. Any critically ill patient who develops bradycardia with rates below 40 or who has second- or third-degree heart block should have a temporary transvenous pacemaker catheter inserted from the external jugular vein into the right ventricle of the heart. Cardiac arrest due to asystole can be prevented, and patients can be paced to improve cardiac output. It has been shown that by pacing patients at rates of 150 beats per minute, ventricular irritability can be decreased. Some patients with repetitive episodes of ventricular tachycardia have been effectively treated by pacing with a transvenous pacer.

CONTROL OF CONTRACTILITY.—Augmentation of cardiac contractility is a vital part of myocardial support. One method of augmenting cardiac contractility is to administer large volumes of intravenous fluid in an attempt to take advantage of the Starling mechanism and increase stroke volume and cardiac output. This method of treatment should be utilized in any shock patient with a normal or low central venous pressure. Even patients in cardiogenic shock following myocardial infarction may be improved by this form of therapy. Careful monitoring of the patient's lung for moist rales and of central venous pressure may reduce the danger of pulmonary edema. The most common method of augmenting cardiac output is the use of beta adrenergic stimulating drugs of which isoproterenol is the prototype. This drug, administered at 5–10 μg per minute, may markedly increase the force of contraction. Unfortunately, increased oxygen consumption by the myocardium and increased ventricular irritability frequently accompany the administration of beta adrenergic drugs. Most vasopressors, such as aramine and levophed, have some beta adrenergic stimulating properties and enhance myocardial contractility in a manner similar to that of intravenous isoproterenol. Recently, the administration of glucagon by intravenous drip has been advocated as a method of augmenting cardiac contractility. Although this drug possesses positive inotropic properties, its effect is weak. Thus, only a small augmentation of cardiac contractility and cardiac output can be anticipated from the administration of intravenous glucagon. Glucagon has the additional disadvantage of causing nausea and vomiting.

CARDIAC ARREST.—Two types of cardiac arrest are seen. These are ventricular fibrillation and ventricular asystole. Clinically, both of these types have an identical appearance. Both may occur suddenly in the critically ill patient and will result in irreversible brain damage to the patient after 3–4 minutes. No detectable pulse, heart sounds, or blood pressure are present with either ventricular fibrillation or asystole. The only method of distinguishing these two types is an electrocardiogram (Fig. 7-3). With

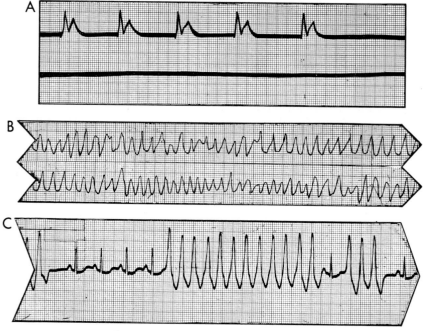

Fig. 7–3.—A, ventricular asystole, B, ventricular fibrillation, C, ventricular tachycardia.

ventricular asystole, the EKG monitor shows a straight-line response. Ventricular fibrillation, on the other hand, shows a chaotic pattern of electrical activity without any definite QRS complexes.

The initial treatment for either form of cardiac arrest is identical. The patient must be given external cardiac massage and must be ventilated within 2–3 minutes after the cardiac arrest. This support must be maintained until the patient's arrest has been corrected. Liberal amounts of IV sodium bicarbonate must be administered every 5 minutes. Usually 40–50 mEq of IV sodium bicarbonate per 5-minute period of arrest is required. If no EKG can be obtained, the patient should be defibrillated using either nonsynchronous direct current countershock or alternating current shock. If the patient has ventricular fibrillation, this shock may be effective in stopping the fibrillation and restoring sinus rhythm. If a patient has asystole, the application of external shock will not prove detrimental. Usually, the defibrillator is set to provide maximum power, e.g., 400 watt seconds. Repeated attempts to electrically defibrillate a patient may be necessary. The administration of intravenous epinephrine is effective in converting fine ventricular fibrillation to a coarse ventricular fibrillation which may then be easier to defibrillate. The administration of IV bretylium (300 mg) may also increase the ease of defibrillation. While attempts to defibrillate will not be harmful to the patient with asystole, they will not prove beneficial. Occasionally, a sharp blow on the chest will cause a cardiac contraction and terminate the asystole. Intravenous or intracardiac catecholamines such as epinephrine (1 cc of 1 to 1,000 solution) or isoproterenol (0.5 mg) may be effective in stimulating electrical and mechanical activity. If all attempts to terminate asystole fail, a temporary transvenous pacemaker should be inserted in the right ventricle and attached to a power source. Occasionally, this is effective in resuming electrical and mechanical activity in a patient with cardiac asystole. Properly performed, external cardiac massage and assisted ventilation can maintain a patient without brain damage for a period of several hours while attempts are made to correct asystole or to terminate ventricular fibrillation.

MECHANICAL SUPPORT OF THE HEART.—Three methods of mechanically assisting the failing heart have recently been devised. The first method reduces the amount of blood the left ventricle ejects. Thus, preload is reduced by shunting venous blood away from the heart, as is done with cardiac bypass. When 80% or more of the cardiac output is bypassed, a significant decrease in cardiac work is achieved. The second method of mechanically assisting the circulation in shock is to use the principle of counterpulsation to reduce the afterload of the left ventricle and increase diastolic pressure. A third method combines principles of the first two. Blood drawn from the venous system is used to augment the stroke volume of the pump and is synchronized with the cardiac cycle.

The advantage of counterpulsation is that it reduces the systolic pressure against which the left ventricle must pump and it augments coronary blood flow by elevation of the aortic diastolic pressure. By synchronous phasic pumping, the systolic pressure in the root of the aorta is reduced during cardiac systole and elevated during cardiac diastole.

It has been shown that coronary blood flow can be increased 25–40% by such techniques. When left ventricular work is reduced by decreasing the afterload of the left ventricle, myocardial oxygen consumption is markedly decreased. In addition, there is evidence that counterpulsation may enhance the rapid development of coronary collateral circulation. In experimental cardiogenic shock, 2 hours of counterpulsation immediately after coronary embolization reduced anticipated mortality 30%. One method of achieving counterpulsation is by increasing and decreasing the volume of blood in the aorta. A balloon introduced into the femoral artery and thoracic aorta is inflated during cardiac diastole and deflated during cardiac systole. Kantrowitz reported a 40% survival rate for 15 patients in cardiogenic shock using counterpulsation by aortic balloon. Soroff has reported on the hemodynamic results of counterpulsation in 7 patients with cardiogenic shock. Counterpulsation was performed an average of 51 minutes. Although only 1 of the 7 patients survived, counterpulsation was followed by a temporary improvement in peripheral perfusion. Soroff mentions that the major limitation to the application of counterpulsation via an intraaortic balloon has been diseased femoral vessels.

Other methods of mechanically assisting the circulation have included synchronous regional pressure variation; for example, an external sleeve to compress the hind quarters of the dog. External synchronous pressure has been used in 2 patients in cardiogenic shock with moderate increases in cardiac output and in diastolic pressure. Intracorporeal pumps have also been used to augment cardiac output. Clot formation remains the most serious problem associated with the chronic implantation of such devices. Efforts at mechanical support of the failing heart are currently in a stage of infancy, but their approach offers great prospects for the future.

PHARMACOLOGY OF DIGITALIS.—This drug is of such importance in providing cardiac support that a detailed consideration of its action is warranted.

In cardiac failure, digitalis produces an increase in the force of systolic contraction, a decrease in heart size, a lengthening of the refractory period, a slowing of conduction through the A-V node and bundle of His, and an increase in automaticity of ventricular muscle. It is apparent that digitalis has both inotropic and chronotropic effects. Recent work has indicated that the selective stimulant effect of cardiac glycosides on the myocardium may be due to their action on the cell membrane. The cardiac cell membrane separates a high concentration of potassium inside the cell from a low concentration outside.

The reverse applies to sodium. An active transport mechanism extrudes sodium ion from the cell and creates an electrical potential gradient and concentration gradient across the cell membrane. At the initiation of the action potential, the membrane is depolarized so that the sodium ion rushes into the cell and potassium ion flows out. The active transport system then extrudes sodium ion and potassium ion returns. It has been well demonstrated that cardiac glycosides inhibit this transport of sodium ion and potassium ion across the cell membrane. There is good experimental evidence to demonstrate that digitalis produces significant inhibition of ATPase. This inhibition of sodium-potassium-ATPase results in an intracellular increase in sodium ion concentration and a decrease in potassium ion and suggests a chemical mode of action of the cardiac glycosides. It is apparent that serum concentrations of various cations may have significant effects on the action of digitalis.

Although the cardiac glycosides are basically similar in action, there are critically important differences in absorption, rapidity of onset, and persistence of action between the various preparations. Digitoxin has proved to be the slowest, and thevetin the most rapid, in onset of action. Other cardiac glycosides fall in intermediate positions. In the treatment of critically ill patients, intravenous digoxin has full activity in 2 hours and some effect within 20–30 minutes. Intravenous ouabain demonstrates full effects within 60 minutes and some effect within 10–15 minutes following intravenous administration. Intravenous digitoxin may require 8 hours for full activity following intravenous administration and is usually too slow for use in a critically ill patient.

CONTRAINDICATIONS TO THE USE OF DIGITALIS.—There are probably no absolute contraindications to the use of digitalis. In the presence of significant congestive heart failure, digitalis has repeatedly been effective in augmenting cardiac performance. Nevertheless, a number of conditions may make the use of digitalis less effective or somewhat hazardous. It is generally agreed that hypertrophic subaortic stenosis is frequently worsened by the administration of digitalis. This drug apparently increases the degree of outflow obstruction to the left ventricle by decreasing the cardiac size. This disease is uncommon, but it should be considered when patients appear to become worse following the administration of digitalis. Other investigators have suggested that in the presence of constrictive pericarditis digitalis may be harmful since it may further decrease diastolic relaxation. In the presence of myocarditis, digitalis may have very little benefit. Castor et al. have listed factors that predispose to the development of digitalis toxicity and include old age, acute myocardial infarction or myocarditis, diuretic-induced potassium depletion, advanced heart disease with severe congestive failure, cor pulmonale, recent cardiac surgery, hypothyroidism, and hemodialysis. The difficulty in many of these conditions is that digitalis, while of benefit, cannot completely reverse the underlying disease and is given to the point of excess. In many conditions that already predispose to ventricular arrhythmias, digitalis may increase the cardiac automaticity. Nevertheless, this is an argument in favor of using smaller doses of digitalis rather than abandoning its use entirely. Using tritiated digoxin, Daugherty has demonstrated that in the presence of impaired cardiac function, hypothyroidism, or cor pulmonale digitalis may still be effective, but smaller maintenance doses are required to avoid cardiac intoxication. Since digitalis slows conduction through the A-V node, the administration of digitalis to a patient who has first- or second-degree heart block may be detrimental in that a higher degree of block may result. Under these circumstances, it may be advisable to insert a temporary transvenous pacemaker into the right ventricle before giving the patient digitalis. Patients with complete heart block may benefit strikingly from the administration of digitalis, and occasionally the degree of block may actually lessen in such patients. On the other hand, patients experiencing ventricular tachycardia and short runs of ventricular premature contractions may be worsened by the administration of digitalis since it may increase ventricular automaticity and irritability.

EFFECTS OF CALCIUM ION CONCENTRATION.—Many of the properties of cardiac glycosides can be imitated by alterations in the calcium ion concentration surrounding cardiac muscle cells. In isolated frog heart preparations, both the therapeutic and toxic effects of ouabain are potentiated by high calcium ion concentrations. Most investigators feel that polarization of the cell membrane mobilizes calcium ion intracellularly without influencing the total content of calcium in the muscle or producing a measurable efflux or influx of calcium ion. It is likely that therapeutic doses of cardiac glycosides influence this action inside the membrane. Gross changes in calcium ion flux occur with much larger toxic doses of digitalis. There are numerous basic observations to the effect that calcium ion increases ventricular excitability. An excess of calcium can produce toxic synergism with digitalis. This has therapeutic implications since malignancy with metastatic bone disease may result in hypercalcemia. Such patients are extremely sensitive to the administration of digitalis. Similarly, a patient already intoxicated with digitalis may be improved by the intravenous infusion of the chelating drug sodium versenate, which lowers the serum concentration of calcium.

POTASSIUM ION CONCENTRATION.—Decrease in plasma and intracellular potassium favors the development of digitalis arrhythmias. Furthermore, toxic doses of digitalis decrease the potassium concentration in heart muscle. Since many critically ill patients may be hypokalemic, for various reasons, it is important to measure the concentration of serum potassium before administering digitalis to these patients. It is generally agreed that therapy with oral or intravenous potassium may inhibit the toxic action of digitalis on the heart by depressing cardiac irritability or by replacing potassium lost from the ventricle. A critically ill patient who has recently been given digitalis and is experiencing frequent ventricular premature contractions should receive supplementary potassium if his serum concentration is low or at a low normal range. Usually 80 mEq of potassium chloride administered intravenously per 24 hours is an adequate dose.

DIGITALIS THERAPY IN THE ANURIC OR OLIGURIC PATIENT

Recently, Jelliff has proposed a rational scheme for digoxin therapy in patients with reduced renal function. The average measured half-time of tritiated digoxin is 1.6 days for patients with normal renal function. In such patients, 65% of a loading dose of digoxin will be present in the body one day later and 35% will have been lost by various routes. Since the subsequent daily maintenance dose is intended to replace daily loss, the proper daily maintenance dose should be 35% of the loading dose if the loading dose was a proper one. When renal function is reduced, digoxin disappears more slowly from the body, and its half-time in the body is prolonged. Consequently, the daily maintenance dose must be correspondingly reduced. The half-time of digoxin in an anuric patient is prolonged to approximately 4.4 days. The proper maintenance dose for an anuric patient should therefore be reduced to 14% of the initial loading dose. Since daily non-urinary losses are 14% of the initial loading dose, daily urinary losses are proportional to endogenous creatinine clearance and should be added to the total loss when calculating a proper daily maintenance dose. Thus, for a creatinine clearance of 120 cc per minute, the digoxin half-life is approximately 1.6 days. For a creatinine clearance of 60 cc per minute the digoxin half-life is approximately 2 days. The daily maintenance of digoxin should be 35% of the loading dose with a creatinine clearance of 100 cc per minute, 25% of loading dose with a clearance of 50 cc per minute, and 20% of loading dose with a creatinine clearance of 25 cc per minute. Similarly, based on blood-urea-nitrogen concentrations, daily maintenance doses of digoxin are as follows: BUN 30 mg% maintenance dose 34%; BUN 50 mg% maintenance dose 26%; BUN 70 mg% maintenance dose 20%. For BUN values in excess of 100 mg% or for endogenous creatinine clearances of 0, the daily maintenance dose should be 14% of the loading dose. The usual dose of intravenous digoxin is between 1 and 2 mg%. In patients with borderline renal function it is probably safer to use a loading dose between 1 and 1.5 mg digoxin and calculate the daily maintenance dose requirement.

Pulmonary Support

GENERAL CONSIDERATIONS

After any severe injury and especially in shock, measurements of arterial blood gases reveal a surprising degree of hypoxemia in spite of hyperventilation and a low Pco_2. The interstitial edema, atelectasis and finally, pulmonary edema which form the anatomic basis for these findings, have already been discussed in Chapter 3 and the several approaches to therapy are diagrammed in Figure 7-4. In essence, the broad objective of pulmonary support is to increase the number of functioning alveoli in order to restore a balance between ventilation and perfusion which results in acceptable blood gas exchange. In addition, no further damage must be done to the lung. In general, when the patient is assisted by a ventilator, the tidal volume and rate must be increased above normal levels to achieve adequate oxygenation but often at the cost of further reduction in Pco_2. A desirable goal is to adjust the tidal volume, rate and FI_{O_2} to the minimum needed to produce a Pa_{O_2} of between 70 and 90 mm Hg and a Pco_2 of between 32 and 40. The peak airway pressure should be maintained at the lowest level commensurate with adequate ventilation since the use of high tidal volumes increases airway pressure, reduces venous return, and further damages the lungs. In the advanced respiratory distress syndrome these goals are difficult, and sometimes impossible to achieve.

In the respiratory distress syndrome, the various families of alveoli that may be envisaged are shown in Figure 3-16. It is clear that at least two approaches to therapy may be taken: (1) the inspired oxygen concentration may be raised (this usually raises the Pa_{O_2} and hemoglobin to 96% saturation), but this therapeutic approach is self-defeating in that it may further damage the remaining functioning alveoli by exposure to high oxygen tension; (2) far more rewarding is an approach aimed at increasing the number of functioning alveolar units. This approach is stressed in Figure 7-4.

Positive-pressure ventilation itself may expand some atelectatic alveoli; adequate humidification will reduce the viscosity of secretions and open obstructed segments of the lung to ventilation. Support of the heart reduces left-sided cardiac failure and reduces pulmonary edema. The shock or injured patient is frequently excessively loaded with fluid by the time he develops problems in pulmonary gas exchange. Judicious restriction of fluid intake and the use of a diuretic, such as ethacrinic acid, returns fluid-filled alveoli to a functional state, thereby reducing the venous admixture. In addition, proper antibiotic treatment resolves inflammatory exudates filling the alveoli. Similarly, better perfusion due to improved myocardial function and the spontaneous lysis of microemboli with improved perfusion brings dead-space alveoli into a functioning state. In spite of all such measures, however, it may be necessary to use high oxygen concentrations to produce sufficient arterial saturation to maintain life. When there is progressive increase in venous admixture, in spite of adequate therapy, the mortality rate is extremely high. In the respiratory distress syndrome, monitoring of arterial blood gases and ventilatory measurements are mandatory, but in addition, calculation of the venous admixture or simple measurement of A-a DO_2 gives a very useful measure of the effectiveness of therapy. When the Pa_{O_2} is less than 60 mm Hg on 100% oxygen, a shunt of

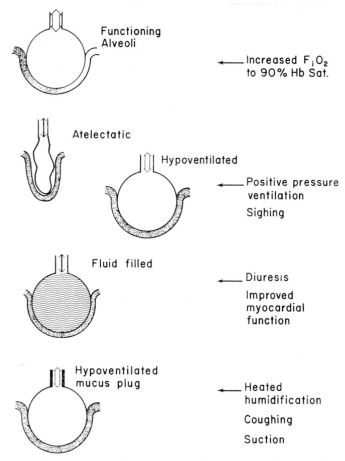

Functioning
Alveoli

Increased F_iO_2
to 90% Hb Sat.

Atelectatic

Hypoventilated

Positive pressure
ventilation

Sighing

Fluid filled

Diuresis

Improved
myocardial
function

Hypoventilated
mucus plug

Heated
humidification

Coughing

Suction

Fig. 7–4.—An approach to the treatment of the respiratory distress syndrome.

30–50% is usually evident and unless pulmonary gas exchange can be improved rapidly, lung damage progresses and death follows.

Patients with adequate ventilation but mild desaturation may be managed for short periods of time by a nasal oxygen catheter or a loose-fitting mask. Using a flow of approximately 5–8 liters per minute of oxygen, 35–40% levels of inspired oxygen can be achieved by these methods. As the system is closed (by tight masking) and the oxygen flow further increased, the inspired oxygen concentration may be driven toward 100%. This approach, however, is not a satisfactory solution to the problem of the severe ventilation-perfusion imbalance seen in the shock patient since it disguises rather than treats the underlying pulmonary lesion.

VENTILATOR SUPPORT

For the patient in respiratory failure, mechanical ventilatory support using positive pressure may be beneficial in many respects. The recruitment of alveoli has been mentioned earlier, and when there is an insufficient alveolar ventilation, tidal volume or rate may be increased. Part or most of the work of respiration may be transferred from the patient to the machine when large minute volumes are needed to maintain arterial saturation. For the patient requiring enriched O_2 mixtures, the ventilator is a convenient method for regulating the inspired oxygen concentration.

INDICATIONS FOR ASSISTED OR CONTROLLED VENTILATION.—Ventilatory support should not be reserved for the near-terminal patient but should be begun early in the course of illness once it becomes clear that the respiratory work load is excessive or that satisfactory gas exchange is not being achieved.

Hypoventilation. This is most commonly seen after the use of muscle relaxants in postanesthesia patients or in the extremely obese. The Bennett PR-2 respirator is well suited for the short-term assistance needed in the former group of patients.

Chest injury. When the chest wall is crushed, the underlying lung can no longer be expanded and tracheostomy with assisted or controlled ventilation becomes a lifesaving treatment.

The respiratory distress syndrome. This is particularly common in the shock patient as well as after fat embolism or other extensive trauma, after burns, and following fluid overload. It is characterized by the inability of the patient to maintain a 90% arterial hemoglobin saturation in spite of increased inspired oxygen concentrations. (This does not apply, of course, to patients with congenital right-to-left shunts or the shunting associated with chronic inflammatory lung disease. It also does not include patients with easily correctable conditions producing atelectasis, such as obstructing bronchial plugs, pneumothorax, or intrapleural fluid accumulations.) When all these conditions are removed from consideration, there remain a number of patients who, in spite of their ability to move either normal or even excessive volumes of air, are unable to maintain effective pulmonary gas exchange due to ventilation-perfusion abnormalities.

NASOTRACHEAL INTUBATION AND TRACHEOSTOMY.—Patients requiring ventilator support must undergo tracheal intubation. The nasotracheal or orotracheal route is preferred for initial support prior to performing tracheostomy or for short-term problems. Currently, these routes are being used for longer and longer periods of support in preference to tracheostomy. Safar's study shows some vocal cord and laryngeal damage after 72 hours of nasotracheal intubation, but support by these routes is usually well tolerated for as long as 7–10 days.

A disadvantage of this approach is that tracheobronchial suctioning may be difficult through the relatively small-bore, long nasotracheal tube. Also, these long tubes have the habit of advancing into a main-stem bronchus. When long-term ventilator support is contemplated, tracheostomy is often necessary. The operation may be hazardous and carry a risk of cardiac arrest when performed without adequate assistance and lighting in a struggling cyanotic patient. Ideally, tracheostomy should be prefaced by orotracheal or nasotracheal intubation. After the tracheobronchial tree is suctioned and the patient thoroughly ventilated with oxygen-rich mixtures if necessary, tracheostomy is performed unhurriedly, precisely, and with complete safety in a stable, well-oxygenated, and sedated patient.

Satisfactory tracheostomy tubes have not yet been developed for long-term ventilator support. All the commonly used cuffed tracheostomy tubes are damaging to the trachea when employed for prolonged periods, or even for short periods when excessive pressure is used on the cuff. To avoid tracheal damage, the cuff should be underinflated to allow a small air leak and, where possible, the cuff should be deflated hourly and the position of the balloon moved. When the patient's condition improves to the point that respirator support may be given intermittently, the cuff should be maintained in the deflated position. Failure to take proper care of the tracheostomy tube results in mucosal sloughing, softening of cartilage at the point of pressure contact, and leads ultimately to perforation or stenosis. After insertion of the nasotracheal or endotracheal tube, both sides of the chest should be auscultated and a chest x-ray inspected to avoid the possibility of unilateral bronchial cannulation.

CHOICE OF VENTILATOR.—The pressure-limited ventilators are triggered by the patient's inspiratory effort and continue to inflate the lungs until a preset pressure has been reached. Some major problems exist in the use of these ventilators: (1) there may be a change in the lung compliance resulting in inadequate ventilation at the pressure set, and (2) a central respiratory drive seen in many shock patients may be exaggerated by the respirator producing extreme degrees of hypocarbia and respiratory alkalosis. Pressure-limited ventilators, triggered by the patient's own respiratory effort, are far more readily tolerated by the conscious patient and are used for assisted ventilation, especially in the hypoventilating patient recovering from anesthesia.

The volume respirator, which operates on the piston or bag reservoir principle, is used for assisted or controlled ventilation and can be regulated to maintain constant tidal and minute volumes, regardless of changes in pulmonary compliance and airway resistance. If a leak develops in the system, however, a patient may be hypoventilated. The ventilators with which we have had some experience will now be discussed.

The Bennett PR-2 ventilator.—This pressure ventilator is used for assisted ventilation and is powered by compressed air or oxygen. The cycling pressure is adjusted to the 15–20 cm range. The expiration time control set on normal gives a ratio of inspiration to expiration of 1;1.5. Advancing the expiration time control increases the duration of expiration. Altering the sensitivity valve determines whether the machine is used for assistance or control. With increased sensitivity, the assistance features of the machine are brought out. Experience with this machine indicates that an erroneous value for inspired oxygen concentration is obtained when the machine is set on air dilution. Various measurements have given from 40 to 90% oxygen with the dilution valve open. The humidifying device supplied originally with the instrument generally fails to give the degree of humidification necessary even when a heating rod is inserted. Accordingly, when the instrument is used, an effective heated humidifier such as the Bennett Cascade Humidifier should be added to it. While this machine represents one of the early generations of ventilators in general usage and has the merit of simplicity of operation, it has several disadvantages. Two of these have already been mentioned: namely, the danger of using, inadvertently, high concentrations of oxygen when the air dilution valve is open and the inadequacy of the humidification system and, even more importantly, the tendency to drive patients who are already hyperventilating into a state of severe hypocarbia. The original model had no spirometer, but this can readily be added to give a measure of the tidal and minute volume.

The Emerson postoperative ventilator.—This instrument is used only for controlled ventilation. It is extremely reliable over long periods of usage and the mechanism is simple. An electric motor operates the piston-driven volume generator. The volume of the cylinder can be adjusted to the desired tidal volume and the cycling is controlled electronically, giving precise adjustment of duration of inspiration and expiration separately. An alarm system and an accessory spirometer for measuring expired tidal volume are generally included. Other important features include an excellent humidification system which consists, in essence, of a pressure cooker from which the humidified gas passes through a reflux condensor filled with copper which is thought to have a bacteriostatic function. In fact, the humidification equipment, while functioning exceptionally well, is rather inconvenient to maintain. Accordingly, we have modified the instrument by substituting a Bennett Cascade Humidifier on the outside housing. This is a great convenience for the nurse or inhalation therapist.

Another important feature of the Emerson ventilator is an automatic sighing device which can be adjusted to sigh a large volume at varying time intervals. Our experience with this ventilator has been very satisfactory. However, it has no assist feature to enable the patient to set his own rate. Thus, the patient must often, at least initially, be heavily sedated to follow the control of the ventilator. Again, careful adjustment of rate and volume are needed to prevent the development of severe degrees of hypocarbia. This ventilator is also readily adapted to controlled positive-pressure breathing by adding a variable resistance at the outflow port. Unless special measures are adopted, it is impossible to obtain an inspired oxygen concentration over 70%. While this constitutes, in fact, a safety feature of the machine, in very advanced lung injury, it is sometimes necessary to use 100% oxygen. To do this, a ventilation bag can be applied to the end of the air-inlet chamber. This modification is also necessary for calculating A-a DO_2 or the shunt equation. While FI_{O_2} can be roughly gauged, measurement with the Beckman D2 unit (Fig. 7-5) gives a precise measurement.

Fig. 7–5.—The Beckman D2 Oxygen Analyzer provides a simple method for measurement of inspired oxygen concentration.

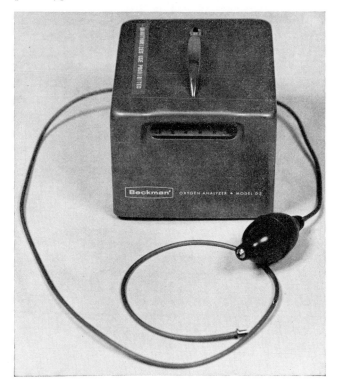

The Bennett MA-1 ventilator.—This new ventilator may be used for either controlled or assisted ventilation and may also be adapted to controlled positive-pressure ventilation. While this machine is expensive, it has certain advantages, the most important of which is an accurate mixing valve. Thus, the settings 20, 40, 60, 80, and 100% oxygen give a fairly reliable measure of $F_{I_{O_2}}$. There is an attached expired air spirometer for measuring tidal volume and a gauge to measure peak airway pressure. A manually operated or automatic sighing device is an important feature. The humidification is entirely adequate utilizing the Cascade humidifier. In using the ventilator, there is a tendency on the part of personnel to utilize only the assist features of the machine since this offers an easier way of managing a patient in ventilatory difficulty. However, this again carries

Fig. 7–6.—Mechanical dead space volume (V_{DM}) required to raise Pa_{CO_2} to approximately 40 mm Hg can be predicted from this nomogram. Pa_{CO_2} is the observed arterial carbon dioxide tension before introduction of the mechanical deadspace, V_T is tidal volume, and V_{Dan} is anatomical deadspace. For the patient with normal pulmonary and circulatory status, the line in the middle gives the required value for V_{DM}. In the presence of pulmonary disease or circulatory failure, a correction must be made by connecting the points on the (Pa_{CO_2}–PE_{CO_2}) line and the V_{DM} line, then extending it to the right. Read the value on the (V_{DM}) corr. line. V_{Dan} is two-thirds of body weight (lb) plus deadspace of the tracheostomy tube and the ventilator. (From Suwa, K., Geffin, B., Pontoppidan, H., and Bendixen, H. H.: A nomogram for dead-space requirement during prolonged artificial ventilation, Anesthesiology 29:1208, 1968.)

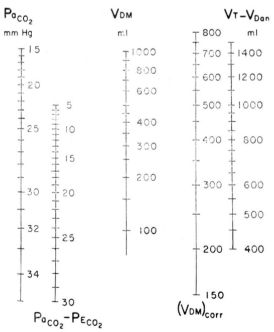

the hazard of excessive ventilation. In the seriously ill patient who tends to hyperventilate naturally, there is a real advantage to controlled rather than assisted ventilation. It is often necessary to add a dead-space extension to raise the P_{CO_2} to the 30–35 mm range. The volume of the dead space needed may be roughly gauged from Pontoppidan's nomogram (see Fig. 7-6).

CARE OF THE PATIENT ON VENTILATOR SUPPORT.—Patients receiving ventilator support should be under constant observation by trained personnel (intensive care unit nurses or inhalation therapists). The risks of positive-pressure ventilation should be well understood (Table 7-3). A running record must be kept of tidal volume, respiratory rate, peak airway pressures, and other measurements (Fig. 7-7). Increasing peak airway pressure at a constant tidal volume suggests stiffening of the lung but this may also be seen when the patient is fighting the ventilator, as shown by the wide swings in negative pressure. Intravenous sedation with morphine is very useful under these circumstances to restore synchrony. Arterial blood gases are the most sensitive indicator of the adequacy of ventilation. The inspired oxygen concentration is adjusted to give an arterial P_{O_2} between 70 and 90 mm Hg and P_{CO_2} of 30 to 40 mm Hg. A common problem in the management of patients on the ventilator is that in order to achieve satisfactory oxygenation, hyperventilation is required, resulting in hypocarbia with the complications to be referred to later.

Because a patient who has undergone tracheostomy has an ineffective cough and cannot mobilize secretions, he must be suctioned regularly. Careful aseptic precautions must be used in suctioning and care of the patient with a tracheostomy. Perhaps one of the most significant recent developments in the care of this patient has been the recognition of the importance of adequate humidification. When the patient is ventilated through a heated humidifier delivering a saturated gas stream at body temperature, the lung passages are adequately humidified. Approximately

---

TABLE 7-3.—TEN COMPLICATIONS OF POSITIVE-PRESSURE VENTILATION

Hypocarbia and severe respiratory alkalosis
Mechanical lung damage by overinflation
Atelectasis by underinflation and lack of large sighing volumes
Reduction in cardiac output by high tidal volume and high airway pressure
Water retention
Lung damage by high oxygen concentration
Bacterial contamination of the lung
Tracheostomy tube complication including tracheal stenosis
    and tracheal perforation
Mechanical failure
Desiccation of the trachea–bronchial tree by inadequate humidification

---

Page _____

CONTINUOUS VENTILATOR CHECK SHEET

Patient _____ Unit Number _____ Diagnosis _____

Attending Physician _____ Resident _____ Date Started _____

Date _____ Order _____

Time												
Tidal Volume												
Respiratory Rate												
Minute Volume												
Airway Pressure												
Sigh Vol. /Pres.												
Oxygen %												
Suctioning												
Cuff Deflate												
Pre-oxygenate												
Humidifier												
Manifold Temp.												
Filled												
Nebulization												
Equipment Changed												
Settings Altered (by whom)												
Technician												
Gas Analysis												
Time												
pH												
p_{O_2}												
p_{CO_2}												
HCO_3												
Sat.												

Fig. 7–7.—Ventilator check sheet maintained by inhalation therapist.

50 mg of water is needed per liter of gas flow to provide full saturation at body temperature. This is best provided by an effective heating device, and the temperature of the inspired gas should be measured near the endotracheal tube. Gas simply bubbled through water at room temperature provides not more than 10 mg per liter and results in desiccation and the formation of obstructing mucus plugs.

A recently recognized complication of prolonged positive pressure ventilation is a tendency to retain water. Daily accurate body-weight measurements point to this complication. Judicious fluid restriction and the use of diuretics may reverse this tendency to develop pulmonary edema.

ADJUSTMENT OF THE VENTILATOR.—When controlled ventilation is used, it is essential that the patient accept the rhythm of the ventilator even if heavy sedation with morphine is initially necessary. Breathing against the ventilator results in turbulent airflow and high airway resistance which, in turn, leads to interference with venous return to the heart. The volume and rate are adjusted on the basis of patient size and ventilatory needs. The Radford nomogram grossly underestimates tidal volume requirements for patients with lung damage. Generally, tidal volumes near 1 liter are needed in the adult. The tidal volume should be adjusted to give a peak airway pressure of less than 25 mm Hg. However, stiffened lungs may require a higher peak pressure for ventilation. Again, emphasis is placed on arterial blood gas measurements. In normal lungs, the Pa_{CO_2} is the best guide to ventilation. In damaged lungs, shunting may lead to such a degree of arterial desaturation that the FI_{O_2} and minute volume must be increased to maintain a Pa_{CO_2} between 70 and 90 mm Hg. Under these conditions, hypocarbia becomes an unwanted but tolerable side effect.

THE PROBLEM OF HYPOCARBIA

The intense respiratory drive developing in patients after peripheral trauma, head injury, and in shock results in hypocarbia which is exaggerated when the patient is assisted rather than controlled by the ventilator. Once a severe level of hypocarbia has existed for some time, a new setting of the capnostat causes a hyperventilatory drive even at low P_{CO_2} and normal P_{O_2} levels and in the absence of metabolic acidosis. These patients with an excessive ventilatory drive, in spite of adequate arterial oxygen saturation, may be very difficult to control without heavy sedation or even the use of curare. The addition of dead space using the nomogram of Pontoppidan in the less-responsive patient will often bring the arterial P_{CO_2} to the desired level. In the responsive patient, however, this merely evokes a further hyperventilatory response and defeats its purpose. While some feel that respiratory alkalosis is harmless and best not treated, clinical experience and certain theoretical considerations suggest that hypocarbia is best avoided in the first instance and corrected when it develops.

SIGHING.—Constant volume respiration over prolonged periods often results in atelectasis. Most modern volume ventilators are now equipped with automatic sighing devices which can be cycled for various time intervals. The tendency for postoperative surgical patients to adopt a shallow, regular pattern of ventilation which leads to atelectasis is dramatically shown in Figure 3-19. To avoid atelectasis, training in deep breathing should be given preoperatively; and postoperatively, patients should be sighed by encouragement, if possible, or by the use of the Ambu bag, if necessary.

Antibiotic Therapy

When the diagnosis of septic shock is made, the identity of the causative microorganisms and their antibiotic sensitivities are usually not available, but in the vast majority of cases, gram-negative bacilli are responsible. McCabe and Jackson report an experience comprising 1,845 patients with gram-negative sepsis. *Escherichia coli* was responsible for 473 cases of septic shock; *Proteus* for 427; *Aerobacter*, 409; *Pseudomonas*, 278; and *Paracolon*, now subdivided into many others (e.g., Serratia, Hafnia, Providence, etc.), 58.

In surgical infections, mixtures of several species are often found. Infection with Pseudomonas is often superimposed on a severe underlying illness such as burns, leukemia, and leaking intestinal anastomoses, and is also often responsible for infections from indwelling intravenous catheters.

Antibiotic treatment therefore should be selected to cover the most probable pathogens involved in gram-negative sepsis before cultures and sensitivities reveal the definitive course of antibiotic therapy. Ampicillin demonstrates in vitro effectiveness against 85% or more of the strains of *E. coli* and 90% of *Proteus mirabilis* strains, but is ineffective against Aerobacter, Pseudomonas, and a majority of Klebsiella. Colistimethate sodium or polymyxin B is effective against 90% of Pseudomonas, and most of the *Klebsiella-Enterobacter* group and *E. coli*, but is totally ineffective against Proteus. Gentamicin is active against most Pseudomonas and Proteus, but is ineffective against intestinal anaerobes. A combination of kanamycin and colistimethate or polymyxin B was found to cover 95% of the gram-negative bacteremias. It is clear therefore that no single antibiotic has a sufficiently broad spectrum to cover all infectious causes of septic shock.

Before any antibiotic therapy is started, cultures of blood, urine, and any exudate should be obtained. A special problem exists in shock patients because there is often associated renal damage with oliguria or anuria. Consequently, antibiotic dosage must be adjusted according to Table 7-4 to prevent toxic accumulation. In patients requiring drug treatment for more than one week, it is advisable to obtain serum drug levels if the creatinine clearance is less than 10 ml/minute and the antibiotic being used is excreted solely by the kidney.

Martin *et al.* conducted prospective controlled clinical trials designed to

TABLE 7-4.—Suggested Doses of Certain Antimicrobial Agents
in Patients with Renal Failure

AGENT	LOADING DOSE	SUBSEQUENT DOSE	INTERVAL BETWEEN DOSES OLIGURIA[*]	AZOTEMIA[†]
Kanamycin sulfate	15 mg/kg	7.5 mg/kg	3–4 days	2 days
Streptomycin	15 mg/kg	7.5 mg/kg	3–4 days	2 days
Colistimethate sodium	5 mg/kg	2.5 mg/kg	3–4 days	2 days
Polymyxin B sulfate	2.5 mg/kg	1.25 mg/kg	3–4 days	2 days
Tetracycline	0.5 gm	0.25 gm	3–4 days	2 days
Chloramphenicol	0.5 gm	0.5 gm[‡]	6 hr	6 hr
Ampicillin	0.5 gm	0.25 gm	12 hr	6 hr
Cephalothin sodium	1.0–2.0 gm	0.5–1.0 gm	24 hr	12 hr
Gentamicin	5 mg/kg	2.5 mg/kg	3–4 days	2 days

[*]Creatinine clearance < 10 ml/minute.
[†]Creatinine clearance > 10 ml/minute.
[‡]Reduce dose in patients with severe liver disease.
From Barnett, J. A., and Sanford, J. P.: Bacterial shock, J.A.M.A. 209:1516, 1969.

compare the efficacy and toxicity of six proposed initial therapies on serious, acute infection of presumed gram-negative rod etiology pending precise definition of the pathogen and its sensitivities. Trial drugs were discontinued when antimicrobial sensitivities of the infecting pathogen were determined. The regimens studied were kanamycin plus polymyxin B or sodium colistimethate, cephaloridine plus polymyxin B or colistimethate, and gentamicin plus or minus cephaloridine. Prior to therapy, 34 patients were in shock. In these patients, the treatable disease mortality rate was lowest in those receiving gentamicin plus or minus cephaloridine (25%). The difference between this mortality and that in the highly comparable pool of patients on non-gentamicin therapy (67%) was thought to be statistically significant.

Nephrotoxicity was most common in patients receiving kanamycin plus a polymyxin (21%), compared with the gentamicin plus or minus the cephaloridine group (6%). This renal insufficiency generally proved to be reversible within 2 to 4 weeks. In all groups, mortality rates were consistently lower in the patients receiving gentamicin plus cephaloridine. In our patients, cephalothin rather than cephaloridine is usually given because of the greater safety of the former. But in patients with normal renal function, cephaloridine is quite satisfactory. It is effective against many anaerobes, most gram-positive organisms (except staphylococci with *marked* B lactamase production), most commonly recovered gram-negative organisms except *Pseudomonas, Serratia,* and non-mirabilis *Proteus.*

The studies by McCabe and Jackson highlight a number of important factors in gram-negative sepsis of which the nature of the underlying disease process was most significant in determining recovery or death. They separate gram-negative sepsis into three groups, depending on the underlying host disease. When the underlying disease process was rapidly fatal, the septic episode terminated fatally in 91% of the patients. When it was ultimately fatal, 66% died during the episode of sepsis. However, when the underlying disease process in itself was nonfatal, only 11% of the patients died as a result of gram-negative sepsis. For example, 31 of 35 patients with leukemia or lymphoma experiencing gram-negative sepsis succumbed, whereas the over-all fatality rate in 115 patients with nonneoplastic disease was 25%, and the lowest fatality rate was among 56 patients with genitourinary disease. These findings make it imperative that host factors be carefully analyzed in determining response to therapy. Severe host disease frequently led to pseudomonas (fatality rate 69%) or mixed species bacteremia (fatality rate 72%). At the other end of the scale, patients with chronic pyelonephritis and bacteremia had extremely low fatality rates. In another study by these authors, shock was observed in 37% of patients with gram-negative bacteremia and usually occurred at the time of, or immediately after, the initial temperature rise. Shock developing later in the course of bacteremia appeared to be the result of persistent infection and vital organ failure rather than a specific manifestation of gram-negative bacteremia. In half the patients, transient oliguria was seen; three patients had frank renal shutdown with persistence of oliguria longer than 3 days, and two of these had experienced an episode of shock.

The use of adrenal steroids in septic shock continues to be a contested issue. When comparing steroid-treated patients with those receiving no steroids, 50% of patients in the former group died as against 24% in the latter. This impression that steroids did not improve the outcome and, in fact, may have contributed to the high fatality rate is borne out when the underlying disease process is categorized according to its severity. A recent study by Freid and Vosty confirms this. As Kass and Finland have emphasized, the lethality of experimental bacterial infection is usually increased by steroid administration. Another double-blind study revealed no advantage in the use of hydrocortisone in the severely ill septic patient. The dose of steroids used, however, was considerably less than the "pharmacologic dose" (50 mg per kilogram of hydrocortisone or equivalent) currently advocated by protagonists of steroid therapy in septic shock. To settle this issue, a prospective double-blind study using the pharmacologic steroid dosage is needed. The results will only be meaningful if cases are carefully matched according to the nature and severity of the underlying disease process.

The current regimen used in the University of Kansas Medical Center for antibiotic therapy in gram-negative sepsis before return of cultures is cephalothin or ampicillin, 8–12 gm per day intravenously, plus gentamicin, 3–5 mg per kilogram per day intravenously. Tetracycline and chloramphenicol are not ordinarily first-line drugs because of decreased effectiveness in patients who have previously received antimicrobial agents. But the anaerobic organism most commonly involved in septic shock, bacteroides, can usually be eradicated by treatment with chloramphenicol or tetracycline. In general, ampicillin and cephalothin are given by intermittent (5–30 min.) infusions every 2–3 hours. Gentamicin, polymyxin, and kanamycin are given by constant drip in 6 or 8 hour schedules. All drugs should be given intravenously in the shock patient, but these drugs can be given intramuscularly later. After return of cultures, drugs are chosen on the basis of specific sensitivities. If *Pseudomonas aeruginosa* is diagnosed, polymyxin B, colistin, or gentamicin is used. With *Proteus mirabilis* infection, ampicillin, cephalothin, cephaloridine, kanamycin, or gentamycin may be used, but only the latter two drugs are likely to be effective in infections caused by indole-positive *Proteus*. The antibiotic therapy should be continued for 7–10 days *after* defervescence. If renal function is normal, kanamycin should be limited to 15 mg per kilogram per day (1.5 gm per day) for not longer than 12 days; polymyxin to 2.5 mg per kilogram per day (200 mg per day), and gentamicin to 5 mg per kilogram per day.

Renal Support

Volume Expansion and Cardiac Support

The most common causes of oliguria and renal damage following operation, trauma, or sepsis are hypovolemia and hypotension. Every effort must therefore be made to ensure adequate hydration with appropriate fluids in high-risk patients in order to prevent oliguria and renal damage. In the hypovolemic patient with hypotension, fluids should be administered rapidly until the filling pressure of the heart is adequate to restore blood pressure. If, however, oliguria persists after re-establishment of cardiac output and blood pressure, a final test with fluid loading and diuretics should be made. If this fails, a fluid restrictive regimen should be adopted.

Diuretics

Mannitol, a hexahydric alcohol, is an osmotic diuretic which is neither metabolized nor absorbed from the renal tubules. After intravenous injection, it is distributed throughout the extracellular space. The chief value of mannitol is in the prevention of renal damage in conditions in which hemolysis or temporary hypotension is likely to occur. It appears to have particular merit during resections of abdominal aortic aneurysms. By increasing tubular urine flow, inspissation of tubular contents is prevented. For this purpose, 25 gm of mannitol is given by slow drip throughout the operation in 500 ml of glucose water. Mannitol should be given separately from blood. The admixture causes severe red cell crenation resulting in aggregates that may impact in the pulmonary vessels.

Mannitol also has some value in identifying renal damage in shock. The patient who has had adequate fluid replacement and blood pressure and still has oliguria should be given a trial with mannitol. If 25 gm of mannitol given over a 10–30 minute period in 100–500 ml of glucose water does not improve urine output, it may be assumed that renal damage has occurred. The therapeutic regimen should then be switched to one of fluid restriction. Further use of mannitol under these conditions may result in fatal pulmonary edema.

Furosemide is a powerful diuretic which inhibits the active reabsorption of sodium in the proximal tubule, ascending loop of Henle, and possibly the distal tubule. A dosage of 20–40 mg may be safely administered intravenously over a period of 1–2 minutes to the oliguric patient after blood pressure and volume have been restored. If diuresis does not occur within 5–10 minutes, renal damage is very likely present. Like mannitol, furosemide may have value in preventing tubular stasis and plugging in transfusion reactions and other conditions. The large loss of fluid and electrolytes in the urine with furosemide must be continually replaced to avoid hypovolemia.

Test of Renal Function

Numerous tests are available to evaluate renal function in the oliguric shock patient (Table 7-5). Unfortunately, most of these tests are qualitative at best and must be combined with a total evaluation of the patient to determine whether renal damage has occurred. More quantitative methods of evaluating the kidney under these conditions, such as creatinine or inulin clearance, are neither practical nor accurate.

The patient with a history of shock, transfusion reaction, or other predisposing condition which causes renal damage with persistent oliguria in the face of a normal blood pressure and adequate central venous pressure most likely has renal damage. Lack of diuresis to a test dose of mannitol or furosemide further substantiates the diagnosis of acute renal insufficiency. A urine osmolality near that of plasma, urine sodium concentrations greater than 60 mEq per liter, and alkaline urine or urine/plasma urea ratio of 10/1 or less strongly suggest renal damage. Finally, a rising

TABLE 7-5.—Test of Renal Function in the Oliguric Patient
with Normal Blood Pressure

Test	Value	Interpretation
CENTRAL VENOUS PRESSURE	Low (0–5 cm H_2O)	HYPOVOLEMIA
	High (10–30 cm H_2O)	FLUID OVERLOAD, HEART FAILURE
Mannitol (25 gm) or furosemide (20–40 mg)	Continued oliguria	Acute renal failure
	Diuresis	Hypovolemia
Urine analysis	Renal tubular cell cast	Acute tubular necrosis
	Erythrocytes or protein (3–4+)	Altered glomerular membrane permeability
	Myoglobin or hemoglobin cast	Myoglobinuria or hemoglobinuria
Urine osmolality	Low (250–300 mOm)	Ability of renal tubular cells to conserve solute lost
	High (700–1000 mOm)	Ability of renal tubular cells to conserve H_2O and concentrate solute intact. Suggests hypovolemia
Urine sodium	Low (0–30 mEq/L)	Ability of renal tubular cells to conserve sodium intact
	High (>60 mEq/L)	Ability of renal tubular cells to conserve sodium lost
Blood urea nitrogen	High (30–100 mg%)	Dehydration or acute renal failure
Serum creatinine	High (5–10 mg%)	Acute renal failure
Serum potassium	High (6–10 mEq/L)	Acute renal failure

blood-urea nitrogen, serum creatinine, and the presence of renal tubular cell casts confirms the diagnosis of acute renal damage and insufficiency.

Treatment of Hyperkalemia

Severe hyperkalemia is a common complication in patients with acute renal failure and marked oliguria, especially following sepsis and breakdown of large tissue masses. Without prompt therapy, various arrhythmias and, finally, cardiac arrest can occur as the potassium level rises above 7 mEq per liter.

Treatment is based on measures to restrict potassium intake and removal of potassium from the extracellular fluid. When marked oliguria occurs, potassium intake must be absolutely curtailed. Sources of potassium, often unrecognized, are banked whole blood (10–30 mEq K^+ per liter of serum) and potassium penicillin (1.2 mEq K^+ per million units of penicillin). Despite early recognition of the oliguric state and restriction of potassium intake, the serum potassium may continue to increase in acute renal failure, especially with severe acidosis and after crushing injury to the large muscle masses. Under these conditions, emergency measures are necessary to reduce high extracellular potassium levels.

Alkalosis generally reduces the serum potassium level due to intracellular shifts of this ion, and acidosis increases serum potassium levels for the opposite reason. Hyperkalemia is exaggerated in the shock patient with severe metabolic acidosis. Sodium bicarbonate, given to correct the acidosis, may dramatically reduce the serum potassium concentration due to relocation of this ion within the cell.

The serum potassium may also be temporarily reduced by administering 100 gm of 50% glucose with 20 units of regular insulin. As the glucose is deposited in the cells in the form of glycogen, potassium is bound intracellularly and serum concentration decreases. In extreme emergencies, in addition to withholding exogenous potassium, correcting acidosis and administering glucose and insulin it may be necessary to antagonize the cardiotoxic effect of hyperkalemia by administering calcium salts. For this purpose, 2–4 gm of either calcium gluconate or lactate can be given slowly in 500 ml of 5% glucose solution. Administration of calcium salts with sodium bicarbonate should be avoided due to precipitation of these salts.

Potassium can be permanently bound and removed from the body by giving the cation exchange resin, sodium polystyrene sulfonate, Kayexalate. This substance will bind approximately 1 mEq of potassium for each gram of resin. In acute situations, it is usually given as a retention enema in a suspension containing 50 gm of Kayexalate in 200 ml of 5% dextrose in water. After 2–4 hours, this can be removed and another 50 gm given on a 24 hour basis. This substance can also be administered orally at a dose of 50–100 gm of resin in 200–300 ml of fluid. Cathartics such as castor oil help to reduce the transit time of this resin through the gut and allow more frequent administration. If the above measures are not effective in reducing high potassium levels, peritoneal or hemodialysis may be necessary to prevent the lethal effects of potassium intoxication.

INDICATIONS FOR DIALYSIS.—The use of dialysis is largely based on clinical experience. Frequently, in uncomplicated acute renal failure where the BUN increases only 10 mg% per day or less, conservative measures such as a low-protein diet, use of the resin, Kayexalate, and other measures are adequate to keep the patient in good condition. In the severely oliguric patient with sepsis or tissue necrosis in whom the BUN increases from 30 to 50 mg% per day, dialysis is usually necessary to prevent severe acidosis, potassium intoxication, and the cerebral, gastrointestinal, and cardiovascular effects of severe uremia. With greater experience and availability of dialysis units throughout the country, dialysis is used more to prevent complications and maintain the patient in good condition rather than to treat life-threatening complications.

The type of dialysis used (peritoneal or hemodialysis) depends upon the facilities available, personnel, and associated disease. For example, hemodialysis requires an arteriovenous shunt and heparinization of the patient. This is an additional hazard in patients with bleeding gastrointestinal lesions, and peritoneal dialysis may be preferable. In situations in which fresh intestinal anastomosis is present, vascular grafts and other intraperitoneal problems, hemodialysis is preferable. Use of either type of dialysis is fraught with complications, and anyone undertaking these procedures should be familiar with them.

Pulmonary edema and sepsis pose a special problem in the patient with acute renal failure. Since excess fluid cannot be removed readily with the usual treatment, phlebotomy or peritoneal dialysis with a hypertonic glucose solution may be necessary to remove fluid in acute situations. Rarely is it necessary to choose other than the optimal antibiotics for the treatment of infection merely because of impaired renal function. Antibiotics should be administered in an adjusted dosage to avoid greater than therapeutic serum levels of the drugs.

DIET IN ACUTE RENAL FAILURE.—The diet in patients with acute renal failure and oliguria is planned to reduce acidosis, azotemia, hyperkalemia and fluid overload while maintaining nitrogen balance. Only enough fluid is given to replace that lost in the feces, urine, sweat, and the lungs. To accomplish this goal, daily body weights are essential. In general, about 40 gm of protein per day is necessary to prevent negative nitrogen balance and to maintain nutrition. This amount can be given without causing severe acidosis and azotemia. In order to obtain the maximum protein sparing effect, it is necessary to provide about 150 nonprotein calories for each gram of protein or 50–60 kilocalories per kilogram of body weight per day. Most patients with renal failure and azotemia cannot take this amount of calories orally due to gastrointestinal distress. Under these conditions, it may be necessary to administer a portion of the calories intravenously or reduce the caloric intake to about 30 calories per kilogram per day.

Adrenergic Drugs

In Chapter 3, some of the general circulatory and metabolic effects of catecholamines were discussed along with Ahlquist's classification. Some of the specific circulatory effects and the clinical experience with these drugs will now be outlined. All the clinical data are complicated by many uncontrolled variables. These include the nature of the underlying disease process, depth and duration of shock, the almost uniform use of a number of different forms of treatment concurrently, and the obvious lack of adequate controls. For these reasons, survival rates between different series cannot be compared at the present time, and the value of any particular agent can only be surmised until extensive clinical hemodynamic and biochemical data have been collected.

The use of the various adrenergic agents will be considered in relation to the different types of shock, although recent studies make it clear that cases of advanced shock may move from one category to another.

Methoxamine

Methoxamine (Vasoxyl) is for all practical purposes a pure alpha adrenergic receptor stimulating agent. It is a potent vasopressor with little if any direct effect on the heart. Administration of this agent causes a rise in arterial blood pressure, but at the expense of peripheral perfusion and cardiac output. The reduced cardiac output results from the reflex bradycardia and negative inotropic effects of the vagus on the heart. Blood flow to most organs, with the exception of the heart and brain, is decreased. An increase in central venous pressure and pulmonary artery pressure is commonly observed with this drug due to the increase in left atrial pressure. Increased venous tone in peripheral veins has been demonstrated with a redistribution of venous blood to the central circulation. An interesting effect of this drug is that when the reflex vagal slowing of the heart is blocked with atropine, methoxamine will further slow the heart. This may be due to the partial beta receptor blocking ability which this drug seems to exhibit in man and the dog, since it prolongs ventricular muscle action potentials and the refractory period and slows A-V conduction.

Norepinephrine

Norepinephrine (Levarterenol) is the chemical transmitter of the postganglionic sympathetic nerve endings. It functions in man as a primary alpha adrenergic receptor stimulant on the peripheral circulation, but it also has beta adrenergic activity on the heart and metabolism. The pharmacologic interpretation of the cardiac effects of norepinephrine have been debated. Some investigators feel that norepinephrine is purely an alpha adrenergic receptor stimulant and explain its action on the heart by postulating that the heart has undifferentiated receptors. Others feel that norepinephrine, like epinephrine, has both alpha and beta adrenergic receptor stimulating properties since its alpha and beta effects can be selectively blocked by the alpha and beta adrenergic blocking agents. In the intact individual, norepinephrine is primarily a vasoconstrictor and its action is exerted on the blood vessels of the kidney, splanchnic organs, the cutaneous area, skeletal muscles, and the lung. The coronary vessels are dilated predominantly due to metabolic factors.

This generalized vasoconstrictor action leads to an increase in total peripheral resistance and arterial blood pressure. A reflex bradycardia results which can be blocked by atropine. Cardiac output is usually decreased with administration of this agent in man. This is probably due to the reflex bradycardia and the increase in total peripheral resistance. Some confusion has arisen in the literature since both norepinephrine and epinephrine have positive inotropic effects on isolated heart preparations, whereas only epinephrine in low concentrations increases cardiac output greatly in intact man. This confusion has been resolved since it has been demonstrated that norepinephrine increases cardiac output in the human after vagus blockade. Norepinephrine, having a more potent peripheral vasoconstrictor effect and causing a greater elevation in blood pressure than does epinephrine in low doses, induces an intense reflex bradycardia. Thus the negative chronotropic effects of the vagal reflex mask the direct stimulating effects of norepinephrine on the heart, and cardiac output changes very little. Norepinephrine has also been shown to increase cardiac output considerably in man and in the dog after alpha adrenergic blockade with phenoxybenzamine. In large concentrations, it increases pulmonary artery pressure in intact dog and man due to an increase in left atrial pressure. There is a rise in venous tone and a shift of blood centrally to the lungs in the dog and possibly in man.

METARAMINOL

Metaraminol (Aramine) is a potent vasopressor and functions to deplete norepinephrine by displacement. Therefore, its actions are almost identical to those of norepinephrine with the exception that metaraminol appears not to reduce renal blood flow as much as norepinephrine in man. It has been shown to liberate norepinephrine and is itself taken up by the postganglionic sympathetic nerve endings and the heart in place of norepinephrine. Pretreatment of subjects with norepinephrine-releasing drugs such as reserpine attenuates or abolishes the action of metaraminol and prolonged administration of metaraminol leads to a state of refractoriness to its vasopressor actions and can cause hypotension. Because of this effect, some investigators have used it to treat hypertension. This phenomenon probably represents a false transmitter action similar to that seen with alpha-methyldopa or may be due to norepinephrine depletion. It has been shown that metaraminol, like norepinephrine, is released by norepinephrine-releasing drugs (reserpine, guanethidine), whereas uptake of metaraminol is inhibited by drugs inhibiting norepinephrine uptake (imipramine, guanethidine). Metaraminol like norepinephrine may be released from the heart by sympathetic nerve stimulation.

Sarnoff showed that the vasoconstrictor and myocardial stimulant effects of metaraminol were separate and dissociated with small doses in the dog. Clearly, myocardial contractility was improved without vasopressor effects when small doses were used.

DOPAMINE

Dopamine is one of the intermediates in the synthesis of norepinephrine and epinephrine and has norepinephrine-like effects. Recent studies, however, have begun to suggest that there are several important differences. In intact animals both norepinephrine and dopamine cause vasoconstriction in skeletal muscle, the kidneys, and splanchnic organs. Norepinephrine, however, appears to be considerably more powerful than dopamine in its vasoconstrictor properties.

Administration of norepinephrine and dopamine into these vascular beds after alpha adrenergic receptor blockade with phenoxybenzamine results in vasodilation (unmasking of the beta adrenergic receptor stimulating properties). This vasodilation in skeletal muscle to both dopamine and norepinephrine after alpha blockade can be blocked with the beta adrenergic receptor blocking agent propranolol. In the kidneys and splanchnic organs, only the norepinephrine-induced vasodilation can be blocked with propranolol, whereas the vasodilation secondary to dopamine cannot be blocked. This has led to the current hypothesis that dopamine receptors exist in the kidneys and splanchnic organs. These dopamine receptors can be blocked with haloperidal and chlorpromazine.

Recently, several clinical reports have suggested that dopamine may be an effective agent in increasing myocardial contractility without excessive peripheral vasoconstrictor effects. Experimental evidence in endotoxin shock preparations suggests that this agent may be effective in reducing splanchnic pooling. Only further studies will clarify the role of dopamine in the support of the shock patient.

EPINEPHRINE

Epinephrine (Adrenalin) is one of the oldest known adrenergic stimulants. Oliver and Schafer, in 1895, showed the pressor action of extracts from the suprarenal gland (predominant site of endogenous production of epinephrine). It is predominantly a beta adrenergic stimulant at low doses, although it does possess potent alpha-mimetic effects in high doses. When infused intravenously, epinephrine causes an increase in heart rate (chronotropic effects). This is the result of the direct action of epinephrine on the sinoatrial node. Also, it has been shown to increase the rate conduction through the atrioventricular node and shorten the refractory period of cardiac muscle. In a standard normotensive preparation, stroke volume increases as a result of the direct effects of epinephrine on the force of myocardial contractility (inotropic effects). Thus, cardiac output increases as a result of the increased stroke volume and heart rate. Total peripheral resistance falls with physiologic doses only, although systolic pressure increases and diastolic pressure remains unchanged or increased slightly, causing a moderate increase in mean blood pressure. Coronary, cerebral, splanchnic, and skeletal muscle blood flow increase, whereas renal blood flow and blood flow through skin and mucous membrane decrease. Increased venous tone has been demonstrated in the extremities in man and throughout the systemic venous bed in the dog causing a shift of blood centrally in the dog and possibly in man. Central venous pressure and pulmonary artery pressure in intact man and animal usually increases with large doses of epinephrine.

ISOPROTERENOL

Isoproterenol (Isuprel) is a pure beta adrenergic receptor stimulating agent. Its effects are similar to that seen with epinephrine in physiologic concentration or with norepinephrine and epinephrine in large doses after alpha adrenergic receptor blockade. The drug increases the rate of firing of the S-A node, the rate of A-V node conduction, and reduces the refractory period of cardiac muscle. This results in a tachycardia which is accompanied by increased myocardial contractility. Cardiac output is increased while mean blood pressure decreases. The reduction in total peripheral resistance is due to the active vasodilation induced by this agent. Blood flow to all organs is increased with the exception, perhaps, of the brain. Increased venous tone is also noted with transfer of venous blood from the peripheral capacitance system to the central circulation. Central venous pressure usually falls, however, due to the positive inotropic and chronotropic effects of this drug on the heart. Of considerable interest are the recent findings that isoproterenol in large doses can act as a beta adrenergic receptor blocking agent like its dichloro analogue dichloroisoproterenol (DCI).

Mephentermine

Mephentermine (Wyamine) appears to be an alpha and beta adrenergic receptor stimulant but its over-all effects are beta-mimetic in nature. Its action on the heart appears to be dependent upon endogenous norepinephrine, since prior treatment of dogs with reserpine abolishes the cardiotonic effects of mephentermine. Prolonged administration of this drug leads to a state of myocardial refractoriness, possibly because of norepinephrine depletion of the heart or other factors not clear at present. When infused, mephentermine increases heart rate and myocardial contractility and increases output. Mephentermine seems to act like isoproterenol on the peripheral circulation by decreasing total peripheral resistance, whereas the arterial pressure remains the same or is decreased slightly. Large doses of mephentermine, in contrast to isoproterenol, does cause vasoconstriction. It appears to increase venous tone since it has been shown in the dog to increase venous return to the heart when cardiac output is maintained constant by right-heart bypass. Antiarrhythmia effects have also been reported for this agent, perhaps due to the catecholamine depletion of the heart.

Alpha-Methyl Tyrosine

Alpha-methyl tyrosine, a congener of tyrosine, blocks the activity of tyrosine hydroxylase, the enzyme responsible for the conversion of tyrosine to dopa. Tyrosine hydroxylase appears to be the rate-regulating enzyme for catecholamine synthesis. It apparently blocks catecholamine synthesis and has been used effectively in controlling pheochromocytoma. Tyrosine hydroxylase inhibitors will have wide use in studies of adrenergic mechanisms, and potentially in clinical therapeutics.

Phenoxybenzamine (Dibenzyline)

Several drugs having alpha adrenergic receptor blocking properties have been developed. First to be recognized were the ergot alkaloids, but these were considerably less specific than the more recently developed drugs. The synthesis of dibenamine and, later, phenoxybenzamine provided long-acting drugs of the halo-alkylamine group. Phentolamine (Regitine), an imidazoline, is probably not as specific as the longer-acting alpha blocking drugs, and it has a short duration of action. Knowledge of the pharmacological properties and early clinical experiences with phenoxybenzamine in shock patients stems from the work of Nickerson.

Phenoxybenzamine or dibenamine given intravenously into healthy, recumbent, normovolemic patients or animals causes minor changes in systolic blood pressure, although diastolic pressure decreases. A reflex tachycardia results from the mild hypotension and decreased baroceptor activity on the vasomotor center. Cardiac output usually increases due to the tachycardia and the effects of endogenous catecholamines on a heart not inhibited by the baroceptor reflex. Blood flow to most organs is not changed under these conditions since little peripheral sympathetic activity exists in normovolemic supine man. Exceptions are resting skeletal muscle or skin exposed to a cool environment (room temperature). The increase in cardiac output seen in resting states is probably accommodated by these organs. Little change in blood flow in warm skin or exercising skeletal muscle occurs since the sympathetic nervous system exerts little control over these organs under these conditions.

Considerable shifting of fluid from the interstitial compartment into the vascular tree occurs with administration of this drug, thereby increasing plasma volume and reducing hematocrit. The mechanisms for these fluid shifts have not been well worked out, but alteration of Starling's forces at the capillary level are most likely involved. Another possibility for the fall in hematocrit after phenoxybenzamine administration is the vasodilation of small vessels with low hematocrit. It is well known that considerable plasma skimming occurs in the microcirculation and that many microvessels contain plasma almost exclusively. Opening up these small channels and perfusion with red-cell containing perfusate would flush out considerable plasma and result in a decrease in hematocrit. Marked shifts of blood also occur from the central circulation (predominantly the lungs) to the systemic vascular bed due to a reduction in systemic venous tone. This phenomenon is responsible for the main hazards in the use of this drug in a hypovolemic patient. Vascular collapse can occur rapidly and be avoided only by massive infusions of fluid.

The effects of phenoxybenzamine differ greatly in an upright individual or in a patient with hypovolemia or excess sympathetic activity due to stress or other factors. Orthostatic hypotension is common and may exist for 24 or more hours after administration of this drug. Administration of this agent to a patient with hypovolemia or pheochromocytoma usually results in a marked tachycardia, hypotension, and variable changes in cardiac output. This hypotension can be reversed only with large volumes of fluid or administration of the octapeptide angiotensin II (Hypertensin). The vasoconstricting effects of angiotensin II are not blocked with the alpha adrenergic blocking agents since it is not an adrenergic receptor stimulating agent.

The alpha adrenergic receptor stimulant properties (vasoconstriction) of norepinephrine and epinephrine are abolished with phenoxybenzamine. Selective efforts on a particular vascular bed may be produced experimentally. Moyer *et al.* and, more recently, Gump and Thal have investigated the effects of selective blockade of the vascular bed of the kidney using phenoxybenzamine. These investigators have confirmed previous in vitro studies demonstrating that dibenzyline becomes firmly and rapidly bound to receptor sites in tissues. Using this approach may protect organs sensitive to ischemia, such as the kidney, during periods of intense sympathetic activity; this finding raises several interesting therapeutic and experimental implications. The chronotropic and inotropic effects of epinephrine and norepinephrine are enhanced by the alpha adrenergic blocking agents due to the impairment of the baroceptor reflex. The tachycardia seen commonly with epinephrine is increased. The bradycardia usually seen with norepinephrine is reversed. Phenoxybenzamine can cause heat loss secondary to cutaneous vasodilation. This agent reaches a maximum activity in 1–2 hours and alpha adrenergic receptor blockade can be demonstrated for 12–36 hours.

PROPRANOLOL (INDERAL)

A number of beta receptor blocking drugs have recently been developed and studied such as dichloroisoproterenol (DCI), pronethalol (Nethalide, Alderline), and propranolol (Inderal). Dichloroisoproterenol is the oldest beta adrenergic agent and has been widely studied in laboratory animals. Since it has intrinsic beta adrenergic receptor stimulating action (positive inotropic and chronotropic effects) in addition to its beta blocking ability, and has not been used clinically, it will not be discussed further. Pronethalol and propranolol, the new beta adrenergic blocking agents, have been widely studied clinically. They have similar effects except that propranolol is ten times as potent on a weight basis as pronethalol. The latter has been shown to cause tumor formation in laboratory animals and, therefore, has been removed from the market.

The systemic effects of propranolol, like phenoxybenzamine, depend upon the existing sympathetic activity at the time of administration. In a healthy, resting patient, beta adrenergic blockade of the heart can be carried out with little measurable effects on heart function. This suggests that the sympathetic nervous system has little stimulating effect on the myocardial tissue in the supine resting man. The concept that resting man has predominantly a vagally controlled heart and under stress a sympathetically controlled heart is borne out by these observations and the observation that atropine blockade of the vagus results in a tachycardia in resting man. If, however, the effects of drugs such as isoproterenol or norepinephrine on the circulation are tested under these conditions, the peripheral vasodilation and cardiac accelerator effects of isoproterenol are blocked, and the peripheral vasoconstrictor effects of norepinephrine are usually enhanced.

Beta adrenergic receptor blockade in conditions in which sympathetic activity to the heart is increased, such as in exercise and in congestive heart failure, results in dramatic impairment of heart function. Observation on individuals exercised to exhaustion reveal the endurance time to be curtailed; cardiac output, mean blood pressure, and left ventricular work significantly decreased over values observed in the same patients undergoing exercise without beta blockade. Thus it is evident that beta adrenergic receptor blockade of the heart severely limits myocardial performance in stress states and restricts the use of propranolol in certain situations. The chief hazard of this drug is the precipitation of heart failure in a marginally compensated individual. Glucagon may be the drug of choice to augment the heart under the influence of propranolol.

In numerous conditions myocardial function is impaired because of excessive sympathetic activity, such as in paroxysmal ventricular tachycardia, hypertrophic subaortic stenosis, and other disorders. Propranolol is effective in the treatment of these disease states. In addition, propranolol is now widely used in the treatment of angina pectoris and various arrhythmias.

Recent developments in the pharmacology of propranolol reveal that its anti-arrhythmic effects after digitalis and anesthetics may be entirely distinct from its tendency to reduce myocardial performance. Propranolol now available is a mixture of the d-l isomers. Pure preparations of d-propranolol is a very weak beta adrenergic receptor blocking agent, whereas, it is as effective as d-l propranolol in preventing arrhythmias due to digitalis and anesthetic agents. The d-isomer of propranolol is not effective in controlling heart rate in supraventricular arrhythmias, however. In contrast l-propranolol which retains beta adrenergic blocking ability is effective in reducing the ventricular response to supraventricular arrhythmias by altering S-A and A-V nodal firing and conduction velocity. These studies suggest that the effects of propranolol (d-l isomer) on the S-A and A-V node are secondary to blockade of the beta receptors, whereas its ability to suppress ectopic arrhythmias, digitalis, and anesthetic-induced arrhythmias is due to an entirely different mechanism, perhaps secondary to its quinidine-like effect .

The potential importance of these observations is obvious since the pure d-isomer preparations of propranolol could be used to control certain arrhythmias without impairing the contractile ability of the heart.

Propranolol has not been used widely in the clinical treatment of shock. Berk has carried out experiments in canine endotoxin and hemorrhagic shock models and has shown increased survival rates with propranolol treatment. He has proposed an interesting concept that vascular pooling of blood and the amount of nonnutrient tissue perfusion in shock states is secondary to beta adrenergic receptor stimulation.

USE OF ADRENERGIC DRUGS IN HYPOVOLEMIC SHOCK

Hypovolemic shock in its early stages responds well to blood, colloid, and balanced saline, but when treatment is delayed or inadequate, what starts as a simple phenomenon of fluid lack becomes complicated by intense vasoconstriction and myocardial failure which is refractory to fluid replacement alone. It is under these circumstances that vasodilator and inotropic drugs appear to be of value. Predominantly vasoconstrictor agents such as methoxamine, metaraminol, and norepinephrine clearly have detrimental effects under these conditions and will not be discussed further.

Nickerson was the first to use phenoxybenzamine and fluids in cases of refractory hypovolemic shock. Blood pressure, pulse rate, and urine output were markedly improved in these patients and clinical evidence of peripheral sympathetic overactivity was reversed with this agent. Lillehei has also treated a number of patients in hypovolemic shock with phenoxybenzamines and fluids. In general, cardiac output could be increased, total peripheral resistance reduced, urine output augmented, and evidence of peripheral vasoconstriction reversed. Wilson, Jablonski, and Thal treated several cases of hypovolemic shock exhibiting a high total peripheral resistance, low cardiac output, and high central venous pressure with 1 mg per kilogram phenoxybenzamine. All these cases were in advanced hypovolemic shock and had manifestations of cardiac failure which prevented further fluid therapy. Most of these patients were young and responded favorably to phenoxybenzamine with a marked fall in central venous pressure and total peripheral resistance, allowing cardiac output to be increased by fluid loading. Further augmentation of cardiac output could be obtained if norepinephrine was given along with the fluids and phenoxybenzamine.

McLean et al. used the inotropic and vasodilator agent isoproterenol in the treatment of advanced and complicated hypovolemic shock. Although survival figures were not encouraging, hemodynamic studies indicated that central venous pressure was decreased, urine output increased, and cardiac output augmented. Other investigators have confirmed the effectiveness of isoproterenol in increasing cardiac output and reducing total peripheral resistance in patients with advanced hypovolemic shock with cardiac failure who have been nonresponsive to fluid loading. Far-advanced hypovolemic shock associated with cardiac failure, low cardiac output, high peripheral resistance, and venous pressures appears to be a prime indication for the use of either phenoxybenzamine or isoproterenol and fluid therapy.

The value of the alpha adrenergic receptor blocking agent phenoxybenzamine in hypovolemic shock has been a matter of some contention, however, because of work on laboratory animals. Muhm and Shumacker studied the effects of phenoxybenzamine, Arfonad, and Apresoline on renal blood flow in normovolemic and moderately hypovolemic states in dogs. They showed that vasodilator agents reduced renal blood flow. Mandelbaum, Silbert, and Berry examined a similar problem during extracorporeal circulation. These workers maintained a constant pump output and measured renal blood flow directly before and after the administration of large doses of phenoxybenzamine. There was a significant fall in renal vascular resistance after alpha adrenergic blockade, but the total peripheral resistance declined to an even greater degree, resulting in a diversion of blood away from the kidney to the regions of lowest resistance. These studies clearly point out the hazards of using these drugs in the presence of hypovolemia without concomitant expansion of the vascular space. Impairment of baroceptor reflexes results in perfusion of nonessential skin and muscular compartments, thereby reducing flow to vital structures.

These studies have been essentially duplicated for other organs by Pollock et al. studying regional blood flow in dogs which were hypovolemic. They found no difference in organ blood flow when phenoxybenzamine treated animals were compared to non-drug-treated animals. Baue et al. studied mesenteric blood flow and oxygen consumption in dogs in hemorrhagic shock treated with phenoxybenzamine and found cardiac output and systemic oxygen consumption to be increased but without a corresponding increase in mesenteric blood flow; moreover, mesenteric oxygen consumption decreased with phenoxybenzamine treatment. Rush et al. found that phenoxybenzamine given during hemorrhagic shock was associated with decreased oxygen consumption, increased oxygen debt, and increased metabolic acidosis. Again, in none of these studies was adequate volume replacement carried out, thereby creating experimental conditions at variance with the current clinical use of the drug. The vasoconstrictive response in shock is at least initially a vital survival mechanism aimed at the redistribution of blood flow from the nonessential muscle masses, skin, gut, and kidneys to the essential cerebral and coronary circulations. To abrogate this response by unselective vasodilation in the face of continuing hypovolemia would seem to be undesirable, and clinical observations tend to confirm this inference. Vasodilation in the face of a continuing low cardiac output is disastrous.

Current clinical usage of phenoxybenzamine in shock is predicated on the prior demonstration of an adequate or increased atrial filling pressure and continuous intravenous infusion to expand intravascular volume. It also seems clear that beneficial results from generalized vasodilation may be anticipated in clinical shock only when considerable increases in total blood flow can be secured by increased venous return to compensate for diversion to less critical regions. The use of norepinephrine, or other inotropic drugs, to increase cardiac output in patients treated with phenoxybenzamine and fluids may be necessary to accomplish this goal in far-advanced shock. Another alternative is the use of phenoxybenzamine in a selective regional fashion as discussed previously.

One question that needs answering is: What precisely are the microcirculatory pathways opened up after alpha adrenergic receptor blockade with phenoxybenzamine? Are these nutritive or bypass channels? The metabolic acidosis frequently seen after using dibenzyline in the vasoconstricted shocked human or animal is thought to be due to washout of lactic acid from the muscle masses and skin and other organs previously isolated by vasoconstriction. This is only transient and is reversed in a matter of minutes with effective circulation. Another possibility is that phenoxybenzamine opens up nonnutrient vessels and results in peripheral shunting. To a large extent, the drug has been used as a last-ditch resort in near-terminal patients; and while tissue perfusion has often appeared better, it seems doubtful that there has been an increase in survival.

CLINICAL USE OF ADRENERGIC DRUGS IN CARDIOGENIC SHOCK

Primary failure of left ventricular ejection is most commonly seen as a result of extensive myocardial infarction, but sometimes it follows cardiac arrhythmias with a rapid ventricular response. The cardiac output reaches low levels as the stroke volume declines, and the calculated total peripheral resistance generally rises to levels higher than is seen in other forms of shock. The intense activity of the sympathetic nervous system in these patients may result in severe vasoconstriction in the extremities with a relatively high central aortic pressure. This, in itself, may further impair myocardial function by increasing the pressure work of the heart.

When the fall in cardiac output occurs gradually over a long period, as in advanced mitral stenosis, a cardiac output well within the levels found in severe shock may be tolerated at rest. When the damage in shock is sudden and severe, circulatory readjustments occur, producing diversion of the circulation from the periphery to the coronary and cerebral areas. The venous pressure is either raised or rises rapidly with relatively small infusions of fluid. This state is tolerated for only relatively short periods, and the mortality rate following myocardial infarction with shock varies between 70 and 100%. Secondary cardiac failure is common and compli-cates many forms of severe shock, regardless of origin. Drug therapy has been used to accomplish seemingly opposite ends. Clearly, coronary per-fusion pressure must be maintained. Yet, the intense vasoconstriction is already present and the use of vasoconstrictor drugs further adds to the work load of the heart as well as increasing its metabolic demands. Con-versely, vasodilator drugs, while lowering total peripheral resistance, may theoretically reduce cerebral and coronary perfusion below critical levels. This dilemma has not yet been resolved.

The literature is replete with clinical reports that provide testimonials to the value of vasopressor agents in temporarily elevating the blood pressure in the majority of patients in cardiogenic shock. Few of these reports make any attempt at measuring myocardial function and tissue perfusion. A few representative current studies in which hemodynamic measurements have been made with various agents will be discussed. Smulyan *et al.* evaluated the effects of norepinephrine and metaraminol administered to 7 patients in shock due to myocardial infarction. Results from these studies showed that cardiac output was consistently decreased and total peripheral re-sistance increased from baseline hemodynamic measurements. Increasing the dosage of these drugs further decreased the cardiac output and in-creased total peripheral resistance. Shubin and Weil, studying the effects of these drugs in patients in cardiogenic shock, confirmed the findings of Smulyan *et al.* but suggested that if the arterial pressure was maintained at a level approximately 30 mm Hg below "normal" systolic blood pressure, excessive vasoconstriction could be avoided and cardiotonic effects ob-served. These studies point out that excessive vasoconstriction resulting from the infusion of norepinephrine or metaraminol will further decrease an already low cardiac output in cardiogenic shock. These conclusions were further substantiated by Gunnar *et al.* when they observed that the pure vasoconstrictor agent, methoxamine, given to patients in shock sec-ondary to acute myocardial infarction caused significant decreases in car-diac output and increases in peripheral resistance as well as clinical deterioration of the patient.

Epinephrine has been used by several investigators in the treatment of low-flow states following cardiac surgery and in myocardial infarction. In general, this agent has effects similar to norepinephrine and metaraminol. Small doses are effective in stimulating the heart without excessive periph-eral vasoconstriction, whereas larger doses result in an elevated central aortic blood pressure, reflex slowing of the heart, decreased cardiac out-put, and intense vasoconstriction. Udhoji and Weil observed similar results with the drug mephentermine in a few patients treated for cardiogenic shock. Cardiac output and blood pressure could be elevated without excessive peripheral vasoconstriction when small amounts were administered. MacLean *et al.*, Smith *et al.*, and numerous other investigators have studied the circulatory effects of isoproterenol in cardiogenic shock and have clearly shown that cardiac output can be increased, blood pressure elevated after administration of isoproterenol, and peripheral perfusion improved with this drug. Excessive vasoconstriction is not a problem with this drug since it causes active vasodilation.

These studies have made it clear that the alpha adrenergic receptor stimulating agents such as methoxamine are not effective in supporting the heart and circulation in cardiogenic shock. Vasoconstrictor agents that are void of inotropic effects, therefore, have virtually no place in the management of a patient in cardiogenic shock. The mixed alpha and beta adrenergic receptor stimulating agents with predominantly alpha-mimetic effects, such as norepinephrine and metaraminol, are effective in supporting pressure but again, like methoxamine, they increase total peripheral resistance and usually decrease cardiac output, particularly in large doses. Central venous pressure frequently rises and the patient deteriorates despite the increase in blood pressure. Small infusions of these drugs are effective in supporting the heart and circulation without excessive increases in total peripheral resistance. The other mixed alpha and beta adrenergic receptor stimulating agents with predominantly beta-mimetic effects, in low doses, such as epinephrine and mephentermine, may also be of some value. And, finally, the pure beta adrenergic stimulating agent isoproterenol is very effective in supporting the heart and circulation without excessive increases in vascular resistance.

None of these agents is without dangerous side effects, however. All are capable of provoking serious arrhythmias. The beta-mimetic agents appear to be more prone to produce arrhythmias than the alpha-beta mixed agents. All patients receiving these agents must be monitored continuously, and if signs of myocardial irritability are evident, they must be stopped. The beta-mimetic agents are notorious in producing a marked tachycardia, and candidates for these drugs usually already have a rapid heart rate, again limiting their use. Prolonged use of any of these agents, particularly isoproterenol, may produce focal myocarditis and further aggravate the pre-existing infarction of the heart.

The final and, perhaps, most important question that must be raised with the use of the adrenergic stimulating agents in shock concerns their metabolic effects. It is known that adrenergic stimulating agents have a calorigenic effect and increase oxygen demands by about 20%. Possibly, the metabolic deficits commonly seen in shock patients may be further aggravated even though the cardiovascular performance and tissue perfusion is improved. Drucker *et al.* have shown that the metabolic deficits are further aggravated and that tolerance to hypovolemia is reduced if norepinephrine is given prior to repletion of blood volume. It seems almost paradoxical to administer agents that increase oxygen demand of tissues when the whole organism is in a state of severe oxygen debt. Clearly, survival under these conditions is limited to cases in which the improvement in oxygen transport and exchange offsets the increased demands for oxygen induced by the drug.

Various attempts have been made to use the alpha adrenergic receptor blocking agents in the treatment of cardiogenic shock. Wilson, Jablonski, and Thal studied the effects of phenoxybenzamine in the treatment of several patients in cardiogenic shock. In general, total peripheral resistance could be reduced and central venous pressure decreased with relief of pulmonary edema, but cardiac output only increased modestly. If norepinephrine was added to the regimen, however, cardiac output could be augmented. While a few patients showed dramatic recovery, the majority eventually died in spite of a transient improvement in hemodynamic measurements.

Use of the Adrenergic Drugs in Septic Shock

At present, septic shock represents a confusing entity which differs from other forms in several vital particulars. While initial hemodynamic studies indicated that septic shock, like hypovolemic and cardiogenic shock, was characterized by a low cardiac output and increased peripheral resistance, subsequent measurements have revealed a far more complex picture. Our early studies identified several hemodynamic patterns. Most interesting of all, and quite commonly seen, was a hyperdynamic form in which the hypotension was associated with a normal or high cardiac output. Also, as judged by the response to fluids, a relative hypovolemia was often present and, in addition, some cases revealed a dominant element of associated cardiac failure. The majority of patients destined to survive responded to fluid and antibiotic therapy coupled with cardiopulmonary support and drainage of abscesses where indicated. The mortality rate in those failing to respond to these primary forms of treatment is approximately 75%. Clearly, in so heterogenous a group of patients, support with vasoconstrictor, inotropic, or vasodilator drugs must be based upon hemodynamic measurement. For example, the low cardiac output group might be expected to respond to drugs such as isoproterenol and phenoxybenzamine; our studies, as well as the more recent reports of Hardaway and other investigators, confirm this. Conversely, the use of these drugs, in the presence of the high cardiac output form of sepsis, would appear to be contraindicated.

Gilbert *et al.*, in 1955, reported one of the first hemodynamic studies in patients with septic shock. They found that the control cardiac output was normal or high and the total peripheral resistance low. With the infusion of norepinephrine into 4 of these patients, a rise in arterial blood pressure and fall in the cardiac output occurred in three instances. Smulyan *et al.* studied the effects of norepinephrine and metaraminol on 8 patients in septic shock. Control cardiac output was normal or low in these patients, and total peripheral resistance was normal or low. After infusion of these agents, cardiac output was increased in half of these patients along with blood pressure and total peripheral resistance. If large dosages of these agents were given, cardiac output seemed to deteriorate while total peripheral resistance further increased. These investigators also consistently observed that the largest increases in peripheral vascular resistance occurred when resistance was already high, and that cardiac output was raised when it was highest and close to normal. In patients who had low cardiac output and total peripheral resistance where, theoretically, an increase in cardiac output and total peripheral resistance would be desirable, the former usually decreased and the latter increased excessively. These studies point out that cardiac failure is common in septic patients and, therefore, augmentation of cardiac output can be accomplished only with these drugs if the heart is capable of being stimulated. These best results are obtained when the dosage of norepinephrine and metaraminol is held to a minimum.

Recent work using canine septic-leg models by Weidner and Clowes, Hopkins *et al.*, and Hermreck and Thal has pointed out several interesting effects of sepsis on the distribution of blood flow. Clowes originally suggested that blood flow was considerably increased through the septic region, and Hopkins *et al.* and our studies confirm and quantitate this observation. In addition, Hopkins *et al.* and our studies have demonstrated that blood flow through this hyperemic septic region can be markedly reduced without creating a local oxygen debt with either systemic or local administration of norepinephrine. These laboratory studies suggest that the altered systemic distribution of blood flow in sepsis can be regulated with small amounts of norepinephrine. This approach may have value in supporting patients with hyperdynamic septic hypotension.

MacLean *et al.* and several other workers have evaluated the effects of the isoproterenol in patients in septic shock. In general, many of these patients were in heart failure and isoproterenol was effective in augmenting the cardiac output, reducing central venous pressure, and increasing hourly urine output. Siegel, Greenspan, and Del Guercio recently studied several patients in septic shock and found that oxygen consumption was usually decreased, tissue oxygen uptake impaired, and ventricular function hypodynamic or hyperdynamic. Isoproterenol was used in a few of these patients and clearly improved myocardial performance, but it had little effect on improving tissue oxygen uptake.

It would appear that isoproterenol and phenoxybenzamine are best suited to support septic shock patients in a state of low cardiac output and high total peripheral resistance. The use of isoproterenol in the high cardiac output, vasodilated state can result in further vasodilation of already high flow regions with aggravation of the abnormal circulatory state, and the effects of phenoxybenzamine under these conditions also appears to be deleterious.

It is obvious that the ideal therapy is not at hand. What one can hope to accomplish with the stimulating or blocking adrenergic agents, with our present state of knowledge, is to tide over the critically ill patients until sepsis is controlled. Control of sepsis, cardiac, pulmonary, and renal support coupled with titrative use of adrenergic agents, despite their limitations, still remain standbys of therapy.

Steroids

Melby, Spink, and others have found no evidence of impaired adrenal steroid production in either experimental or clinical shock. Nevertheless, pre-treatment with steroids shows a clear-cut protective effect against many forms of experimental shock. The mechanism for this is unknown, and similar protection can be shown with a number of other unrelated agents. Several possible beneficial effects of steroids have been proposed; in the isolated heart preparation, they appear to have an inotropic effect on the heart. There is also a suggestion that they may produce a mild alpha adrenergic blockade, thereby improving tissue perfusion, and Weissman has demonstrated that steroids stabilize the mitochondrial membrane and diminish the intracellular release of lysosomal enzymes. Nevertheless, evidence for any special value of steroids in the treatment of shock in general, and septic shock in particular, is debatable.

The spread of sepsis and the development of septic shock are seen in patients receiving steroids for immunosuppression, and a cooperative study using a double-blind technique suggests that hydrocortisone may actually aid in the spread of infection. From the study by Freid and Vosty it is apparent that the results of treatment are very difficult to evaluate because of the heterogeneous nature of the underlying disease process. The proponents of steroid therapy use pharmacologic doses, preferably Dexamethasone, 40 mg intravenously followed by 20 mg every 4–6 hours. Treatment should not be continued for more than 24 hours in order to avoid depression of the immune mechanism and also to avoid the danger of upper gastrointestinal hemorrhage. An ever-present danger is that steroids may be given in place of effective fluid, cardiac, and ventilatory support.

Hypothermia in the Treatment of Shock

It is generally accepted that the fundamental defect in shock is an inadequate supply of oxygen to meet the energy requirements of the cell. The concept of reducing metabolic needs, therefore, appears to be sound and is the basis for the survival of the hibernating animal. It is known that metabolic rate can be reduced considerably by means of total body hypothermia. As a rough guide, the metabolic requirements can be reduced almost 50% by depressing the body temperature by 10°C. In practice, however, reduction of the body temperature below 32°C results in marked cardiac slowing and a fall in cardiac output. The danger of ventricular fibrillation is enhanced, blood viscosity increases, and tissue perfusion is impaired. At the present time, deep hypothermia does not appear to be of value in the management of the shock patient. On the other hand, reduction of high fever to normal or levels slightly lower than normal is often a useful adjunctive measure.

The most effective management of severe degrees of fever is by the use of a hypothermia blanket kept at from 5° to 10°C. This measure is assisted by the administration of drugs such as chlorpromazine to reduce compensatory shivering and cutaneous vasoconstriction. Unfortunately, the cooling blanket is often used in the conscious patient for minor or transient rises in temperature, producing considerable discomfort and shivering, thus increasing metabolic need.

Salicylates, considered previously only in the light of their analgesic and antipyretic actions, have recently been shown to have important effects in inhibiting the release of plasma kinins. The antipyretic effect appears to be directly on the central nervous system. Part of this effect is related to their ability to induce sweating. With larger doses, this drug is also capable of increasing oxygen consumption, apparently by uncoupling oxidative phosphorylation and, in this respect, high doses may actually be fever producing, particularly in infants.

Treatment of the Complications of Shock

Upper Gastrointestinal Bleeding

Greater or lesser degrees of upper gastrointestinal bleeding are extremely common consequences of shock and are especially prone to occur after septic shock. Operative and postmortem examination of the stomach and upper gastrointestinal tract in these patients commonly shows superficial gastritis or multiple superficial erosions along the lesser curvature of the stomach. Esophageal erosion and ulceration of the first portion of the duodenum are less common but may be encountered as the chief source of bleeding. The origins of this complication are still far from clear.

Several possibilities have been suggested. These include reduction in splanchnic blood flow during and after episodes of shock, alteration in gastric mucosal blood flow, and excess acid production. Also, there is evidence to suggest that bypass of nutritive channels may deprive the gastric mucosa of its circulation and impairment of oxidative phosphorylation in the antral mucosa may diminish the active synthesis of gastric mucin. Stress, steroids, and aspirin are thought to have a similar depressing effect on the synthesis of gastric mucin. In addition, cerebral edema and the cerebritis which accompany septic shock may induce hypersecretion of acid.

It is likely that a host of other unknown factors must be considered in the pathogenesis. Also, exaggerating this tendency to bleed from the gastrointestinal tract is the coagulopathy associated with the shock state. The seriousness of massive gastrointestinal hemorrhage as a complication of shock can scarcely be overestimated. It is a common cause of death in patients who survive the initial episode of shock. Treatment is usually begun by irrigating the stomach with cold saline, using the Ewald tube by preference, because of the large clots forming in the stomach. But even this tube is usually inadequate to remove the large leathery clots that line the bleeding surface. Approximately 50% of patients respond to initial treatment with lavage and blood replacement. Operative treatment used in the remainder has, in general, been disappointing. Kirtley and Scott, however, have reported a success rate of 66% using vagotomy and pyloroplasty. However, others have reported re-bleeding in approximately 70% of patients treated in this way. In the patient bleeding massively with diffuse gastritis, the operation of choice appears to be vagotomy with high or even total gastric resection. Since sepsis is so commonly related to "stress" ulceration, appropriate antibiotic treatment and the drainage of abscesses are fundamentals in the prophylaxis and treatment of this condition.

INFECTION

Impairment of the ability of the reticuloendothelial system to clear bacteria and particulate matter has been well documented after shock in both man and the experimental animal. The severity of the reticuloendothelial dysfunction appears to be directly related to the duration and degree of shock. Patients who have experienced an episode of shock are particularly prone to develop pneumonia and infection of wounds, breakdown of surgical anastomoses, and septicemias. Wound healing appears to be interfered with and, for all these reasons, the shock patient (regardless of the origin of the illness) should be placed on prophylactic, broad-coverage antibiotic therapy by the intravenous route in high doses. Blood cultures should be taken frequently and a continuous search made for loculated abscesses. The presence of infection, as indicated earlier, considerably raises cardiac work and, to a lesser degree, the oxygen demands.

THROMBOSIS

The older patient with diseased blood vessels is particularly liable to develop cerebral, coronary or peripheral vascular thrombosis following a period of hypotension and diminished perfusion. Efforts toward maintaining blood pressure and thus increasing cerebral and coronary flow must be undertaken even if the temporary use of vasopressor drugs in titrative amounts becomes necessary. Some have proposed the use of heparin as a prophylactic to prevent the disseminated intravascular coagulation which occurs in severe shock, but this has not received adequate clinical trial because of its obvious hazards in the posttraumatic or postoperative patient.

REFERENCES

PROPHYLAXIS

Dripps, R. D., Strong, M. J., and Price, H. L.: The heart and general anesthesia, Mod. Concepts Cardiovas. Dis. 32:805, 1963.
Smith, N. T., Eger, E. I., Stoelting, R. K., and Whitcher, C.: Cardiovascular effects of Halothane in man, J.A.M.A. 206:1495, 1968.

FLUID REPLACEMENT

Adamson, J., and Hillman, R. S.: Blood volume and plasma protein replacement following acute blood loss in normal man, J.A.M.A. 205:63, 1968.
Baue, A. E., Tragus, E. T., Wolfson, S. K., Cary, A. L., and Parkins, S. M.: Hemodynamic and metabolic effects of Ringer's lactate solution in hemorrhagic shock, Ann. Surg. 166:29, 1967.
Bunker, J. P., Bendixon, H. H., and Murphy, A. J.: Hemodynamic effects of intravenously administered sodium citrate, New England J. Med. 266:372, 1962.
Bunker, J. P., Stetson, J. B., Coe, R. C., Grillo, H. C., and Murphy, A. J.: Citric acid intoxication, J.A.M.A. 157:1361, 1955.
Crenshaw, C. A., Canizaro, P. C., Shires, G. T., and Allsman, A.: Changes in extracellular fluid during acute hemorrhagic shock in man. Unpublished data.
Dillon, J., Lynch, L. J., Myers, R., Butcher, H. R., and Moyer, C. A.: A bioassay of the treatment of hemorrhagic shock. I. The roles of blood, Ringer's solution with lactate,

and macromolecules (Dextran and Hydroxyethyl Starch) in the treatment of hemorrhagic shock in anesthetized dog, Arch. Surg. 93:537, 1966.

Einheber, A., and Carter, D.: Failure of ten per cent low molecular weight dextran as a blood substitute after oligemic shock in primates, J. Trauma 6:630, 1966.

Gelin, L. E.: Fluid Substitution in Shock, in Bock, K. D. (ed.): Shock: Pathogenesis and Therapy, Ciba Foundation International Symposium (Berlin: Springer-Verlag, 1962), p. 332.

Goetz, R. H., Selmonosky, C. A., and State, D.: Effect of amine buffer tris (hydroxymethyl) amino methane (THAM) on renal blood flow during hemorrhagic shock, Surg. Gynec. & Obst. 117:715, 1963.

Howland, W. S., Bellville, J. W., Zucker, M. B., Boyan, P., and Cliffton, E. E.: Massive blood replacement: V. Failure to observe citrate intoxication, Surg. Gynec. & Obst. 105:529, 1957.

Linman, J. W.: Physiologic and pathophysiologic effects of anemia, New England J. Med. 279:812, 1968.

Moore, F. D.: The effects of hemorrhage on body composition, New England J. Med. 273:567, 1965.

Moore, F. D., and Bernhard, W. F.: Efficacy of Tris buffer in the management of metabolic lacticacidosis accompanying prolonged hypothermic perfusions, Surgery 52:905, 1962.

Moore, F. D., and Shires, G. T.: Moderation, Ann. Surg. 166:300, 1967.

Roth, E., Lax, L. C., and Maloney, J. V.: Ringer's lactate solution and extracellular fluid volume in the surgical patient: A critical analysis, Ann. Surg. 169:149, 1969.

Rush, B., and Eiseman, B.: Limits of non-colloid solution replacement in experimental hemorrhagic shock, Ann. Surg. 165:977, 1967.

Shires, T., Brown, F. T., Canizaro, P. C., and Somerville, N.: Distributional changes in extracellular fluid during acute hemorrhagic shock, Surg. Forum 11:115, 1960.

Shires, T., Williams, J., and Brown, F.: Acute change in extracellular fluids associated with major surgical procedures, Ann. Surg. 154:803, 1961.

Myocardial Support

Ackerman, G., Doherty, J., and Flanigan, W.: Peritoneal dialysis and hemodialysis of triturated digoxin, Ann. Int. Med. 67:718, 1967.

Binder, N. J.: Evaluation of therapy in shock following acute myocardial infarction, Am. J. Med. 18:622, 1955.

Corday, E., and Lillehei, R.: Pressor agents in cardiogenic shock, Am. J. Cardiol. 23: 900, 1969.

DiPalma, J. (ed.): Drill's Pharmacology in Medicine (3rd ed., New York: McGraw-Hill Book Company, 1965).

Doherty, J., and Perkins, W.: Digoxin metabolism in hypo- and hyperthyroidism, Ann. Int. Med. 64:489, 1966.

Guyton, A. C.: Regulation of cardiac output, New England J. Med. 277:805, 1967.

Jelliffee, R. W.: An improved method of digoxin therapy, Ann. Int. Med. 69:703, 1968.

Kastor, J., and Yurchak, P.: Recognition of digitalis intoxication in the presence of atrial fibrilation, Ann. Int. Med. 67:1045, 1967.

MacLean, L. D., Duff, J. H., Scott, H. M., and Peretz, D. I.: Treatment of shock in man based on hemodynamic diagnosis, Surg. Gynec. & Obst. 120:1, 1965.

Nixon, P. G., Ikram, H., and Morton, S.: Cardiogenic shock treated with infusion of dextrose solution, Am. Heart J. 73:843, 1967.

Shubin, H., and Weil, H. H.: The treatment of shock complicating acute myocardial infarction, Progr. Cardiovas. Dis. 10:30, 1967.

Soroff, H. S.: Physiologic support of heart action, New England J. Med. 280:693, 1969.

Thorp, R., and Cobbin, L.: Cardiac Stimulant Substances (New York: Academic Press, 1967), pp. 103-133.

Pulmonary Support

Catterall, M., Kazantizis, G., and Hodges, M.: The performance of nasal catheters and a face mask in oxygen therapy, Lancet 1:415, 1967.
Frank, H. A., and Fine, J.: Traumatic shock: Study of effect of oxygen on hemorrhagic shock, J. Clin. Invest. 22:305, 1943.
Haddad, C., and Richards, C. C.: Mechanical ventilation of infants: Significance and elimination of ventilator compression volume, Anesthesiology 29:365, 1968.
Hedley-Whyte, J., Pontoppidan, H., and Morris, M. J.: The response of patients with respiratory failure and cardiopulmonary disease to different levels of constant volume ventilation, J. Clin. Invest. 45:1543, 1966.
Kilburn, K. H.: Shock, seizures, and coma with alkalosis during mechanical ventilation, Ann. Int. Med. 65:977, 1966.
Mills, M., McFee, A. S., and Baisch, B. F.: The postresuscitation wet lung syndrome, Ann. Thoracic Surg. 3:182, 1967.
Robbins, L., Crocker, D., and Smith, R. M.: Tidal volume losses of volume-limited ventilators, Anesth. & Analg. 46:428, 1967.
Simmons, D. H., Nicoloff, J., and Guze, L. B.: Hyperventilation and respiratory alkalosis as signs of gram-negative bacteremia, J.A.M.A. 174:2196, 1960.
Singer, M. M.: On the selection of respirators, Anesthesiology 28:485, 1967.
Yong, H. H., and Lowe, H. J.: Humidification of inspired air, J.A.M.A. 205:907, 1968.

Antibiotics

Freid, M. A., and Vosti, K. L.: The importance of underlying disease in patients with gram-negative bacteremia, Arch. Int. Med. 121:418, 1968.
McCabe, W. R., and Jackson, G. G.: Gram-negative bacteremia I and II, Arch. Int. Med. 110:847, 1963.
Martin, C. M., Cuomo, A. J., Geraghty, M. J., Zager, J. R., and Mandes, T. C.: Gram-negative rod bacteremia, J. Infect. Dis. 119:506, 1969.
Talbot, J. H. (ed.): Gram-negative bacteremia, J.A.M.A. 205:92, 1968.

Renal Support

Auger, R. G., Dayton, D. A., Harrison, C. E., Tucker, R. M., and Anderson, C. F.: Use of ethacrynic acid in mannitol-resistant oliguric renal failure, J.A.M.A. 206:891, 1968.
Merrill, J. P.: Dialytic Methods of Treatment, in Strauss, M. B., and Welt, L. G. (eds.) *Diseases of the Kidney* (Boston: Little, Brown and Company, 1963).
Miller, R. B., and Tassistro, C. R.: Peritoneal dialysis, New England J. Med. 281:945, 1969.
Roberts, B. E., and Smith, P. H.: Hazards of mannitol infusions, Lancet 2:421, 1966.
Seldin, D. W., Corter, N. W., and Rector, F. C., Jr.: Consequences of Renal Failure and Their Management, in Strauss, M. B., and Welt, L. G. (eds.): *Diseases of the Kidney* (Boston: Little, Brown and Company, 1963).

Adrenergic Drugs

General
Baue, A. E.: The treatment of septic shock: A problem intensified by advancing science, Surgery 65:850, 1969.
Baue, A. E.: Recent developments in the study and treatment of shock, Surg. Gynec. & Obst. 127:849, 1968.
Epstein, S. E., and Braunwald, E.: Beta-adrenergic receptor blocking drugs. Mechanisms of action and clinical applications, New England J. Med. 275:1106, 1966.

Hermreck, A. S., and Thal, A. P.: The Adrenergic Drugs and Their Use in Shock Therapy, in *Current Problems in Surgery* (Chicago: Year Book Medical Publishers, Inc., July, 1968).

Innes, I. R., and Nickerson, M.: Drugs Acting on Postganglionic Adrenergic Nerve Endings and Structures Innervated by Them (Sympathomimetic Drugs), in Goodman, L. S., and Gilman, A. (eds.): *The Pharmacological Basis of Therapeutics* (3d ed., New York: The Macmillan Company, 1965), Chap. 24.

Koelle, G. B.: Drugs Acting at Synaptic and Neuroeffector Junctional Sites, in Goodman, L. S., and Gilman, A. (eds.): *The Pharmacological Basis of Therapeutics* (3d ed., New York: The Macmillan Company, 1965), Chap. 21.

Nickerson, M.: Drugs Inhibiting Adrenergic Nerves and Structures Innervated by Them, in Goodman, L. S., and Gilman, A. (eds.): *The Pharmacological Basis of Therapeutics* (3d ed., New York: The Macmillan Company, 1965), Chap. 26.

Pitt, B., and Ross, R. S.: Beta adrenergic blockade in cardiovascular therapy, Mod. Concepts Cardiov. Dis. 38:47, 1969.

Clinical

Anderson, R. W., James, P. M., Bredenger, C., and Hardaway, R. M.: Phenoxybenzamine in septic shock, Ann. Surg. 165:341, 1967.

Coffin, L. H., Ankeney, J. L., and Beheler, E. M.: Experimental study and clinical use of epinephrine for treatment of low cardiac syndrome, Circulation 33 (Supp. 1):1, 1966.

Cohn, J. D., Greenspan, M., Goldstein, C. R., Gudwin, A. L., Siegel, J. H., and Del Guercio, L. R. M.: Arteriovenous shunting in high cardiac output shock syndromes, Surg. Gynec. & Obst. 127:282, 1968.

Dietzman, R. H., Block, J. H., Feemster, J. A., Idezuki, Y., and Lillehei, R. C.: Mechanisms in the production of shock, Surgery 62:645, 1967.

Gilbert, R. P., Honig, K. P., Griffin, J. A., Becker, R. J., and Adelson, B. H.: Hemodynamics of shock due to infection, Stanford M. Bull. 13:239, 1955.

Goldberg, L. I., MacCannel, K. L., McNay, J. L., Meyer, M. B.: The use of dopamine in the treatment of hypotension and shock after myocardial infarction or cardiac surgery, Am. Heart J. 72:568, 1966.

Gunnar, R. M., Cruz, A., Boswell, J., Co, B. S., Pietras, J., and Tobin, J. R.: Myocardial infarction with shock: Hemodynamic studies and results of therapy, Circulation 33:753, 1966.

Kardos, G. G.: Isoproterenol in the treatment of shock due to bacteremia with gram-negative pathogens, New England J. Med. 274:868, 1966.

Lillehei, R. C., Longerbean, J. K., Block, J. H., and Manax, W. G.: The nature of irreversible shock: Experimental and clinical observations, Ann. Surg. 160:682, 1964.

MacLean, L. D., Duff, J. H., Scott, J. M., and Peretz, D. I.: Treatment of shock in man based on hemodynamic diagnosis, Surg. Gynec. & Obst. 120:1, 1965.

MacLean, L. D., Mulligan, W. G., McLean, A. P. H., and Duff, J. H.: Patterns of septic shock in man—A detailed study of 56 patients, Ann. Surg. 167:543, 1967.

Nickerson, M.: Drug Therapy of Shock, in Bock, K. D. (ed.): *Shock, Pathogenesis and Therapy* (Berlin: Springer-Verlag, 1962), p. 356.

Nickerson, M., and Carter, S. A.: Protection against acute trauma and traumatic shock by vasodilators, Canad. J. Biochem. 37:1161, 1959.

Nickerson, M., and Gourzis, J. T.: Blockade of sympathetic vasoconstriction in the treatment of shock, J. Trauma 2:399, 1962.

Shubin, H., and Weil, M. H.: Hemodynamic Alterations in Patients after Myocardial Infarction, in Mills, L. D., and Moyer, J. H. (eds.): *Shock and Hypotension: Pathogenesis and Treatment—A Hahnemann Symposium* (New York: Grune & Stratton, Inc., 1965), p. 499.

Siegel, J. H., Greenspan, M., Del Guercio, L. R. M.: Abnormal vascular tone, defective oxygen transport and myocardial failure in human septic shock, Ann. Surg. 165:504, 1967.

Skillman, J. J., Eltringham, W. K., Zollinger, R. M., Jr., Lauler, D. P., and Moore, F. D.: Phenoxybenzamine-induced vasodilation: A stimulus to increased plasma volume with reduced central venous pressure and aldosterone hypersecretion in man, Surgery 64:368, 1968.

Smith, H. J., Oriol, A., Morch, J., and McGregor, M.: Hemodynamic studies in cardiogenic shock: Treatment with Isoproterenol and Metaraminol, Circulation 35:1084, 1964.

Smulyan, H., Cuddy, R. P., and Eich, R. H.: Hemodynamic effects of pressor agents in septic and myocardial infarction shock, J.A.M.A. 190:188, 1964.

Udhoji, V. N., and Weil, M. H.: Vasodilator action of a "pressor amine" Mephentermine (Wyamine), in circulatory shock, Am. J. Cardiol. 16:841, 1965.

Wessler, S., and Avioli, L. V.: Propranolol therapy in patients with cardiac disease, J.A.M.A., #2, 206:357, 1968.

Wilson, R. F., Jablonski, D. V., and Thal, A. P.: Usage of Dibenzyline in human shock, Surgery 56:172, 1964.

Wilson, R. F., Sukhnanden, R., and Thal, A. P.: Combined use of norepinephrine and Dibenzyline in clinical shock, Surg. Forum 15:30, 1964.

Wilson, R. F., Thal, A. P., Kindling, P. H., Grifka, T., and Ackerman, E.: Hemodynamic measurements in septic shock, Arch. Surg. 91:121, 1965.

Experimental

Albrecht, M., and Clowes, G. H. S., Jr.: The increase of circulatory requirements in the presence of inflammation, Surgery 56:158, 1964.

Baue, A. E., Johnson, D. G., and Parkins, W. M.: Blood flow and oxygen consumption with adrenergic blockade in hemorrhagic shock, Am. J. Physiol. 211:354, 1966.

Baue, A. E., Jones, E. F., and Parkins, W. M.: The effects of beta-adrenergic receptor stimulation on blood flow, oxidative metabolism and survival in hemorrhagic shock, Ann. Surg. 167:403, 1968.

Berk, J. L., Hagen, J. F., Beyer, W. H., Dochat, G. R., and LaPointe, R.: The treatment of hemorrhagic shock by beta adrenergic receptor blockade, Surg. Gynec. & Obst. 125:311, 1967.

Berk, J. L., Hagen, J. F., Beyer, W. H., Gerber, M. J., and Dochat, G. R.: The treatment of endotoxin shock by beta adrenergic blockade, Ann. Surg. 169:74, 1969.

Drucker, W. R., Kingsbury, B., and Graham, L.: Metabolic effects of vasopressors in hemorrhagic shock, Surg. Forum 13:16, 1962.

Gump, F. E., Magill, T., Thal, A. P., and Kinney, J. M.: Regional adrenergic blockade by intra-arterial injection of phenoxybenzamine, Surg. Gynec. & Obst. 127:319, 1968.

Hermreck, A. S., and Thal, A. P.: Mechanisms for the high circulatory requirements in sepsis and septic shock, Ann. Surg. 170:677, 1969.

Hermreck, A. S., and Thal, A. P.: Effects of vasoactive drugs on blood flow and oxygen utilization by septic tissue, Surg. Forum 20:17, 1969.

Hopkins, R. W., Pauly, R. P., Peters, T. E., and Simeone, F. A.: Effects of levarterenol on blood flow in inflammation, Arch. Surg. 97:1032, 1968.

McNay, J. L., and Goldberg, L. I.: Comparison of the effects of Dopamine, Isoproterenol, norepinephrine and bradykinin on canine renal and femoral blood flow, J. Pharmacol. & Exper. Therap. 151:23, 1966.

Mandelbaum, I., Silbert, M., and Berry, J.: Phenoxybenzamine and renal blood flow during extracorporeal circulation, Surg. Forum 16:40, 1965.

Moyer, J. H., Morris, G., and Beazley, L. H.: Renal hemodynamic response to vasopressor agents in the treatment of shock, Circulation 12:96, 1955.

Muhm, H. Y., and Shumacker, H. B.: Effects of adrenergic blocking agents on renal blood flow in normovolemic and moderately hypovolemic states, Surg. Forum 16:1, 1965.

Pollock, L., Kjartansson, K. B., Delin, N. A., and Schenk, W. G.: Regional blood flow alterations, Arch. Surg. 89:344, 1964.

Rush, B. F., Rosenberg, J. G., and Spencer, F. C.: The effects of treatment with Dibenzyline on cardiac dynamics and oxidative metabolism in hemorrhagic shock, Ann. Surg. 162:1013, 1965.

Sarnoff, S. J., Case, R. B., Berglund, E., and Sarnoff, L. C.: Ventricular function V. The circulatory effects of Aramine: Mechanism of action of "vasopressor" drugs in cardiogenic shock, Circulation 10:84, 1954.

STEROIDS

Melby, J. C., and Spink, W. W.: Comparative studies on adrenal cortical function and cortisol metabolism in healthy adults and patients with shock due to infection, J. Clin. Invest. 37:1791, 1958.

Sambhi, M. P., Weil, M. H., Udhoji, V. N., and Shubin, H.: Adrenocorticoids in management of shock, Internat. Anesth. Clin. 2:421, 1964.

TREATMENT OF THE COMPLICATIONS OF SHOCK

Edlick, R. F., Goodale, R. L., Lande, A. J., Kuphal, J. E., and Wangensteen, O. H.: Gastric tamponade as an adjunct to cooling for massive upper gastrointestinal tract hemorrhage: A preliminary report of a new technique, Surgery 66:699, 1969.

Kirtley, J. A., Scott, H. S., Jr., Sawhers, J. L., Graves, H. A., and Lawler, M. R.: The surgical management of stress ulcers, Ann. Surg. 169:801, 1969.

Penner, A., and Bernheim, A. I.: Acute postoperative esophageal, gastric and duodenal ulcerations, Arch. Path. 28:129, 1939.

Singh, G. B., Sharma, J. N., Kar, K.: Pathogenesis of gastric ulceration produced under stress, J. Path. Bact. 94:375, 1967.

Index